Study Guide for

Maternal-Child Nursing

Fifth Edition

Emily Slone McKinney
Susan Rowen James
Sharon Smith Murray
Kristine Ann Nelson
Jean Weiler Ashwill
Vanessa Flannery
Kari Mau
Jennifer Rodriquez
Dawn Piacenza
Karen Holub
Grace Moodt
Jacqueline Carroll

Prepared by:

Jennifer T. Alderman, MSN, RNC-OB, CNL
Assistant Professor
School of Nursing
University of North Carolina at Chapel Hill
Chapel Hill, North Carolina

Stephanie C. Evans, PhD, RN, CPNP-PC, CLC
Assistant Professor
Harris College of Nursing and Health Sciences
Texas Christian University
Fort Worth, Texas

ELSEVIER

ELSEVIER

3251 Riverport Lane
St. Louis, Missouri 63043

STUDY GUIDE FOR MATERNAL-CHILD NURSING,
FIFTH EDITION

ISBN: 978-0-323-47869-4

Notices

Knowledge and best practice in this field are constantly changing. As new research and experience broaden our understanding, changes in research methods, professional practices, or medical treatment may become necessary.

Practitioners and researchers must always rely on their own experience and knowledge in evaluating and using any information, methods, compounds, or experiments described herein. In using such information or methods, they should be mindful of their own safety and the safety of others, including parties for whom they have a professional responsibility.

With respect to any drug or pharmaceutical products identified, readers are advised to check the most current information provided (i) on procedures featured or (ii) by the manufacturer of each product to be administered and to verify the recommended dose or formula, the method and duration of administration, and contraindications. It is the responsibility of practitioners, relying on their own experience and knowledge of their patients, to make diagnoses, to determine dosages and the best treatment for each individual patient, and to take all appropriate safety precautions.

To the fullest extent of the law, neither the Publisher nor the authors, contributors, or editors assume any liability for any injury and/or damage to persons or property as a matter of products liability, negligence or otherwise, or from any use or operation of any methods, products, instructions, or ideas contained in the material herein.

Senior Content Strategist: Sandra Clark
Senior Content Development Manager: Laurie Gower
Content Development Specialist: Jennifer Wade
Publishing Services Manager: Deepthi Unni
Project Manager: Apoorva V
Designer: Muthukumaran Thangaraj

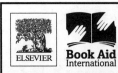

Working together
to grow libraries in
developing countries

www.elsevier.com • www.bookaid.org

Printed in the United States of America

Last digit is the print number: 9 8 7 6 5 4 3 2

Introduction

This *Study Guide* is designed to help students effectively use the textbook, *Maternal-Child Nursing,* fifth edition. In addition to reviewing content of the text, this *Study Guide* encourages students to think critically in applying their knowledge.

Activities are provided in a variety of formats—matching, true/false, and short answer—and focus on recall and application of concepts and essential content of each chapter.

Critical Thinking Exercises, Case Studies, Student Learning Applications, and **Suggested Learning Activities** help apply knowledge to solve problems, make decisions about care management, and provide responses to a patient's questions and concerns. **Review Questions** test knowledge and understanding of the content in each chapter.

Answers to all activities are provided at the back of this *Study Guide.*

Contents

1 Foundations of Maternity, Women's Health, and Child Health Nursing

HELPFUL HINT

A fundamentals-of-nursing textbook can provide additional information on many topics covered in the chapter as they relate to the nursing profession.

MATCHING KEY TERMS

Match the term with the correct definition.

1. _____ Advocacy
2. _____ Morbidity
3. _____ Malpractice
4. _____ Neonatal mortality
5. _____ Birth centers
6. _____ Ethics
7. _____ Bioethics
8. _____ Negligence

a. Infant deaths that occur in the first 28 days of life

b. Speaking or arguing in support of a policy or person's rights

c. Negligence of a professional person

d. Provide maternity care outside acute-care settings for low-risk pregnant women

e. Ratio of sick-to-well persons in a defined population

f. Application of ethics to health care

g. Rules or principles that govern conduct

h. Failure to act in the way a reasonable, prudent person of a similar background would act in a similar circumstance

HISTORICAL PERSPECTIVES

Maternity Nursing

1. Identify the three basic principles of family-centered maternity care.

    a. _____

    b. _____

    c. _____

2. Describe each of these settings for childbirth.

    a. The traditional hospital setting

    b. Labor, delivery, and recovery (LDR) rooms

c. Labor, delivery, recovery, and postpartum (LDRP) rooms

d. Birth centers

e. Home births

Pediatric Nursing

Answer as either true (T) or false (F).

1. _____ Throughout history, children have been valued and protected by society.

2. _____ During the 19th century, the most serious child health problems were directly related to poverty and over-crowding.

3. _____ The first public health program for mothers and children was initiated by Lillian Wald.

4. _____ Hospital policies have changed in response to an awareness of children's emotional and psychologic needs.

CURRENT TRENDS IN MATERNITY AND PEDIATRIC CARE

1. How has cost containment affected maternity and pediatric care?

Answer as either true (T) or false (F).

2. _____ Special Supplemental Nutrition Program for Women, Infants, and Children (WIC) provides supplemental food supplies to bottle-fed children but not to breastfeeding mothers.

3. _____ Premature births have increased in the past two decades.

4. _____ African-American women have lower maternal mortality rates than Caucasian women.

5. _____ Infant mortality rates have continued to drop since 1950 as a result of better neonatal care.

6. _____ Unintentional injuries are the leading cause of death in children aged 1 to 19 years.

7. _____ There is no link between children living in poverty and poorer health outcomes.

ETHICAL PERSPECTIVES ON MATERNAL AND CHILD NURSING

1. Four of the most important ethical principles are _____, _____,

_____, and _____.

LEGAL ISSUES

1. What are the four elements of negligence/malpractice?

   a. _____

   b. _____

   c. _____

   d. _____

2. Identify the four requirements of informed consent.

a. _____

b. _____

c. _____

d. _____

SUGGESTED LEARNING ACTIVITIES

1. Gather additional information about one of the health care assistance programs (e.g., WIC; Medicaid's Early Periodic Screening, Diagnosis, and Treatment [EPSDT] program; Public Law 99-457; or the Healthy Start program) presented in this chapter.

2. Research agencies available in your town that offer assistance, such as health care, food, clothing, or emotional support, to pregnant women who are unable to pay for such assistance.

CRITICAL THINKING EXERCISES

1. Share with other students any legal situations you have encountered or read about that have involved nurses and maternity or pediatric patients.

2. Discuss the following situation with fellow students: Sally, who is 23 years old, is 24 weeks pregnant with her first child. She admits to her nurse-midwife that she continues to use several illegal drugs on a weekly basis. What are the nurse-midwife's legal and ethical responsibilities to the mother and fetus?

REVIEW QUESTIONS

Choose the correct answer.

1. Lillian Wald is recognized for which contribution to nursing?
   a. She discouraged the practice of tightly swaddling infants in three layers of clothing.
   b. She initiated public health nursing at the Henry Street Settlement.
   c. She promoted family-centered care for hospitalized children.
   d. She developed infection control procedures in hospitals and foundling homes.

2. What was identified in the chapter as a societal issue that affects maternity and pediatric nursing?
   a. Fewer children are living in poverty.
   b. Violence in schools has decreased.
   c. Families are the fastest growing group of homeless people.
   d. The number of uninsured American children has decreased.

3. A practice model that uses a systematic approach to identify specific patients and manage patient care is:
   a. case management.
   b. the nursing process.
   c. a clinical pathway.
   d. a health maintenance organization.

4. Which statement about family-centered maternity care is correct?
   a. Family-centered care decreases the responsibility of maternity nurses.
   b. Although the settings have changed, childbirth is still viewed as a medical event.
   c. Care is adapted to meet the physical and psychologic needs of the family.
   d. Maternal–infant bonding is the primary focus of family-centered care.

2 The Nurse's Role in Maternity, Women's Health, and Pediatric Nursing

A fundamentals-of-nursing textbook can provide additional information on professional nursing roles and processes.

THE ROLE OF THE PROFESSIONAL NURSE

Answer as either true (T) or false (F).

1. _____ The professional nurse has a responsibility to provide high-quality care to all patients.

2. _____ Standards of practice describe the level of performance expected of a professional nurse.

3. _____ Maternity nurse practitioners usually assist with childbirth.

KEY CONCEPTS

4. List six roles of maternity and pediatric nurses.

   a. _____   d. _____

   b. _____   e. _____

   c. _____   f. _____

5. List the factors that influence learning.

6. Describe the education and services that each type of advanced practice nurse is qualified to deliver.

   a. Certified nurse-midwives _____

_____

_____

   b. Nurse practitioners _____

_____

_____

   c. Clinical nurse specialists _____

_____

_____

IMPLICATIONS OF CHANGING ROLES FOR NURSES

1. How does therapeutic communication differ from social communication?

2. When using active listening, the nurse attends to _____ and _____.

3. In the following situations, identify the communication block illustrated by the nurse's response. Provide an alternative nursing response.

   a. A child is crying and resisting as the nurse is about to administer an intramuscular injection. The nurse says, "This will not hurt a bit. You will be just fine."

   Communication block: _____

   Alternative response: _____

   b. A pregnant woman, on strict bed rest, tells the nurse, "I do not think I can stand much more of this. I did not think my pregnancy would be like this." The nurse responds, "Rest up now. You will not get this much rest again in your life."

   Communication block: _____

   Alternative response: _____

4. The primary purpose of critical thinking in nursing is: _____

   _____.

5. Identify the five steps of the critical thinking process.

   a. _____

   b. _____

   c. _____

   d. _____

   e. _____

Answer as either true (T) or false (F).

6. _____ A body posture that facilitates nurse–patient communication is talking with the arms crossed over the chest.

7. _____ Cultural differences do not affect communication.

8. _____ Nonverbal behaviors may communicate a more powerful message to a patient than spoken words.

THE NURSING PROCESS IN MATERNITY AND PEDIATRIC CARE

1. Describe the difference between a screening (database) assessment and a focused assessment.

2. For each broad goal, write at least three outcome criteria that are patient focused, use measurable verbs, have a time frame, and are realistic.

   a. Following a cesarean birth, the woman will have increased mobility.

   b. The pregnant woman will have adequate nutrition.

   c. The child with leukemia will not get an infection.

5

SUGGESTED LEARNING ACTIVITIES

1. Arrange to observe a nurse-midwife, nurse practitioner, or clinical nurse specialist. What educational preparation was needed for this advanced practice? What did you find most interesting about this experience?

2. Research the effects of various herbal remedies on pregnant women and children. What difficulties did you have in obtaining scientific research on the herbal remedies?

CRITICAL THINKING EXERCISES

1. In a clinical setting, select a topic that a patient and/or family needs to learn. Use at least four of the principles of teaching and learning in your presentation. Explain how you used each principle in your teaching.

2. Recall a conversation you had with a patient. Which therapeutic communication techniques did you use in your dialogue? Give examples from your conversation. What would you do differently to improve your therapeutic communication skills?

REVIEW QUESTIONS

Choose the correct answer.

1. Your friend says she is not sure she wants a doctor to deliver her second baby because she believes doctors are too busy to talk with her when she has check-ups. The best alternative professional for you to suggest is the:
   a. maternity nurse practitioner.
   b. certified nurse-midwife.
   c. lay midwife.
   d. clinical nurse specialist.

2. A primary difference between social and therapeutic communications is that therapeutic communication is:
   a. designed to obtain information in a minimum amount of time.
   b. the only appropriate professional communication.
   c. focused on achieving a relevant goal for the patient.
   d. limited to the information necessary for safe care.

3. A pregnant woman tells the nurse, "I am so confused. My husband wants me to have my tubes tied after the baby comes, but what if something happens to the baby?" The nurse replies, "You are afraid of having permanent contraception before you know if your baby is well." The nurse's response is an example of:
   a. directing.
   b. paraphrasing.
   c. summarizing.
   d. pinpointing.

4. A nursing diagnosis differs from a collaborative problem primarily regarding whether the nurse:
   a. can prescribe definitive treatment for the problem.
   b. identifies a patient's strength or weakness.
   c. determines that an actual or a potential problem exists.
   d. can evaluate the patient's response to treatment.

3 The Childbearing and Child-Rearing Family

HELPFUL HINT

Review stress and coping information in a fundamentals-of-nursing textbook.

MATCHING KEY TERMS

Match the term with the correct definition.

1. _____ Coping

2. _____ Culture

3. _____ Discipline

4. _____ Ethnocentrism

5. _____ Fatalism

6. _____ Nuclear family

7. _____ Stress

a. Designed to teach a child how to effectively function in a society

b. Belief that events are predestined

c. Efforts directed toward managing or solving various events, problems, or stressors

d. Any situation, positive or negative, requiring an adjustment on the part of individuals, families, or groups

e. Family headed by two parents who are motivated to learn about parenting

f. The opinion that the beliefs and customs of one's own ethnic group are superior to those of others

g. The sum of the values, beliefs, and practices of a group of people that are transmitted from one generation to the next

THE FAMILY AND NURSING CARE

1. List some potential problems that may be encountered by each of the following types of families:

   a. Dual income

   b. Single parent

   c. Blended

   d. Adoptive

   e. Multigenerational

f. Same-sex parents

g. Adolescent parents

h. Families with substance abuse

i. Families with special needs children

2. In front of each family coping strategy, place an "I" if the strategy is internal or "E" if the strategy is external.

a. _____ Role flexibility

b. _____ Being open and honest

c. _____ Social support system

d. _____ Joint (family) problem solving

e. _____ Using humor

f. _____ Seeking information from clergy

g. _____ Seeing spiritual meaning in events

h. _____ Joining self-help groups

CULTURAL INFLUENCES ON MATERNITY AND PEDIATRIC NURSING

Explain how the characteristics of cultural groups affect nursing communication.

1. Southeast Asians

   a. Voice tone

   b. Eye contact

2. Hispanics: conversational methods

3. Middle-Easterners

   a. Interpreters

   b. Paternalism

8

PARENTING

Answer as either true (T) or false (F).

1. _____ An authoritarian parent discusses the household rules with the child.

2. _____ Children of authoritarian parents tend to lack self-confidence.

3. _____ Authoritarian parents permit compromises about rules.

4. _____ Permissive parents tend to inconsistently discipline their children.

Briefly describe each of the following discipline measures:

5. Redirection

6. Reasoning

7. Time-out

8. Consequences

9. Behavior modification

10. Corporal punishment

SUGGESTED LEARNING ACTIVITIES

1. Interview a classmate who is from a cultural background different from yours. How do your health beliefs differ? How are they similar?

2. Interview a classmate from a similar cultural background. How do your health beliefs differ? How are they similar?

CRITICAL THINKING EXERCISES

A family is a single-income family consisting of the natural parents and their two sons, aged 4 and 2 years. The parents are in the process of getting a divorce. The mother will have custody of the boys, and they will move in with her parents so that she will be able to go back to work full-time. The boys will spend every other weekend and one night each week with their father.

1. What stressors may the following experience?

   Father

   Mother

   Children

   Grandparents

2. How can the children be helped through this transition?

REVIEW QUESTIONS

Choose the correct answer.

1. A Muslim woman is admitted to the postpartum unit after delivering a baby girl. Considering the cultural needs of this patient, what should be included in her plan of care?
   a. Inclusion of meat with every meal
   b. Having only female nurses care for the patient
   c. Not putting ice in the bedside water pitcher
   d. Assessment for herbal use

2. The purpose of discipline is to:
   a. teach a child how to effectively function in a society.
   b. establish the self-fulfilling prophecy.
   c. assert parental control over the child.
   d. transmit the family's culture.

3. An example of a family that is classified as *high risk* is a (an):
   a. traditional family.
   b. single-parent family.
   c. adoptive family.
   d. family headed by adolescents.

4. A nurse reacts with anger because a woman who did not have prenatal care explains that she does not see pregnancy as an illness requiring medical care. The nurse's reaction demonstrates:
   a. cultural diversity.
   b. ethnicity.
   c. ethnocentrism.
   d. fatalism.

5. A mother tells the nurse that she puts her 3-year-old son in a time-out chair in a corner for 3 minutes when he misbehaves. She asks the nurse if this is correct. The nurse responds:
   a. "You are correctly using the time-out."
   b. "You should put the time-out chair in the center of family activity."
   c. "I would increase the time-out to 5 minutes."
   d. "Do you talk about the misbehavior while he is in the chair?"

6. A statement that uses effective reasoning techniques is:
   a. "You are not being very nice when you throw toys at your friend."
   b. "I would not throw that toy if I were you."
   c. "I feel embarrassed when you throw toys at someone."
   d. "I will not let you play at your friend's house if you throw toys."

7. An 8-year-old child hit by a car has been in the intensive care unit (ICU) for a week. She has a lengthy recovery ahead. Both parents have been at her side since the injury. They have not been properly eating and look exhausted. An appropriate nursing diagnosis for this family would be:
   a. parental role conflict relayed to the change in the environment.
   b. fear related to the child's critical condition.
   c. ineffective family health maintenance management related to the situational crisis.
   d. risk of impaired home maintenance related to a lack of support.

4 Communicating with Children and Families

Review sections on language and cognitive development in Chapters 4 through 9 in your textbook.

MATCHING KEY TERMS

Match the term with the correct definition.

1. _____ Empathy

2. _____ Empowerment

3. _____ Active listening

4. _____ Preparation

5. _____ Sensory information

6. _____ Self-esteem

7. _____ Therapeutic relationship

8. _____ Win–win solution

a. Information obtained from sight, taste, touch, smell, and hearing

b. Personal value that individuals place on themselves

c. Seeing a situation from another person's perspective while remaining objective

d. Provision of information before procedures, treatments, or events

e. Attending to another person to gain an understanding of the actual and implied message

f. Actions taken to enable another person to fully participate in the decision-making

g. Resolution of a conflict that both parties can support

h. Balance between appropriate involvement and professional separation when relating to children and their families

COMPONENTS OF EFFECTIVE COMMUNICATION

Answer as either true (T) or false (F).

1. _____ Communication involves more than expressing words from one person to another.

2. _____ Touch communicates more meaning to a younger child than to an older child.

3. _____ The child or family members may feel intimidated when the nurse stands over them while talking.

4. _____ Research shows that the verbal content of a message conveys more than nonverbal communication.

5. _____ Cultural differences are particularly important to consider with regard to touch and personal space.

6. _____ The nurse can demonstrate attentiveness by maintaining eye contact.

7. _____ The nurse expresses empathy using similar words to restate what the speaker has just said.

8. _____ Active listening requires attentiveness, empathy, an open mind, and clarifying what the speaker says.

9. _____ To listen with impartiality, nurses must hold their personal beliefs and values in abeyance.

10. _____ What we say is often less important than how we say it.

11. _____ Talking to a child with your hands on your hips is an example of a closed body posture.

12. _____ An appropriate time to teach a 4-year-old about surgery is immediately after the parents have gone home.

FAMILY CENTERED COMMUNICATION

1. How can family centered care be achieved?

2. List five key components of open communication in a family centered care environment.

    a. _____

    b. _____

    c. _____

    d. _____

    e. _____

3. Identify seven strategies to manage conflict that may occur between parents and the nurse.

    a. _____

    b. _____

    c. _____

    d. _____

    e. _____

    f. _____

    g. _____

TRANSCULTURAL COMMUNICATION

1. To provide appropriate care for the child and family, during the initial interview, the nurse should gather information about the following five areas:

    a. _____

    b. _____

    c. _____

    d. _____

    e. _____

THERAPEUTIC RELATIONSHIPS: DEVELOPING AND MAINTAINING TRUST

1. List three behaviors that are warning signs of a nurse's overinvolvement.

    a. _____

    b. _____

    c. _____

NURSING CARE: COMMUNICATING WITH CHILDREN AND FAMILIES

Answer as either true (T) or false (F).

1. _____ The optimal time to prepare a toddler for a painful procedure is just before the procedure is performed.

2. _____ Explanations should include what the child will experience through the senses.

3. _____ It is better not to tell a child how long a painful or invasive procedure will take.

4. _____ Once a procedure is completed, it should not be discussed with the child.

5. _____ When talking with toddlers, nurses should use proper technical terms for body parts and processes.

6. _____ Evaluation of the family's understanding is an ongoing process.

COMMUNICATING WITH CHILDREN WHO HAVE SPECIAL NEEDS

1. Suggest three strategies the nurse could use when caring for a child who has a severe visual impairment.

   a. _____

   b. _____

   c. _____

2. Suggest three strategies the nurse could use when caring for a child who is deaf.

   a. _____

   b. _____

   c. _____

SUGGESTED LEARNING ACTIVITIES

1. Review Table 4-4, "Considerations in Choosing Language," in your textbook. Think about the words you use when talking to children. How often have you used potentially ambiguous, difficult to comprehend, or unfamiliar language? Make a conscious effort to use clear, softer, more familiar language. Once you have had the opportunity to try this "new" language, consider its effects. What were the children's reactions to each style of communication?

STUDENT LEARNING APPLICATION

Enhance your learning by discussing your answers with other students.

A mother brings her 4-year-old son to the pediatrician's office for a well-child examination. The physician completes the examination and reminds her that the child is due for immunizations during this visit. The nurse walks into the examining room holding a syringe in her hand. She looks at the child and says, "This shot is so you won't get diphtheria, pertussis, or tetanus. I am going to put the needle in your leg (points to the thigh area). You can cry or yell, but I need you to keep your leg still. It is going to hurt." She administers the injection and says, "Here is a Band-Aid to put on the sore spot. That wasn't too bad, was it?" The nurse leaves before he has a chance to respond.

1. What effective communication techniques were used by this nurse?

2. What communication pitfalls do you recognize in this nurse–child interaction?

3. What suggestions can you offer to make the nurse's communication more effective?

A 3-year-old with a diagnosis of liver failure is hospitalized. She is deaf. Her mother, who is present, primarily speaks Spanish but can understand some English. When the nurse enters the room, the child cries and wants to be held by her mother. The nurse approaches to take vital signs, but the child cries even louder.

1. What does the child's behavior communicate to you?

2. What should the nurse do about measuring vital signs at this time?

3. How can the nurse establish a rapport with the mother and child?

4. What measures should the nurse take to communicate with the mother and child?

REVIEW QUESTIONS

Choose the correct answer.

1. A 5-year-old is scheduled for a computed tomography (CT) scan of her head. What is the best time for her mother to initiate a discussion about the procedure?
   a. Immediately before the procedure begins
   b. Two hours before the procedure
   c. The day before the procedure
   d. A few days before the procedure

2. Which nursing action indicates that the nurse understands the components of effective communication?
   a. The nurse stands right next to the chair where the child is seated.
   b. The nurse asks an adolescent whether she can give her a hug.
   c. The nurse speaks to a child who is aphonic in a loud, clear voice.
   d. The nurse talks with her arms folded across her chest.

3. An adolescent tells the nurse, "I don't like this hospital room." An active listening response to this child's statement is:
   a. "Don't you know this is the best room in the house?"
   b. "Let me see whether there are any other rooms available."
   c. "What's wrong with this room?"
   d. "So, would you prefer a different room?"

4. The developmentally appropriate strategy for the nurse to use when performing preoperative teaching with a 10-year-old is to:
   a. keep explanations under 5 minutes.
   b. sequentially organize information.
   c. use puppets to explain the surgery.
   d. start preoperative teaching 3 hours before the surgery.

5. A child with a hearing impairment needs to have an arm cast. What can the nurse do to facilitate communication with the child throughout the cast application process?
   a. Face the child when speaking.
   b. Speak at a slower pace than usual.
   c. Talk clearly and directly into the child's ear.
   d. Keep gestures to a minimum.

6. Which example describes how a nurse can display an open body posture?
   a. Speaking to a child with head bowed
   b. Frequently shifting weight from one leg to the other while speaking
   c. Leaning away from the child while talking
   d. Talking while the hands are freely moving

7. A child has just been diagnosed with diabetes. The child's father tells the nurse, "My wife will be back in the morning. Before she left, she told me that she has a lot of questions about what to do." What is the most appropriate response for the nurse to make at this time?
   a. "You will be meeting with the clinical specialist tomorrow. Ask her tomorrow."
   b. "Did the clinical specialist give you any papers to read? If not, I'll get a pamphlet for you."
   c. "Your wife might want to write down her questions so she won't forget anything when she comes back tomorrow."
   d. "Why don't you tell me what information you received from the clinical specialist today?"

5 Health Promotion for the Developing Child

HELPFUL HINT

Review growth and development in a developmental psychology textbook.

MATCHING KEY TERMS

Match the term with the correct definition.

1. _____ Cephalocaudal
2. _____ Chronologic age
3. _____ Developmental age
4. _____ Growth spurts
5. _____ Heredity
6. _____ Learning
7. _____ Nutrients
8. _____ Proximodistal
9. _____ Recommended dietary allowance
10. _____ Regression

a. Progression from midline to periphery

b. Age based on functional behavior and ability to adapt to the environment

c. Transmission of genetic characteristics

d. Progression from head to toe

e. Appearance of behavior more appropriate at an earlier stage of development

f. Behavior changes that occur as a result of maturation and experience with the environment

g. Age in years

h. Brief periods of a rapid increase in growth rate

i. Foods that supply the body with elements necessary for metabolism

j. Recommendations for the average amount of nutrients that should be consumed by healthy people in the United States

TYPES OF PLAY

Match each type of play with its description.

1. _____ Dramatic play
2. _____ Familiarization play
3. _____ Symbolic play

a. Children use games and interactions that represent an issue or a concern to be addressed

b. Children use materials associated with health care in creative, playful activities

c. Children act out roles and experiences that happened to them or someone else

OVERVIEW OF GROWTH AND DEVELOPMENT

Fill in the blanks.

1. Nurses need to have an understanding of growth and development to design care plans that:

_____

2. An increase in physical size is referred to as: _____

3. Physical changes in the complexity of body structures that enable a higher-level functioning are known as: _____

_____

4. _____ is an increase in the capabilities resulting from growth, maturation, and learning.

5. Changes in behavior that occur as the result of both maturation and experience with the environment are termed:

_____

6. Nurses must be familiar with normal patterns of growth and development so that

_____ can be detected and treated early.

7. Next to each age, write the corresponding stage of growth and development.

a. 8 years _____   d. 10 months _____

b. 2 years _____   e. 4 years _____

c. 17 years _____   f. 3 weeks _____

8. List three parameters used to measure growth in infants and children.

a. _____

b. _____

c. _____

9. An infant's birth weight typically doubles by _____ and triples by

_____.

10. _____ is an indicator of brain growth.

11. Primary dentition consists of _____ teeth; permanent teeth number

_____.

PRINCIPLES OF GROWTH AND DEVELOPMENT

Match each pattern of growth and development with its example.

1. _____ Cephalocaudal

2. _____ General to specific

3. _____ Proximodistal

4. _____ Simple to complex

a. An infant responds to an earache by flailing the extremities; the toddler responds by tugging at the ear.

b. A toddler can use two-word sentences; a preschooler can tell stories.

c. In the embryo, the development of the bronchus precedes the development of the bronchioles and alveoli.

d. The infant can lift the head before being able to lift the trunk.

Fill in the blanks.

5. Children may regress to earlier developmental levels when they are _____.

6. Define critical period. _____

Answer as either true (T) or false (F).

7. _____ Toys manufactured outside of the United States may have high concentrations of lead.

8. _____ Maternal diabetes can adversely affect fetal development.

Chapter **5**   **Health Promotion for the Developing Child**

9. _____ Children are less susceptible to air pollution than adults because they have a smaller lung capacity.

10. _____ Breastfeeding can expose infants to environmental toxins.

11. _____ A standard growth curve is appropriate for assessing all children regardless of their racial or ethnic backgrounds.

12. _____ A child's temperament can influence how the parents interact with the child.

13. _____ Only inherited diseases can affect the growth and development in the fetus.

THEORIES OF GROWTH AND DEVELOPMENT

Match each stage of Piaget's theory with the example that is characteristic of that stage.

1. _____ Sensorimotor   a. Is able to see another's point of view

2. _____ Preoperational   b. Exhibits magical thinking

3. _____ Concrete operations   c. Develops a sense of object permanence

4. _____ Formal operations   d. Is able to appreciate symbolism

Identify which of Freud's stages of psychosexual development is represented by each of the following:

5. Child explores the world with the mouth: _____

6. Child may initially demonstrate aggression toward the same-sex parent: _____

7. Child develops an adult view of sexuality: _____

8. Child learns to control the elimination processes: _____

9. Child typically prefers same-sex friends: _____

Fill in the blanks in the following statements to complete the developmental tasks of Erikson through adolescence.

10. Trust versus _____

11. _____ versus shame and doubt

12. _____ versus guilt

13. Industry versus _____

14. _____ versus role confusion

Match each level of Kohlberg's theory with its example.

15. _____ Pre-morality   a. "I'll take my medicine to make my nurse happy."

16. _____ Morality of conventional role conformity   b. "I won't hit them because the nurse will yell at me."

17. _____ Morality of self-accepted moral principles   c. "I won't blast my radio. It's not fair to the other patients."

THEORIES OF LANGUAGE DEVELOPMENT

Fill in the blanks.

1. Language development closely parallels _____ development.

2. Receptive language is the ability to: _____.

3. Expressive language is the ability to: _____.

ASSESSMENT OF GROWTH

Fill in the blanks.

1. Why are a child's height, weight, and head circumference plotted on standardized growth charts at every well-child checkup?

   _____

   _____

2. Body mass index measures growth and _____ in children older than 2 years.

3. Why is it important to recognize abnormal growth patterns? _____

   _____

   _____

ASSESSMENT OF DEVELOPMENT

Fill in the blanks.

1. List four methods of assessing development.

   a. _____

   b. _____

   c. _____

   d. _____

2. Name two prescreening tools that have been found to be sensitive and specific for detecting developmental problems.

   a. _____

   b. _____

3. The Denver Developmental Screening Test II (DDST-II) assesses development in which four functional areas?

   a. _____

   b. _____

   c. _____

   d. _____

Answer as either true (T) or false (F).

4. _____ Only nurses who have been trained to administer the DDST-II should conduct formal screenings.

5. _____ The DDST-II is similar to an intelligence quotient (IQ) test.

6. _____ Parents should be present during DDST-II screening.

7. _____ When children younger than 6 years are hospitalized, they should be given the DDST-II.

8. _____ Nurses are able to diagnose developmental delays using the DDST-II.

THE NURSE'S ROLE IN PROMOTING OPTIMAL GROWTH AND DEVELOPMENT

Fill in the blanks.

1. What is anticipatory guidance?

   _____

   _____

THE DEVELOPMENTAL ASSESSMENT

Answer as either true (T) or false (F).

1. _____ Children's developmental needs are the same as their psychosocial needs.

2. _____ When discussing a child's development with parents, considering the family's culture is important.

3. _____ Observing a child in various situations can provide information about the child's development.

Fill in the blanks.

4. Play is considered to be children's _____.

5. Practice play is also known as _____.

6. Symbolic play uses games and interactions to _____.

7. Games include _____.

Match each type of play with its description.

8. _____ Associative   a. Child plays alone

9. _____ Cooperative   b. Child watches others playing

10. _____ Onlooker   c. Children play in groups and establish rules for participating

11. _____ Parallel   d. Children play side-by-side but do not interact with each other

12. _____ Solitary   e. Children play together but without establishing rules and goals

HEALTH PROMOTION

Answer as either true (T) or false (F).

1. _____ Immunizations are effective in decreasing the incidence of childhood infectious diseases.

2. _____ Because all states require immunizations for children attending school, obtaining parental informed consent is not necessary.

3. _____ The preferred site for intramuscular injections in infants is the deltoid.

4. _____ Age-appropriate doses of acetaminophen may be given if the child experiences discomfort following an immunization.

5. _____ When administering more than one injection, the nurse should administer the vaccines using separate syringes at different sites.

6. _____ An otherwise healthy child with a low-grade fever can receive immunizations.

7. _____ Because of the threat of bioterrorism, the American Academy of Pediatrics recommends the routine administration of the smallpox vaccine for all children who are not immunocompromised.

8. _____ The *Haemophilus influenzae* type b (Hib) vaccine has significantly reduced the incidence of seasonal influenza among infants and young children.

20

Fill in the blanks.

9. In general, children who are immunocompromised should not receive _____ vaccines.

10. Because of the possibility of anaphylactic reactions, it is essential to have _____ available while administering immunizations.

Match each nutrient with its function.

11. _____ Carbohydrates

12. _____ Fats

13. _____ Proteins

14. _____ Water

15. _____ Vitamins/minerals

    a. Building and maintaining body tissue

    b. Transporting nutrients to and waste away from cells

    c. The primary dietary source of energy

    d. Regulating metabolic processes

    e. A secondary dietary source of energy

Fill in the blanks.

16. Why is dietary fat intake not restricted in children younger than 2 years? _____

_____

_____

17. After the age of 4 years, fat intake should be between _____ % and _____ % of daily calories.

18. Why is it important to gather data about a hospitalized child's food preferences?

_____

_____

19. List three methods of obtaining a dietary history.

    a. _____

    b. _____

    c. _____

20. What is the leading cause of death in children in the United States?

_____

SUGGESTED LEARNING ACTIVITIES

1. Observe pediatricians or nurse practitioners performing well-child assessments. How did they establish trust with the child and parents? How did they go about assessing the child's growth? How did they assess development? How did they convey their findings to the child's parents? Were they able to effectively work with both the child and parents?

2. Chart the height, weight, and head circumference of at least three children (an infant, a young child, and a school-age child or adolescent) on a standardized growth chart. Write a brief interpretation of your findings.

3. Have a discussion with your peers about how poverty can adversely affect a child's growth and development.

STUDENT LEARNING APPLICATIONS

Enhance your learning by discussing your answers with other students.

Parents have brought their 12-month-old daughter to the pediatrician for a well-baby checkup. They tell you they are concerned because she is not as tall as her brother was at 12 months and because she cannot yet walk. You plot her height, weight, and head circumference and find that these measurements fall within the same growth channel as on her previous visits. You have received training in administering the DDST-II. You perform this assessment and find that the child has no delays. Her immunizations are up to date. From a dietary history, you learn that she is drinking low-fat (2%) milk from a cup.

1. How would you interpret the child's growth charts for the parents?

2. The parents express relief that their child "passed the IQ test" when you interpret the results of the DDST-II for them. How would you respond to that?

3. What immunizations are required at this time?

4. What anticipatory guidance would you give to the parents?

5. How would you determine whether the parents' concerns about their daughter's growth and development have been alleviated?

REVIEW QUESTIONS

Choose the correct answer.

1. Cephalocaudal development follows:
   a. the pattern of myelinization.
   b. the development of the bronchial tree.
   c. language development.
   d. neuromuscular development.

2. An infant responds to an injection by crying and flailing the extremities, whereas a preschooler responds by rubbing the injection site. This is an example of what pattern of development?
   a. Cephalocaudal
   b. Proximodistal
   c. General to specific
   d. Simple to complex

3. A child's growth and development are affected by:
   a. cultural background.
   b. heredity.
   c. socioeconomic status.
   d. all of these.

4. Which theorist described how children learn?
   a. Erikson
   b. Freud
   c. Kohlberg
   d. Piaget

5. Teaching about safety to school-aged children should be geared toward their:
   a. parents.
   b. chronologic age.
   c. cognitive level of development.
   d. ability to answer questions.

6. Parents of a preschooler are concerned because she wants "to marry" her father and has told her mother to "go outside and play in the street and get hit by a car." The nurse realizes that the:
   a. family should seek counseling.
   b. preschooler's behavior is normal.
   c. child has probably been abused by her mother.
   d. parents are not addressing the child's need for initiative.

7. The secondary dietary source of energy is:
   a. carbohydrates.
   b. fats.
   c. proteins.
   d. vitamins.

8. An adolescent who has been losing weight will record everything he eats for three days. This is an example of:
   a. an anthropometric measurement.
   b. cultural influences on diet.
   c. dietary guidelines.
   d. a food diary.

9. Nurses can prevent childhood injuries by:
   a. modeling safety practices.
   b. educating parents through anticipatory guidance.
   c. supporting legislation that advocates safety measures.
   d. all of the above.

10. When children play board games, they learn that taking turns is rewarded and that cheating is not rewarded. This fosters their:
    a. cognitive development.
    b. emotional development.
    c. moral development.
    d. physical development.

11. A 12-month-old child's immunization record indicates that only one set of immunizations was administered at 2 months. The nurse knows that:
    a. the entire series of immunizations must be repeated.
    b. the HPV vaccine should be administered now.
    c. it is dangerous to readminister the hepatitis b vaccine.
    d. the DTaP vaccine, and not the Td vaccine, should be administered.

6 Health Promotion for the Infant

HELPFUL HINT

Review infant development in a developmental psychology textbook.

MATCHING KEY TERMS

Match the term with the correct definition.

1. _____ Asphyxiation
2. _____ Critical milestones
3. _____ Developmental milestones
4. _____ Egocentrism
5. _____ Mistrust
6. _____ Object permanence
7. _____ Parent–infant attachment
8. _____ pincer grasp
9. _____ Sensorimotor stage
10. _____ Stranger anxiety
11. _____ Trust

a. Benchmarks of development that indicate that the child is normally developing

b. Inability to see another person's point of view

c. Emotional foundation on which a healthy personality is built

d. Use of the index finger and thumb to pick up objects

e. State of suffocation that severely compromises oxygen delivery

f. Realization that things continue to exist when out of sight

g. Distress experienced when the infant is separated from caregivers or meets unfamiliar persons

h. Negative resolution of Erikson's first developmental task

i. Developmental benchmarks that, if not reached, necessitate a full developmental assessment

j. Piaget's first stage of cognitive development

k. Sense of connection between the parent and infant

GROWTH AND DEVELOPMENT OF THE INFANT

Next to each activity, write the age at which the behavior generally first appears.
Age Choices

1 to 2 months   3 months   4 to 5 months   6 to 7 months   8 to 9 months   12 months

1. Begins to obey simple commands _____

2. Crying becomes differentiated _____

3. Sits alone _____

4. Smiles in response to others _____

5. Birth weight doubles _____

6. Cruises around the furniture _____

7. Begins to demonstrate stranger anxiety _____

8. Is alert for 1.5 to 2 hours _____

9. Behavior is mostly reflexive _____

10. Can breathe when the nose is obstructed _____

11. Pincer grasp develops _____

12. Birth weight triples _____

13. Turns from the abdomen to the back _____

14. Has a beginning sense of object permanence _____

Fill in the blanks.

15. Infants are vulnerable to respiratory infections because of _____ and _____.

16. During infancy, the heart rate _____, while the blood pressure _____.

17. _____ transmits additional immunoglobulin A (IgA) protection to the infant.

18. At what age does the ability to digest and absorb fats reach adult levels? _____

19. Because infants' renal systems are immature, they are at risk for _____.

Match each substage of Piaget's sensorimotor stage with its description.

20. _____ Reflex activity   a. Actions become intentional.

21. _____ Primary circular reactions   b. Begins to have sense of object permanence

22. _____ Secondary circular reactions   c. Activities become less reflexive and more controlled.

23. _____ Coordination of secondary schemata   d. Behavior is dominated by reflexes.

Answer as either true (T) or false (F).

24. _____ Depth perception is present at birth.

25. _____ Lack of eye muscle control at 2 months requires evaluation.

26. _____ All newborns should be screened for hearing problems.

27. _____ By 10 months, an infant should respond to his or her name.

28. _____ An infant's social smile is a communication tool.

29. _____ Vocalization is a reflexive activity.

30. _____ Infants' expressive language is more advanced than receptive language.

31. Briefly describe how an infant develops a sense of suspicion and mistrust.

_____

_____

_____

_____

32. How is the parent–infant attachment strengthened?

_____

_____

_____

_____

25

33. Why does stranger anxiety begin at approximately 6 to 7 months?

_____

_____

_____

_____

HEALTH PROMOTION FOR THE INFANT AND FAMILY

Fill in the blanks.

1. Transplacental passive immunity lasts approximately _____ months.

2. Infant formula lacks the _____ properties and easy _____ of breast milk.

3. Give three examples of mothers who should not breastfeed their infants.

   a. _____

   b. _____

   c. _____

4. What is weaning?

   _____

5. Describe how to introduce solid foods into an infant's diet.

   _____

   _____

   _____

   _____

Answer as either true (T) or false (F).

6. _____ Infants typically have 12 teeth by their first birthday.

7. _____ Baby aspirin is the drug of choice for alleviating teething discomfort.

8. _____ Parents can use a washcloth and a tiny bit of toothpaste to clean their infant's teeth.

9. _____ Bottle mouth caries are preventable.

10. _____ Botulism is associated with an infant intake of honey.

11. List four recommendations from the American Academy of Pediatrics for preventing Sudden Infant Death Syndrome (SIDS).

   a. _____

   b. _____

   c. _____

   d. _____

Fill in the blanks.

12. When riding in a car, infants weighing less than 20 lb should be placed in the back seat in a _____ facing car safety seat.

13. Sunscreen should be applied to an infant's skin starting at the age of _____.

14. Temperature settings on hot water heaters should be no higher than _____ °F.

15. Gates at the top and bottom of the stairs should be in place when the child starts to _____.

16. List four foods that pose an asphyxiation risk.

    a. _____

    b. _____

    c. _____

    d. _____

17. List four suggestions that may help parents reduce their infants' irritability.

    a. _____

    b. _____

    c. _____

    d. _____

18. Why should parents consult a health care professional before giving their infant chamomile tea for colic?

    _____

    _____

SUGGESTED LEARNING ACTIVITIES

1. Design a safety booklet for parents of infants.

2. Perform a developmental assessment on an infant. Assess fine and gross motor skills, language patterns, and psychosocial interactions. Based on your knowledge of infant growth and development, determine whether the infant is functioning at the expected level.

STUDENT LEARNING APPLICATIONS

Enhance your learning by discussing your answers with other students.

An 8-month-old infant is being hospitalized for 2 weeks to receive intravenous antibiotic therapy.

1. What can the nurse do to facilitate parent–infant attachment during this period?

2. How can the nurse deal with the infant's stranger anxiety?

3. What can the hospital staff do to facilitate the development of trust in the infant?

REVIEW QUESTIONS

Choose the correct answer.

1. According to Piaget, an infant who intentionally shakes a rattle to hear the sound is in what substage?
   a. Reflexive
   b. Primary circular reactions
   c. Secondary circular reactions
   d. Coordination of secondary schemata

2. An 11-month-old infant enjoys picking up pieces of banana one by one with the thumb and index finger and throwing them on the floor. This is an example of:
   a. egocentrism.
   b. pincer grasp.
   c. oral activity.
   d. reflexive activity.

3. An infant should turn her eyes and head toward a sound coming from behind her at:
   a. birth.
   b. 4 months of age.
   c. 6 months of age.
   d. 10 months of age.

4. An infant will develop a sense of mistrust if he is:
   a. adopted.
   b. hospitalized after birth.
   c. consistently ignored.
   d. sent to daycare before 2 months of age.

5. Parent–infant attachment:
   a. is critical for survival.
   b. is essential for normal development.
   c. involves the infant as an active participant in the process.
   d. is all of the above.

6. The parents of a 3-month-old infant with colic explain that because their daughter does not sleep through the night, they feel very frustrated. The nurse's first action is to:
   a. provide information about normal sleep–wake cycles in a 3-month-old infant.
   b. suggest that they practice relaxation techniques.
   c. assure them that they are not bad parents.
   d. demonstrate how to soothe the infant.

7. Which statement suggests that the parent needs more information about infant nutrition?
   a. "I'll change from breast milk to whole milk at approximately 6 months."
   b. "I'll introduce soft foods at approximately 5 months."
   c. "I'll add new foods one at a time."
   d. "I'll gradually introduce drinking from a cup."

8. An appropriate "finger food" for an 11-month-old infant is:
   a. cheerios.
   b. lollipops.
   c. popcorn.
   d. raisins.

9. Which statement about immunity and immunizations is true?
   a. Breastfed infants do not need immunizations until they are weaned.
   b. Infants are prone to infectious diseases because of immature immune systems.
   c. Transplacental passive immunity lasts through the first year of life.
   d. Immunizations offer the infant total protection against infectious diseases.

10. Which infant is at risk for developing lead toxicity?
    a. A 10-month-old whose mother crafts stained glass.
    b. An 8-month-old living in a recently constructed house.
    c. A 9-month-old who plays with toys that are made in the United States.
    d. A 6-month-old whose 9-month-old cousin has lead toxicity.

7 Health Promotion During Early Childhood

HELPFUL HINT

Review toddler and preschool development in a developmental psychology textbook.

MATCHING KEY TERMS

Match the term with the correct definition.

1. _____ Associative play
2. _____ Autonomy
3. _____ Caries
4. _____ Cooperative play
5. _____ Dysfluency
6. _____ Irreversibility
7. _____ Negativism
8. _____ Parallel play
9. _____ Physiologic anorexia
10. _____ Regression
11. _____ Ritualism
12. _____ Symbolic play
13. _____ Symbolic thought
14. _____ Transductive reasoning

a. Return to a behavior characteristic of an earlier stage of development

b. Inability to undo an action that has been performed

c. Reasoning from particular to particular

d. Ability to independently function

e. Playing alongside, but not with, others

f. Tooth decay

g. Ability to allow a mental image to represent something that is not present

h. Decreased appetite related to a decreased caloric need

i. Group play without goals

j. Need to maintain sameness

k. Disorders in the rhythm of speech in which the child knows what to say but is unable to do so

l. Games or play that represents an issue to be addressed

m. Opposition or resistance to the direction of others

n. Organized play with group goals

GROWTH AND DEVELOPMENT DURING EARLY CHILDHOOD

Fill in the blanks.

1. During early childhood, the average weight gain is _____ lbs/yr.

2. Children reach one half of their adult height between the ages of _____ and

_____ years.

3. All 20 deciduous teeth are present by the age of _____ years.

For each of the following, write (T) if the behavior first occurs during toddlerhood or (P) if it first occurs during the preschool years.

4. _____ Learns to walk well

5. _____ May have imaginary friends

6. _____ Handedness clearly established

7. _____ Exhibits negativism as an expression of independence

8. _____ Object permanence firmly established

9. _____ Separation anxiety peaks during this period

10. _____ Gender identity well established

11. _____ May start to use aggressive speech

12. _____ Is in the intuitive substage of Piaget's preoperational stage

13. _____ Masturbation is common

14. _____ Is an avid climber

15. _____ Obeys rules out of self-interest

16. _____ Can brush teeth with supervision

Match each characteristic of preoperational thinking with its example.

17. _____ Animism

18. _____ Centration

19. _____ Egocentrism

20. _____ Irreversibility

21. _____ Magical thought

a. Aaron believes the TV is watching him while he sleeps.

b. Beth took the toy truck apart and cannot put it back together.

c. Carla's brother is in the hospital. She believes she made him sick because she did not want to play with him.

d. Diego can follow only one direction at a time.

e. Elgin took Fatima's toy and cannot understand why Fatima is upset.

HEALTH PROMOTION FOR THE TODDLER OR PRESCHOOLER AND FAMILY

Answer as either true (T) or false (F).

1. _____ Young children should drink two cups of whole milk a day.

2. _____ An appropriate serving size for solid food for the young child is one tablespoon of solid food per year of age.

3. _____ It is appropriate to substitute fruit juice but not fruit drinks for milk.

4. _____ A toddler who eats little solid food but drinks a quart of milk per day is meeting recommended dietary allowances (RDAs).

5. _____ Food jags cause physiologic anorexia.

Fill in the blanks.

6. When should a child first visit the dentist?

_____

7. Why are bedtime rituals important for young children?

_____

_____

8. Explain the difference between nightmares and night terrors.

_____

_____

_____

_____

9. A child learns self-control through _____ and _____.

10. List four discipline techniques appropriate for the preschooler.

    a. _____

    b. _____

    c. _____

    d. _____

11. How can parents prevent drownings?

_____

_____

_____

_____

12. Why is the use of booster seats in the car recommended for preschoolers who weigh more than 40 lbs?

_____

_____

_____

_____

13. What should preschoolers be taught to do in the event that their clothes catch on fire?

_____

_____

_____

_____

14. What do parents need to know about firearm safety?

_____

_____

_____

_____

31

15. What is included in teaching children about sexual abuse?

_____

_____

_____

_____

_____

_____

16. Most children are ready for toilet training by 18 to 24 months. What is the rationale for postponing it until later?

_____

_____

_____

_____

_____

17. List four strategies parents can use to decrease the frequency of temper tantrums.

a. _____

b. _____

c. _____

d. _____

18. How can parents deal with sibling rivalry when a new baby is coming into the household?

_____

_____

_____

_____

_____

19. How can parents help a child who stutters?

_____

_____

_____

_____

_____

SUGGESTED LEARNING ACTIVITY

Interview the parents of a toddler. Discover how they deal with the child's negativism. How did the parents handle toilet training? Was it difficult or easy? If the child has temper tantrums, how do the parents handle them? Ask the parents what information would have been helpful for them to know before their child entered the "terrible twos."

STUDENT LEARNING APPLICATIONS

Enhance your learning by discussing your answers with other students.

A mother has brought her 4-year-old son to the clinic for a well-child checkup. After the physical examination, she seems uncomfortable and hesitant but eventually tells you that she sometimes finds her son masturbating. She finds this very distressing because of her religious beliefs. She says, "I can't believe my little boy picked up such a filthy habit." She tells you that she has punished her son by not letting him play with the other children in their neighborhood.

1. What is your personal reaction to the mother's story?

2. If you have personal misgivings about her actions or reactions, what could you do to help yourself remain nonjudgmental?

3. How would you explain the child's sexuality to his mother while acknowledging the importance of her religious beliefs?

4. How could you use Kohlberg's theory to help the mother understand her son's ability to distinguish right from wrong?

REVIEW QUESTIONS

Choose the correct answer.

1. Which statement indicates that the parents of a toddler need more information about toddler safety?
   a. "We always put her in her car safety seat, even if we only drive down the street."
   b. "We never let her play outside alone."
   c. "We always put our cleaning supplies on the shelves above the sink."
   d. "One of us stays with her the entire time that she is in the bathtub."

2. During a well-child checkup, a father asks the nurse whether his 3-year-old son, who weighs 31 lb, can use the car seatbelt instead of the child car safety seat. The nurse's best response is:
   a. "He's old enough to use a shoulder harness and lap belt."
   b. "He should continue to use the car safety seat."
   c. "It's time to switch to a booster seat."
   d. "He'll be safest in a rear-facing car safety seat."

3. What provides a toddler with a sense of security?
   a. Animism
   b. Egocentrism
   c. Negativism
   d. Ritualism

4. Toddlers have temper tantrums because they:
   a. have limited language ability.
   b. are not getting enough attention.
   c. are unable to distinguish right from wrong.
   d. have poor parent–child attachments.

5. During a well-child checkup, the nurse notices that a toddler's teeth are brownish and speckled with white. The nurse suspects that the child:
   a. does not brush her teeth.
   b. goes to sleep with a bottle of milk.
   c. eats too much candy.
   d. ingests too much fluoride.

6. According to Erikson, preschoolers who are encouraged to try new things and be creative will develop a sense of:
   a. autonomy.
   b. initiative.
   c. industry.
   d. integrity.

7. A parent tells the nurse that she is worried because her preschooler has an imaginary friend. The nurse explains that:
   a. the parent should consider enrolling in parenting classes.
   b. the child would probably benefit from going to daycare a few days a week.
   c. imaginary friends are not unusual during the preschool period.
   d. the parent should try to spend more time with the child.

8. While a 5-year-old is hospitalized for an appendectomy, he tells the nurse that he is in the hospital because he was bad. The nurse should:
   a. suspect child abuse and report it to the authorities.
   b. question the parents about their discipline methods.
   c. explain to the child why he is in the hospital.
   d. ignore the comment.

9. A 3-year-old walks out of the kitchen drinking a bottle of dishwashing liquid. After taking the bottle away from her, the parents should:
   a. call 911.
   b. induce vomiting.
   c. call a poison control center.
   d. give her 4 oz of milk to drink.

10. A hospitalized 5-year-old thinks that the IV pole is a skinny monster that is going to tie her up. This is an example of:
    a. animism.
    b. centration.
    c. hallucinatory delusions.
    d. magical thinking.

11. Which action suggests that a 20-month-old should not yet begin toilet training?
    a. He says "Pee-pee" when his diaper is soiled.
    b. His mother is expecting a baby in 3 weeks.
    c. He is able to remove his pants.
    d. He can sit and walk well.

12. Which action indicates that a 5-year-old is ready for kindergarten?
    a. The child can follow three-part instructions.
    b. The child can wait and take turns.
    c. The child is able to independently go to the bathroom.
    d. All of these indicate readiness for school.

8 Health Promotion for the School-Age Child

HELPFUL HINT

Review school-age development in a developmental psychology textbook.

MATCHING KEY TERMS

Match the term with the correct definition.

1. _____ Caries
2. _____ Conservation
3. _____ Malocclusion
4. _____ Menarche
5. _____ Self-care children

a. Misalignment of teeth
b. Ability to understand that certain properties of objects remain the same despite changes in appearance
c. Children who care for themselves after school
d. Onset of menstruation
e. Tooth decay

GROWTH AND DEVELOPMENT OF THE SCHOOL-AGE CHILD

Answer as either true (T) or false (F).

1. _____ Throughout the school-age years, boys are consistently taller and heavier than girls.
2. _____ The onset of puberty is signaled by the adolescent growth spurt.
3. _____ Tonsil enlargement in the school-age child is considered an abnormal finding.
4. _____ All permanent teeth are in place by the age of 12 years.
5. _____ Menarche occurs later in females who are obese.

Fill in the blanks.

6. Why is active play important for school-age children?

_____

_____

_____

_____

_____

7. Why are children more prone to dehydration than adults?

_____

_____

_____

8. Reversibility allows children in the concrete operational stage to anticipate the results of their _____.

9. Children understand the principle of conservation of _____ before they understand conservation of _____.

35

10. Why is collecting stickers an appropriate activity for school-age children?

_____

_____

_____

_____

_____

11. How do friendships change as school-age children mature?

_____

_____

12. Why do middle ear infections occur less often in school-age children than in younger children?

_____

_____

13. How do children develop a sense of industry?

_____

_____

14. How is the developmental task of industry related to self-esteem?

_____

_____

15. Why are rules important to school-age children?

_____

_____

16. Briefly describe why children obey rules in each of the following stages of moral development.

    a. Preconventional, stage 2: _____

    b. Conventional, stage 3: _____

    c. Conventional, stage 4: _____

17. For parents' moral teaching to be effective, they must:

    a. _____ in accordance with their own values.

    b. Be consistent in their _____ of what the child should do.

    c. Be consistent in administering _____ and _____.

HEALTH PROMOTION FOR THE SCHOOL-AGE CHILD AND FAMILY

Fill in the blanks.

1. School-age children need how many servings of the following foods each day?

    a. _____ oz. of grains

    b. _____ cups of vegetables

    c. _____ cups of fruits

    d. _____ oz. of protein

    e. _____ cups of dairy products

2. A 6-year-old needs approximately _____ hours of sleep, whereas a 12-year-old needs _____ hours.

3. How can parents foster a sense of responsibility in their children?

_____

_____

_____

_____

4. List three strategies parents can use to help their child succeed in school.

   a. _____

   b. _____

   c. _____

5. How can nurses act as advocates for self-care children?

_____

_____

_____

_____

_____

6. What can parents do to prevent childhood obesity?

_____

_____

_____

_____

_____

_____

SUGGESTED LEARNING ACTIVITIES

1. Interview an elementary school teacher. Ask about the common stressors encountered by students in the teacher's class. How does the teacher's perception of student stressors compare with those identified in your textbook? What information does the teacher think school-age children need to help them cope more effectively with stress?

2. Choose one of the topics under "Sources of Stress in Children" in your textbook. Design a teaching plan focused on this topic and intended for a group of 8- to 10-year-old children. What makes this topic stressful? How can children in this age group cope with that stressor?

STUDENT LEARNING APPLICATIONS

Enhance your learning by discussing your answers with other students.

A 7-year-old girl missed a week of school because of nausea and vague abdominal pain on waking in the morning. She felt better after her siblings left for school each morning but had temper tantrums when her parents suggested she go to school in the afternoon. She had no symptoms over the weekend. On Monday morning, her symptoms returned, and her parents made an appointment with the pediatric nurse practitioner (PNP). After a thorough physical examination, the PNP made the tentative diagnosis of school refusal.

1. What in this scenario suggests school refusal?

2. What questions would you ask the child about her relationships with her parents, teachers, siblings, classmates, and friends to discover the "cause" of her school refusal?

3. The father asks, "What should we do if my daughter says she is sick tomorrow?" What suggestions can the PNP give him?

4. Two days later, the father calls to say that his daughter told him that she thinks her math teacher "hates" her. How can the PNP help the family and child deal with this situation?

REVIEW QUESTIONS

1. Sex education for the 9-year-old child should include information about:
   a. anatomy and physiology.
   b. bodily functions.
   c. what to expect during puberty.
   d. all of the above.

2. Children at an increased risk for dental caries include those who:
   a. wear braces.
   b. do not wear mouth protectors during sports activities.
   c. use smokeless tobacco.
   d. do any of the above.

3. Children in the intuitive thought stage:
   a. form hypotheses.
   b. are able to reverse their thinking.
   c. classify objects into categories.
   d. exhibit egocentrism.

4. Parents should limit school-age children's daily television viewing time to:
   a. 1 hour.
   b. 2 hours.
   c. 3 hours.
   d. 4 hours.

5. An appropriate coach for a child's basketball team:
   a. has a win-at-all-costs philosophy.
   b. is courteous to children, referees, and other coaches.
   c. divides the children into teams based on age.
   d. demonstrates all of the above.

6. An example of an activity that develops fine motor skills in the school-age child is:
   a. rollerblading.
   b. playing the guitar.
   c. playing tag.
   d. swimming.

7. An 8-year-old child typically:
   a. solves problems through random guessing.
   b. comprehends historical time.
   c. understands the conservation of mass.
   d. cannot appreciate another person's point of view.

8. *Healthy People 2020* objectives for school-age children include:
   a. increasing the proportion of children with disabilities who spend at least 40% of their time in regular education programs.
   b. reducing the proportion of children with mental health problems.
   c. increasing the proportion of children older than 2 years who consume at least 30% of their calories from fat.
   d. increasing the proportion of children who receive dental sealants on their molar teeth.

9. A child who does not successfully complete the developmental task of industry develops a sense of:
   a. shame and doubt.
   b. guilt.
   c. inferiority.
   d. confusion.

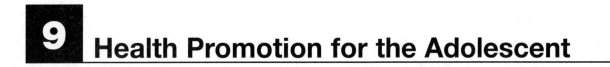

9 Health Promotion for the Adolescent

HELPFUL HINT

Review adolescent development in a developmental psychology text.

MATCHING KEY TERMS

Match the term with the correct definition.

1. _____ Adolescence
2. _____ Autonomy
3. _____ Egocentrism
4. _____ Identity formation
5. _____ Primary sexual characteristics
6. _____ Puberty
7. _____ Pubescence
8. _____ Reproductive maturity
9. _____ Risk-taking behavior
10. _____ Secondary sexual characteristics
11. _____ Sexual maturity rating (SMR)

a. Spermatogenesis in males and menstruation in females
b. Acquisition of psychosocial, sexual, and vocational identity
c. Period before sexual maturity
d. Capacity to be self-governing
e. Transition from childhood to adulthood
f. Internal and external reproductive organs
g. Stages of sexual maturation
h. Behavior that predisposes a person to harm
i. Concern with self
j. Achievement of reproductive maturity
k. Physical characteristics of males and females that have no direct role in reproduction

ADOLESCENT GROWTH AND DEVELOPMENT

Fill in the blanks.

1. Physical maturation in girls occurs with the onset and establishment of _____.

2. Another term for the adolescent growth spurt is: _____.

3. In girls, the appearance of _____ is the first sign of ovarian functioning.

4. Breast enlargement in boys is called: _____.

5. An adolescent's chronologic age provides less information about physical development than does _____.

6. In boys, the first sign of pubertal changes is: _____.

7. The secretion of sex hormones (_____ in girls and _____ in boys) stimulates the development of breast tissue, pubic hair, and genitalia.

8. List five effective strategies the nurse can use when communicating with teens.

   a. _____

   b. _____

   c. _____

d. _____

e. _____

9. In adolescent psychosocial development, what is meant by the "moratorium"?

_____

_____

_____

_____

10. What functions do adolescent peer groups serve?

_____

_____

_____

_____

For questions 11 through 18, identify the period of adolescence (early, middle, or late) during which the described behavior is most likely to occur.

11. Best friends are of the same gender. _____

12. Adolescents react to an imaginary audience. _____

13. Emancipation from parents is a major issue. _____

14. Adolescents overidentify with glamorous role models. _____

15. Conflicts with parents escalate. _____

16. Conformity with a peer group is less important. _____

17. Gang membership brings security. _____

18. This is the most frustrating time for parents. _____

HEALTH PROMOTION FOR THE ADOLESCENT AND FAMILY

Answer as either true (T) or false (F).

1. _____ Lack of self-esteem and peer pressure influence a teen's sexual behavior.

2. _____ Adolescents require fewer calories during peak height velocity (PHV).

3. _____ When transporting an avulsed tooth, place it in a container of milk.

4. _____ Because of PHV, adolescents require at least 10 hours of sleep per night.

5. _____ Regular exercise promotes healthy sleep patterns.

6. _____ More teens die from unintentional injuries than from all other causes of death combined.

7. _____ Adolescents with tattoos may be injured during magnetic resonance imaging.

Fill in the blanks.

8. The USDA recommends an intake of _____ cal/day for adolescent girls and _____ cal/day for adolescent boys.

9. Adolescents who use tanning salons are at risk for _____, _____, and _____.

10. In addition to depression, risk factors for teen suicide include:

_____

_____

_____

_____

Answer as either true (T) or false (F).

11. _____ A teen's cognitive ability affects contraceptive practices.

12. _____ Studies indicate that adolescents believe that engaging in oral sex is more socially acceptable and less risky than vaginal intercourse.

13. _____ Ideally, contraceptive education should include both partners.

14. _____ All threats of suicide by an adolescent should be taken seriously.

15. _____ Violence is an innate human behavior.

16. _____ Homicide is the second leading cause of death among teens aged 15 to 19 years.

SUGGESTED LEARNING ACTIVITY

Visit a teen pregnancy center in your community. Find out what services are offered, how teens are selected for the program, how the program is evaluated, and how it is funded. What other health promotion activities does the program provide for teens? Report your findings to your class.

STUDENT LEARNING APPLICATIONS

Enhance your learning by discussing your answers with other students.

You are invited to address a high school parent–teacher meeting to talk about early adolescent health.

1. Which health topics would you include? Why would you include these?

2. What developmental information would you include? Why?

3. Which topics would you include on psychologic health? Why?

REVIEW QUESTIONS

Choose the correct answer.

1. According to Piaget, most adolescents eventually achieve which stage?
   a. Sensorimotor
   b. Preoperational
   c. Concrete operations
   d. Formal operations

2. In adolescence, sexual activity is usually related to:
   a. risk taking.
   b. alcohol and/or substance abuse.
   c. low self-esteem.
   d. all of these.

3. According to Erikson, a person who has not successfully completed the developmental task of adolescence will experience:
   a. shame and doubt.
   b. identity.
   c. role confusion.
   d. guilt.

4. Which tool is used to assess sexual maturity?
   a. Denver Developmental Screening Test II (DDST-II)
   b. Dubowitz
   c. Tanner
   d. Elkind

5. A hospitalized adolescent has emotional highs followed by emotional lows. The nurse notes that the adolescent:
   a. is a substance abuser.
   b. is emotionally labile.
   c. has access to alcohol.
   d. None of the above.

6. Which is a *Healthy People 2020* objective for adolescents?
   a. Increase high school completion.
   b. Reduce physical fighting.
   c. Reduce pregnancies.
   d. All of the above.

7. In boys, PHV occurs during Tanner stages:
   a. 1 and 2.
   b. 2 and 3.
   c. 3 and 4.
   d. 4 and 5.

8. Gynecomastia:
   a. is always bilateral.
   b. occurs in the majority of adolescent males.
   c. requires surgical intervention.
   d. begins during late adolescence.

10 Heredity and Environmental Influences on Development

HELPFUL HINT

Review the principles of heredity.

MATCHING KEY TERMS

Match the term with the correct definition.

1. _____ Allele   a. Common gene variation

2. _____ Karyotype   b. Cell with an added set of chromosomes

3. _____ Monosomy   c. Alternate gene form

4. _____ Mutation   d. Variation in a gene that affects function

5. _____ Polymorphism   e. Chromosomes arranged from largest to smallest pairs

6. _____ Polyploidy   f. One extra chromosome present in each body cell

7. _____ Somatic cell   g. All or part of a chromosome attached to another

8. _____ Teratogen   h. Body cells other than germ cells

9. _____ Translocation   i. Cells with only one chromosome

10. _____ Trisomy   j. Agent that causes or increases the risk for a birth defect

HEREDITARY INFLUENCES

1. Explain how deoxyribonucleic acid (DNA), genes, and chromosomes are related.

2. What is the Human Genome Project?

3. The explosion of knowledge about the genetic basis for disease raises many legal and ethical issues. How can this knowledge affect the following?

a. Privacy

b. Self-esteem

c. Level of anxiety

d. Health insurance coverage

4. For each type of single-gene abnormality, describe the conditions necessary for a child to be affected and specify any sex differences.

a. Autosomal recessive

b. Autosomal dominant

c. X-linked recessive

Answer as either true (T) or false (F).

5. _____ Sickle cell disease follows an autosomal-recessive pattern of development.

6. _____ Type O blood follows an autosomal-dominant pattern of development.

7. _____ All sons of a father with hemophilia will inherit the disease.

8. _____ Turner syndrome is an example of a numerical abnormality.

9. _____ Fragile X syndrome is the most common form of female intellectual disability.

MULTIFACTORIAL DISORDERS

1. Describe two characteristics typical of multifactorial birth defects.

a. _____

b. _____

2. What factors influence the risk for the occurrence of a multifactorial disorder?

ENVIRONMENTAL INFLUENCES

1. When should a rubella immunization be administered to a woman of childbearing age?

2. In prescribing drugs for pregnant women, what must the nurse practitioner balance?

3. When a pregnant woman requires an urgent X-ray study, her lower abdomen is _____.

4. Why should pregnant women avoid saunas and hot tubs?

GENETIC COUNSELING

Fill in the blanks.

1. Genetic counseling focuses on the entire _____.

2. Genetic counseling is considered _____ because the counselor does not tell the patient what decision to make.

NURSING CARE OF FAMILIES CONCERNED ABOUT BIRTH DEFECTS

1. How do nurses in the following practices provide care related to genetics?

   a. Women's health nurses

   b. Antepartum nurses

   c. Neonatal nurses

   d. Pediatric nurses

SUGGESTED LEARNING ACTIVITIES

1. In the clinical setting, review charts for women or children who were referred for genetic counseling or genetic studies. Why were they referred? Who participated in the counseling? What were the outcomes? Discuss your findings with your classmates.

2. Using the symbols and examples in your textbook as a guideline, draw a three-generation pedigree of your family tree. Note any traits [normal (e.g., blood type) or abnormal] that you know about each person. What patterns emerge?

Choose the correct answer.

1. The nurse notes this information on the chromosomal study of an infant with a birth defect: 46, XY. This means that the infant has:
   a. abnormal genes in all 46 chromosomes.
   b. a normal male chromosome analysis.
   c. an abnormal female chromosome makeup.
   d. Down syndrome (trisomy 21).

2. The nurse should expect a pregnant African-American woman to be offered genetic testing for which disorder?
   a. Cystic fibrosis
   b. Tay–Sachs disease
   c. Rh isoimmunization
   d. Sickle cell disease

3. Parents of a child with an abnormal autosomal-recessive disorder want to know whether the problem is likely to recur if they have another child. The nurse knows that:
   a. it is unlikely that they would ever have another child with the abnormality.
   b. each pregnancy has a one in four (25%) chance of resulting in another affected child.
   c. any pregnancy that occurs before the mother is 40 years old is not likely to have the defect.
   d. their risk for having another child with the defect cannot be exactly calculated.

4. A woman who is 5 weeks pregnant asks the nurse whether she can take a specific medication to relieve her cold symptoms. The nurse's answer is primarily based primarily on:
   a. whether the drug is prescribed or available over-the-counter.
   b. the severity of the woman's respiratory symptoms.
   c. the pregnancy category of the drug.
   d. how long the woman has had the cold.

5. A pediatric nurse is caring for an infant girl with hemophilia A. The nurse realizes that:
   a. both parents must have hemophilia.
   b. the mother is a carrier and the father has hemophilia.
   c. hemophilia is an autosomal-dominant trait.
   d. the infant is misdiagnosed.

11 Reproductive Anatomy and Physiology

MATCHING KEY TERMS

Match the term with the correct definition.

1. _____ Linea terminalis

2. _____ Nocturnal emissions

3. _____ Perineum

4. _____ Rugae

5. _____ Vulva

   a. Imaginary line dividing the upper (false) pelvis from the lower (true) pelvis

   b. Spontaneous release of seminal fluid from the penis during sleep

   c. Small ridges or folds of tissue in the female vagina and on the male scrotum

   d. Collective term for all of the female external reproductive organs

   e. Posterior part of external female reproductive organs

Match each structure with its function(s). Some letters may be used more than once.

6. _____ Acini cells

7. _____ Bartholin's glands

8. _____ Corpus cavernosum

9. _____ Corpus spongiosum

10. _____ Leydig cells

11. _____ Montgomery's tubercles

12. _____ Myoepithelial cells

13. _____ Scrotum

14. _____ Sertoli cells

15. _____ Skene's glands

   a. Enable the erection of the penis for coitus

   b. Nourish sperm during their formation within the testes

   c. Promote the lubrication of the vagina for coitus

   d. Produce milk from substances extracted from blood

   e. Secrete a substance to keep nipples soft during breastfeeding

   f. Regulate the temperature of the testes to promote normal sperm formation

   g. Lubricate the female's urethra

   h. Secrete testosterone in the male

   i. Eject milk into the ductal system of the breast

KEY CONCEPTS

1. What mechanism prevents the onset of puberty before the proper time?

2. The period when reproductive organs become fully functional is called _____. It begins at an approximate age of _____ years in girls and an approximate age of _____ years in boys.

3. The first outward change of puberty in girls is _____. The first outward change of puberty in boys is _____.

4. Girls usually experience their first menstrual period at approximately _____ years after the first outward change associated with puberty.

5. What factors cause the average male to be taller than the average female at physical maturity?

6. Explain the importance of each type of smooth muscle fiber in the myometrium. Where is each type primarily located?

   a. Longitudinal fibers
      - Importance:

      - Location:

   b. Interlacing (figure-eight) fibers
      - Importance:

      - Location:

   c. Circular fibers
      - Importance:

      - Location:

7. Fertilization normally occurs in the _____.

8. When are female gametes formed? When are male gametes formed?

9. Describe events in each phase of the ovarian cycle.

   a. Follicular phase

   b. Ovulatory phase

   c. Luteal phase

10. Describe events in each phase of the endometrial cycle.

a. Proliferative phase

b. Secretory phase

c. Menstrual phase

11. Why might a man who usually wears very tight underwear have a problem with infertility?

REVIEW QUESTIONS

Choose the correct answer.

1. The sex of an infant will be female unless:
   a. two X chromosomes are received from the mother.
   b. the Y chromosome is received from the father.
   c. conception occurs during the last half of the female reproductive cycle.
   d. the mother's ovary produces testosterone early in pregnancy.

2. The primary purpose of gonadotropin-releasing hormone (GnRH) is to stimulate:
   a. the development of the woman's breasts for lactation.
   b. growth of pubic and axillary hair.
   c. breakdown of the endometrium during the menstrual flow.
   d. secretion of follicle-stimulating hormone (FSH) and luteinizing hormone (LH) from the anterior pituitary gland.

3. The first outward change of puberty in girls is:
   a. rapid growth to reach the adult height and weight.
   b. enlargement and development of the breasts.
   c. onset of menstruation.
   d. increase in clear vaginal secretions.

4. Choose the girl who is most likely to have secondary amenorrhea.
   a. Amanda, a 15-year-old, who is approximately 10% above her ideal weight for height.
   b. Brittany, a 17-year-old, who is preparing for competing in a national gymnastic tournament.
   c. Chloe, a 16-year-old, who had her first menstrual period 1 year ago at the age of 15 years.
   d. Deanna, a 16-year-old, who had her first signs of puberty at the age of 10 years.

5. Males are usually taller than females when they reach their adult height because their:
   a. growth in height occurs early in puberty and continues for a short time after puberty.
   b. secretion of testosterone delays the closure of the epiphyses of the long bones.
   c. puberty changes begin approximately 2 years later than in the average female.
   d. rapid increase in height begins later in puberty and continues for a longer time.

6. The layer of uterine muscle that is most active during labor is composed of what kind of fibers?
   a. Longitudinal
   b. Interlacing
   c. Circular

7. The layer of uterine tissue that responds to cyclic changes in hormones that are secreted by the pituitary gland is the:
   a. perimetrium.
   b. myometrium.
   c. endometrium.

8. Conditions that cause the fallopian tubes to be narrower than normal may result in:
   a. excessive cramping and bleeding during menstruation.
   b. increased likelihood of pregnancy during each cycle.
   c. more rapid propulsion of the ovum through the tube.
   d. implantation of a fertilized ovum within the tube (see Chapter 25).

49

9. Extra follicles that remain after ovulation:
   a. release their ovum during the last half of the reproductive cycle.
   b. resume maturation during the next reproductive cycle.
   c. may be fertilized during another reproductive cycle.
   d. are unresponsive to stimulating hormones and do not mature.

10. Menstruation occurs because the:
    a. hormone stimulation from the corpus luteum ceases.
    b. blood vessels in the uterine lining become too long and twisted.
    c. corpus luteum increases estrogen and progesterone production.
    d. ovum has been passed from the woman's body.

11. Milk is manufactured within the _____ of the breast.
    a. lactiferous ducts
    b. alveoli
    c. myoepithelium
    d. Montgomery's tubercles

12. The primary purpose of the cremaster muscle is to:
    a. eject milk into the lactiferous ducts of the breasts.
    b. maintain the uterus in the anteflexed position.
    c. keep the testes cooler than the rest of the body.
    d. expel seminal fluids to nourish the sperm at ejaculation.

12 Conception and Prenatal Development

MATCHING KEY TERMS

Match the term with the correct definition.

1. _____ Autosome
2. _____ Conceptus
3. _____ Corpus luteum
4. _____ Embryo
5. _____ Gamete
6. _____ Mitosis
7. _____ Oogenesis
8. _____ Ovulation
9. _____ Placenta
10. _____ Somatic cell

a. Fertilized ovum
b. Developing baby from weeks 3 to 8
c. Non-sex chromosome
d. Reproductive cell
e. Ordinary body cell
f. Structure that provides nourishment for the developing baby
g. Cells that remain after ovum formation and secrete estrogen and progesterone
h. Formation of female gametes
i. Cell division in body cells
j. Release of the mature ovum from the ovary

KEY CONCEPTS

1. Compare mitosis with meiosis in the following ways:

Factor	Mitosis	Meiosis
Type of cell involved		
Number and type of chromosomes in each resulting cell		

2. Compare oogenesis with spermatogenesis in the following ways:

Factor	Oogenesis	Spermatogenesis
Number and type of chromosomes in each mature gamete		
Number of gametes that result from each primary cell		
When gametogenesis begins and ends during life		

3. What are the two major occurrences immediately after fertilization?

a. _____

b. _____

4. List three reasons that the fundus is the best area for implantation.

a. _____

b. _____

c. _____

5. List the three germ layers and structures that develop from each.

a. _____

b. _____

c. _____

6. When during prenatal development does each event occur?

a. Closure of the neural tube

b. The heart contains four chambers

c. All abdominal organs are within the abdominal cavity

d. External ear development begins

e. Fetal sex is apparent by the external genitalia

f. Fetal movements are felt by the mother

g. Surfactant production begins

7. Describe each of these fetal structures or substances and state their purpose.

a. Vernix caseosa

b. Lanugo

c. Brown fat

d. Surfactant

8. What is the difference between the fertilization and gestational ages?

9. Explain how each of the following mechanisms allows the fetus to thrive in the relatively low-oxygen environment of the uterus.

a. Fetal hemoglobin and hematocrit

b. Relative fetal and maternal blood carbon dioxide levels

10. Describe how the passage of maternal immunoglobulin G (IgG) antibodies can be either beneficial or harmful to the fetus.

a. Beneficial

b. Harmful

11. Explain the function of each placental hormone.

   a. Human chorionic gonadotropin (hCG)

   b. Human placental lactogen (hPL), now called human chorionic somatomammotropin

   c. Estrogen

   d. Progesterone

12. State the three functions of amniotic fluid:

   a. _____

   b. _____

   c. _____

13. Explain the umbilical cord structure and function.

   a. Umbilical vein

   b. Umbilical arteries (two)

   c. Wharton's jelly

14. Explain the factors that cause each of these fetal circulatory shunts to close after birth and the eventual outcome for each.

   a. Foramen ovale

   b. Ductus arteriosus

   c. Ductus venosus

15. Describe monozygotic and dizygotic twinning in the following terms:

Factor	Monozygotic	Dizygotic
Number of ova and sperm involved		
Genetic component		
Sex		
Hereditary tendency		
Number of amnions and chorions		

CRITICAL THINKING EXERCISES

1. A woman thinks she is pregnant but begins "spotting" (light vaginal bleeding). Her hCG levels are very low. What is the likely consequence of the low hCG levels? Why?

2. What is a likely occurrence if a fetus is born with a lecithin-to-sphingomyelin (L/S) ratio of 1:1?

REVIEW QUESTIONS

Choose the correct answer.

1. An important purpose of seminal fluid is to:
   a. digest microorganisms in the female digestive tract.
   b. prevent the premature movement of sperm tails.
   c. protect sperm from the acidic vaginal environment.
   d. transport the sperm into the uterine cavity.

2. Fertilization is complete when:
   a. the fusion of the sperm and ovum nuclei occurs.
   b. a sperm enters the ovum in the fallopian tube.
   c. the fertilized ovum has its first cell division.
   d. the morula fully implants into the uterine lining.

3. The embryo is fully implanted in the uterus on which day after conception?
   a. 3
   b. 6
   c. 10
   d. 15

4. Which fetal circulatory structure carries blood with the highest oxygen concentration?
   a. Umbilical artery
   b. Umbilical vein
   c. Ductus arteriosus
   d. Pulmonary vein

Chapter **12 Conception and Prenatal Development**

13 Adaptations to Pregnancy

MATCHING KEY TERMS

Match the term with the correct definition.

1. _____ Amenorrhea
2. _____ Chloasma
3. _____ Hyperemia
4. _____ Multigravida
5. _____ Physiologic anemia of pregnancy
6. _____ Striae gravidarum
7. _____ Ambivalence
8. _____ Couvades
9. _____ Introversion
10. _____ Mimicry
11. _____ Narcissism
12. _____ Role transition

a. A woman who has been pregnant more than once

b. Mask of pregnancy

c. Congested with blood in a part of the body

d. Irregular reddish streaks caused by lineal tears in the connective tissue; "stretch marks"

e. Decrease in hematocrit that occurs because the plasma volume expands more than the red blood cell volume

f. Absence of menstruation

g. Conflicting feelings

h. Changing from one pattern of behavior to another

i. Concentration on oneself and one's body

j. Preoccupation with self

k. Observing and copying the behaviors of others

l. Pregnancy-related symptoms and behaviors experienced by some prospective fathers

KEY CONCEPTS

1. When during pregnancy, does each of these markers in fundal height occur?

   a. Uterus can first be palpated above the symphysis pubis.

   b. Fundus can be palpated midway between the symphysis pubis and umbilicus.

   c. Fundus is at the umbilicus level.

   d. Fundus is at the xiphoid process.

2. What is the cause of each of the following changes in the cervix during pregnancy?

    a. Chadwick's sign

    b. Goodell's sign

    c. Mucous plug

    d. Bloody show

3. What is the possible result of each of the following changes in the vagina during pregnancy?

    a. Increase in vascularity

    b. Growth of connective tissue

    c. Secretion of increased amounts of glycogen

4. Why is progesterone essential in pregnancy?

5. Progesterone is produced first by the _____ and then by the _____.

6. Why does ovulation cease during pregnancy?

7. What breast changes occur during pregnancy?

8. Describe changes in maternal heart sounds that may occur during pregnancy. When do the changes in the heart sounds occur? Describe common changes in the heart sounds.

9. Complete the table to describe changes in the pregnant woman's blood. Consult a manual of laboratory tests or medical–surgical text for nonpregnant values, if needed.

Component	Nonpregnancy Level	Pregnancy Level	Change
Plasma volume			
Red blood cell volume			
Leukocytes			
Fibrinogen			

10. What is "supine hypotensive syndrome"? What signs and symptoms might a woman with this syndrome display? What should the nurse do to prevent or relieve it?

11. Why does the pregnancy-induced change in fibrinogen levels have a protective effect yet also increase the risk?

12. What nasal changes are common during pregnancy? What causes them?

13. What two factors contribute to a woman's sense of dyspnea?

   a. _____

   b. _____

14. Why are pregnant women more likely to develop gallstones?

15. Why does a pregnant woman's bone mass remain stable, although the fetus requires calcium for skeletal development?

16. What changes in carbohydrate metabolism and in the production, utilization, and breakdown of insulin occur during pregnancy? Why do these changes occur? How does the woman's body normally respond to these changes?

17. Describe edema that is expected during pregnancy and why it occurs. When should it be reported?

18. List the presumptive, probable, and positive indications of pregnancy. What is the difference among the three classifications?

19. List some reasons for a false-negative pregnancy test.

20. At what point in gestation is it possible to hear fetal heart sounds using Doppler?

21. Use Nägele's rule to calculate the estimated dates of delivery (EDDs) for each of these dates representing last normal menstrual period dates.

    a. February 4

    b. August 2

22. Why is a pregnancy risk assessment not a one-time evaluation?

23. What routine urine testing is performed during prenatal visits?

24. How do each of the following differ when a woman has a multifetal pregnancy?

    a. Uterine size

    b. Fetal movements

    c. Weight gain

25. Describe significant maternal changes that occur in a multifetal pregnancy.

    a. Blood volume

b. Cardiac workload

c. Respiratory workload

d. Blood vessel compression

e. Bowels

26. What teaching is appropriate for each common discomfort of pregnancy?
    a. Nausea and vomiting

    b. Heartburn

    c. Backache

    d. Urinary frequency

    e. Varicosities

    f. Hemorrhoids

    g. Constipation

    h. Leg cramps

27. What should the pregnant woman be taught about the following practices during pregnancy? How would you explain this to a woman if you were the nurse?

a. Over-the-counter drugs

b. Tobacco

c. Illegal drugs

d. Hot tubs and saunas

e. Douching

f. Exercise

g. Use of a seatbelt

28. List the typical maternal responses for each trimester of pregnancy.

a. First trimester

b. Second trimester

c. Third trimester

29. What changes occur that make the fetus seem real to the pregnant woman?

30. How might sexual interest and activity change during pregnancy? What factors may increase or decrease interest in either partner of the couple?

61

Chapter **13** **Adaptations to Pregnancy**

31. How does the woman's perception of the baby change during pregnancy?

    a. First trimester

    b. Second trimester

    c. Third trimester

32. What is the significance of quickening in the woman's developing relationship with her fetus?

33. Why might grief have a place during a desired and normal pregnancy?

34. Describe the four maternal tasks of pregnancy, according to Rubin.

    a.

    b.

    c.

    d.

35. Describe the three developmental processes that the expectant father goes through during a pregnancy.

    a.

    b.

    c.

36. Describe three major factors that influence the grandparents' responses to pregnancy and birth.

a.

b.

c.

37. Describe ways to ease the adaptation of siblings to the birth of an infant.

a. Toddlers

b. Preschoolers

c. School-age children

d. Adolescents

38. How may each of these factors influence a woman's psychosocial adaptation to pregnancy?

a. Young age

b. Absence of a partner

c. Multiparity

39. How may health beliefs differ for pregnant patients from the following cultures?

a. Hispanics

b. American Indians

c. Southeast Asians

d. Muslims

e. Russians

40. What do each of these factors have to do with a woman's choice to take childbirth classes?
    a. Income

    b. Desire to participate

    c. Fear

41. List content typically covered in early pregnancy classes.
    a. First trimester

    b. Second trimester

42. List three important precautions for exercise classes during pregnancy.
    a.

    b.

    c.

43. What are important topics to cover in a cesarean birth preparation class?

CRITICAL THINKING EXERCISES

1. Assess a pregnant woman's blood pressure in each of the following ways. Allow at least 2 minutes between readings. Compare the systolic and diastolic blood pressures. Compute the mean arterial pressure (MAP) for each reading.

   a. Lateral recumbent position

   b. Sitting with arm supported

   c. Sitting with arm dependent

   d. Standing

   e. Diastolic pressure at sound muffling (Korotkoff's 4th phase)

   f. Diastolic pressure at disappearance of sounds (Korotkoff's 5th phase)

2. Compare a prenatal clinic's documentation forms for the initial and subsequent antepartal visits with the recommended assessments listed in the text. What is that clinic's usual recommended frequency for follow-up prenatal visits?

3. Talk with nurses at a local prenatal clinic to determine which different cultural groups they typically serve. Ask them how they incorporate cultural beliefs and values into care.

4. Talk to a pregnant woman about her psychologic reactions to pregnancy. Compare her reactions with the typical responses listed in the text.

5. Talk with expectant fathers about when their baby first became real to them.

6. Observe the interactions of the nursing staff with a woman who did not have prenatal care. Do you note any differences from the interactions with women who have had prenatal care?

7. What are the major cultural groups you encounter in the clinical setting? What specific practices or beliefs can you identify that are unique to each group?

8. You may have to help a woman correct her labor breathing or breathe with her while she is in labor, so you must know it well. Practice the breathing techniques until you are comfortable with them. Then teach them to a friend or family member.

9. Try the breathing techniques during a stressful situation. For example, take a cleansing breath when you begin your next nursing test. Breathe slowly as you take the test. Did it help reduce your stress?

10. Prepare a birth plan that you would like, identifying any special preferences you would like to include in a birth experience.

CASE STUDIES

Katherine is making her first prenatal visit on August 15. She has a 2-year-old son who was delivered at 40 weeks, a 5-year-old daughter delivered at 38 weeks, and 7-year-old twin daughters delivered at 35 weeks. She had a spontaneous abortion 3 years ago at 10 weeks. Her last menstrual period was April 5. Her fundal height is at the level of the umbilicus. She denies any major complaints and states that her health has been good.

1. Determine Katherine's gravida and para. Describe her obstetric history with the TPAL acronym.

2. What is Katherine's EDD?

3. What is Katherine's gestation on the day of her first visit?

4. Compare the present fundal height with the gestation of her pregnancy. If there is a discrepancy, what are some possible causes for it?

5. What factors may have influenced Katherine to delay her first antepartum visit?

6. What diagnostic studies should the nurse anticipate?

Sara is a 17-year-old girl who is making her first visit to the prenatal clinic at 24 weeks of gestation with her first pregnancy. She admits that this pregnancy was not planned and that she has little contact with the baby's father. She quit school during her senior year of high school because she was embarrassed about her situation. She has gained 20 pounds and feels that she is unattractive and fat. She is the oldest of six children and lives at home with her parents.

7. What factors may be involved in Sara's delay in seeking prenatal care?

8. What two priority nursing diagnoses are apparent by Sara's situation?

9. What conflicts are likely between Sara and the clinic staff (physicians and nurses)?

10. What services, in addition to prenatal care, is Sara likely to need because of her situation?

11. What long-term consequences are more likely because of Sara's pregnancy at this time in her life? Why?

REVIEW QUESTIONS

Choose the correct answer.

1. A pregnant woman expects to give birth to her first baby in approximately 1 week. She asks the nurse whether she has a bladder infection because she urinates so much, although urination causes no discomfort. The nurse should explain to her that:
   a. urinary tract infections are most common just before birth, so she should have a urine specimen tested.
   b. her fetus is probably lower in her pelvis, putting more pressure on her bladder.
   c. limiting her fluid can reduce the number of times she must interrupt her activity to urinate.
   d. the fetal growth has probably stopped and she should expect to start labor in a few days.

2. A woman having physiologic anemia of pregnancy has hemoglobin and hematocrit levels of at least:
   a. 10 g/dL and 30%.
   b. 10.5 g/dL and 32%.
   c. 11 g/dL and 35%.
   d. 12 g/dL and 38%.

3. Slight respiratory alkalosis during pregnancy enhances:
   a. the growth of the fetal arteries within the placenta.
   b. the decrease in systolic and diastolic blood pressures.
   c. maternal metabolism of food and nutrients.
   d. transfer of fetal carbon dioxide to the maternal blood.

4. A pregnant woman is prone to urinary tract infection primarily because:
   a. a large volume of fetal wastes must be excreted by her kidneys.
   b. urine stasis allows additional time for bacteria to multiply.
   c. the volume of urine excreted is reduced and its specific gravity is high.
   d. reduced blood flow to the urinary tract allows waste to accumulate.

5. A pregnant woman complains that both of her thumbs hurt at times. Neither thumb is inflamed or discolored. The nurse should explain to the woman that:
   a. she probably injured her hand and does not recall doing so.
   b. an undiagnosed fracture may have improperly healed.
   c. osteoarthritis often has its onset during pregnancy.
   d. increased tissue fluid is causing nerve compression.

6. A pregnant woman has a blood glucose screening at 26 weeks of gestation. The result is 128 mg/dL. The nurse should expect that:
   a. no additional glucose testing will be needed.
   b. insulin injections will be needed by 30 weeks of gestation.
   c. oral drugs may be prescribed to lower her glucose level.
   d. more testing is needed to determine additional therapy.

7. A woman who is 12 weeks pregnant begins wearing maternity clothes. This is most likely an example of:
   a. introversion.
   b. mimicry.
   c. narcissism.
   d. fantasy.

8. Choose the maternal behavior that best describes role playing during pregnancy.
   a. The woman shifts from saying, "I am pregnant" to "I am having a baby."
   b. The woman begins calling her fetus by a name rather than "it."
   c. The woman tries to care for infants while an experienced mother watches.
   d. The woman becomes less absorbed in her own needs and focuses on the fetus.

9. The nurse can best help a man assume his role as a parent by:
   a. encouraging him to ask questions about his partner's pregnancy.
   b. referring him to prenatal discussion groups for expectant fathers.
   c. advising the woman to limit discussions of her symptoms during early pregnancy.
   d. enrolling him in childbirth classes to actively involve him in the birth process.

10. Choose the most likely reaction of an 8-year-old to his mother's pregnancy.
    a. Embarrassment or shame at his mother's appearance
    b. Inability to sense the reality of the infant
    c. Desire to role play his big-brother status
    d. Interest in learning about the developing baby

11. The nurse is teaching a Laotian woman about self-care during pregnancy. The nurse can best determine whether she learned the information by:
    a. asking the woman to indicate what teaching she did and did not understand.
    b. observing for the woman's eye contact with the nurse during teaching.
    c. recognizing that nodding while being taught indicates understanding.
    d. having the woman restate the information that is taught.

12. The primary benefit of a preconception class is to:
    a. reduce the risk of having a baby with a birth defect.
    b. begin the pregnancy in an optimal nutritional state.
    c. limit the number of unplanned pregnancies in the community.
    d. encourage the couple to have their baby at that facility.

13. The primary benefit of perinatal education is to help:
    a. reduce the likelihood that the parents will have problems with their infant.
    b. women have a satisfying, medication-free childbirth.
    c. parents become active in health maintenance during pregnancy and birth.
    d. enhance the chance that the prospective parents will return to a hospital.

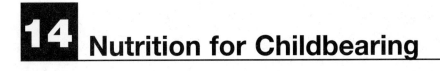

14 Nutrition for Childbearing

MATCHING KEY TERMS

Match the term with the correct definition.

1. _____ Gynecologic age
2. _____ Heme iron
3. _____ Kilocalorie
4. _____ Lactovegetarian
5. _____ Lacto-ovovegetarian
6. _____ Ovovegetarian
7. _____ Pica
8. _____ Nonheme iron
9. _____ Nutrient density
10. _____ Vegetarian
11. _____ Vegan

a. Ingestion of a nonfood substance
b. Measure of the energy value of foods
c. Quality of proteins, vitamins, and minerals per 100 calories
d. Number of years since menarche
e. Iron form most usable by body; obtained from meat, poultry, or fish
f. Iron form less usable by body; obtained from plants
g. One who eats no animal products
h. One whose diet is primarily plant foods and who avoids animal foods
i. Vegetarian who includes milk products in his or her diet
j. Vegetarian who includes eggs in his or her diet
k. Vegetarian who includes milk and eggs in his or her diet

KEY CONCEPTS

1. List four major consequences associated with an inadequate prenatal weight gain.

   a. _____
   b. _____
   c. _____
   d. _____

2. List six major consequences associated with an excessive prenatal weight gain.

   a. _____
   b. _____
   c. _____
   d. _____
   e. _____
   f. _____

3. List the suggested pregnancy weight gains for each category.

   a. Normal prepregnancy body mass index (BMI) 18.5 to 24.9

   b. Prepregnancy (BMI) <18.5

   c. Prepregnancy BMI 25 to 29.9

   d. Prepregnancy BMI >30

4. A general guideline for pregnancy weight gain is _____ kg (_____ pounds) during the first trimester and _____ kg (_____ pounds) per week thereafter.

5. List the kilocalorie content for the following food types.

   a. Carbohydrates _____/g

   b. Proteins _____/g

   c. Fats _____/g

6. After an early pregnancy, the woman should take in approximately _____ kcal/day more than her usual intake.

7. Daily prepregnancy protein needs average _____ g. The amount of protein needed during pregnancy is _____ g/day.

8. Name the four fat-soluble vitamins.

   a. _____

   b. _____

   c. _____

   d. _____

9. List some high-calcium foods other than dairy foods.

10. Why is a routine vitamin–mineral capsule supplementation risky?

11. The recommended fluid intake during pregnancy is _____ cups daily. Which fluids should be limited?

12. What is the recommended number of servings from each food group for pregnant women?

    a. Whole grains

    b. Vegetables and fruits

    c. Dairy foods

    d. Protein foods

    e. Fats, oils, concentrated sugars

13. Explain the influence of "hot" and "cold" (or "yin" and "yang") on the diet of some pregnant women.

14. Describe the childbearing diet preferences typical of Southeast Asian women.

    a. Foods encouraged

    b. Foods discouraged

    c. Postpartum changes

    d. Nutrients commonly deficient in the diet

    e. Increasing nutrient intake with traditional foods

15. Describe the childbearing diet preferences typical of Hispanic women.

    a. Influence of the "hot" and "cold" theory

    b. Common foods

    c. Common problem areas in the diet

16. Describe the eligibility aspects of the WIC (Special Supplemental Nutrition Program for Women, Infants, and Children) program.

17. Which nutrients are usually lacking in the diets of adolescents?

18. Describe the nursing approaches that enhance the likelihood that an adolescent will follow a nutritional diet during pregnancy.

19. Explain how a vegetarian woman can meet the needs of pregnancy for each nutrient listed.

    a. Protein

    b. Calcium

    c. Vitamin B$_{12}$

20. List a nursing teaching that helps a pregnant woman manage nausea and vomiting.

21. What nutritional problems may the multipara have?

22. What additional nutritional needs does the woman with a multifetal pregnancy have?

23. What nutritional needs do women in each of these situations have?

    a. Substance abuse

    b. Smoking

    c. Alcohol abuse

24. How may each of these drugs interfere with nutrition intake during pregnancy?

    a. Marijuana

    b. Heroin

    c. Cocaine

    d. Amphetamine

25. What problems may occur in each of these lactating mothers?

    a. Dieter

    b. Adolescent

    c. Vegan

    d. One who avoids dairy products

26. What are the recommendations for each of these substances during lactation?

    a. Alcohol

    b. Caffeine

    c. Fluid intake

CRITICAL THINKING EXERCISES

1. Select a cultural group prevalent in your clinical agency. Ask the women whether any foods are encouraged or forbidden by their culture during pregnancy and the reasons for each. Ask them how long they have been in the United States and how this influences their food choices.

2. Determine what non-English diet pamphlets and teaching materials are available at your clinical facility.

3. Use a pediatric textbook or growth chart to solve this problem related to a young adolescent weight gain during pregnancy.

   Prepregnancy height: 64 inches (162 cm)
   Prepregnancy weight: 105 pounds (47.7 kg)
   Expected normal weight gain over 40 weeks: _____ pounds (_____ kg)
   Expected weight gain for pregnancy: _____ pounds (_____ kg)

   Total desired weight gain during pregnancy: _____ pounds (_____ kg)

4. Call your local WIC program and tell them you are a nursing student. Ask about the services they provide, eligibility criteria, and the number of women and children served in your area. If possible, observe a counseling session.

5. Complete a 24-hour diet history on yourself. Determine whether you meet the recommended dietary allowances (RDAs) and what, if any, changes you should make.

6. Ask pregnant or postpartum women whether they are aware of food cravings or aversions during pregnancy. What nutritional consequences might result from those you find?

CASE STUDY

Carmen is a 23-year-old Latina who is pregnant with her third baby. She is being seen for the first time in the clinic. Her other two children are 1 and 2 years old. Her last menstrual period was 15 weeks ago. She is 63 inches tall and weighs 152 pounds, 15 pounds more than her prepregnant weight. Her hemoglobin level is 10.5 g/dL. She says she "can't drink milk" but prefers to drink colas. Carmen is married, and her husband works as a gardener.

1. What is Carmen's top-priority nutrition-related problem?

2. What nutritional problems are likely during this pregnancy? What foods help manage these problems?

3. What cultural aspects should the nurse consider?

Choose the correct answer.

1. The recommended total weight gain during pregnancy for a 15-year-old of normal weight for height should be approximately:
   a. 12 pounds.
   b. 20 pounds.
   c. 35 pounds.
   d. 45 pounds.

2. Poor weight gain during early pregnancy is associated with:
   a. pregnancy-induced hypertension.
   b. small-for-gestational-age infants.
   c. preterm labor and birth.
   d. risk for postpartum hemorrhage.

3. To reduce the incidence of neural tube defects such as spina bifida, women of childbearing age are recommended to consume:
   a. at least 0.4 mg folic acid per day in foods and supplements.
   b. 300 extra calories near the expected conception date.
   c. 60 mg of supplemental iron, in addition to high-iron foods.
   d. two added servings of foods high in vitamin C.

4. Choose the correct nursing teaching about a woman's iron supplement during pregnancy.
   a. Take the iron supplement 30 minutes before the first food of the day.
   b. Taking the iron supplement with dairy foods will reduce the gastric side effects.
   c. Stools are somewhat loose and are lighter brown than usual.
   d. A food high in vitamin C may enhance the absorption of iron.

5. A calcium supplement is best taken:
   a. with high-iron foods.
   b. at bedtime.
   c. with meals.
   d. upon arising.

6. When teaching an adolescent about nutrition during pregnancy, the nursing approach should:
   a. focus on the girl's responsibility to her fetus.
   b. provide as many choices as possible from nutritious foods.
   c. ask the girl to limit snacking and fast foods.
   d. explain how a good pregnancy diet will promote her health.

7. The main risk to a woman who practices pica during pregnancy is:
   a. inadequate intake of essential nutrients.
   b. rapid absorption of nutrients such as iron.
   c. reduced fluid intake because of ice consumption.
   d. nonacceptance of the practice by caregivers.

8. Choose the correct nursing approach regarding caffeine use during pregnancy.
   a. Teach that caffeine has not been shown to be a risk.
   b. Limit the total intake of caffeine-containing drinks to four daily.
   c. Discuss the sources of caffeine in addition to coffee and tea.
   d. Drink one additional glass of plain water for each caffeine-containing drink.

9. A non-breastfeeding woman is anxious to lose weight after birth. Which nursing education is most appropriate?
   a. She may immediately begin dieting because she is not breastfeeding.
   b. She should consume a minimum of 1800 calories each day to maintain energy.
   c. She should take her prenatal vitamin–mineral supplement while dieting.
   d. She should wait at least 3 weeks before beginning a diet.

15 Prenatal Diagnostic Tests

Match the term with the correct definition.

1. _____ Alpha-fetoprotein (AFP)

2. _____ Amniocentesis

3. _____ Biophysical profile

4. _____ Chorionic villus sampling (CVS)

5. _____ Lecithin/sphingomyelin ratio

6. _____ Neural tube defect

7. _____ Surfactant

8. _____ Ultrasonography

a. Imaging technique that uses high-frequency sound waves to visualize internal body structures

b. Substance secreted by mature fetal lungs

c. Congenital defect of the spinal cord

d. Method of evaluating fetal well-being

e. Tissue obtained from the fetal side of the developing placenta

f. Ratio used to determine fetal lung maturity

g. Withdrawing amniotic fluid for laboratory examination

h. Fetal proteins used to screen for specific abnormalities

KEY CONCEPTS

1. List typical purposes for an ultrasound examination during the:

   a. First trimester

   b. Second and third trimesters

2. In which type of ultrasound examination is a full bladder needed, transvaginal or transabdominal? What is the reason?

3. Under what circumstances is an accurate gestational age especially important? How is it assessed by ultrasonography? When is the gestational age determination most accurate?

4. What conditions are suggested by alpha-fetoprotein levels that are:

   a. Low

   b. High

5. What is multiple-marker screening and what is its purpose? What follow-up tests may be needed?

6. Chorionic villus sampling (CVS) is done as early as _____ weeks of pregnancy.

7. List four risks of CVS.

   a. _____

   b. _____

   c. _____

   d. _____

8. List the purpose for amniocentesis during the:

   a. Second trimester

   b. Third trimester

9. What lecithin/sphingomyelin (L/S) ratio suggests fetal lung maturity? In what maternal disorder may this ratio not be associated with fetal lung maturity?

10. What is the purpose of testing phosphatidylglycerol (PG) and phosphatidylinositol (PI) in the amniotic fluid?

11. Mid-trimester amniocentesis results are known in approximately _____ weeks.

12. What is the purpose of a vibroacoustic stimulation test (VST)?

13. The basic principle of the contraction stress test is to observe the response of the _____

    to the stress of _____.

14. What two methods are used to cause uterine contractions when conducting a contraction stress test?

    a. _____

    b. _____

15. Describe the possible results and implications of a contraction stress test.

16. The biophysical profile assesses which five fetal parameters?

    a. _____

    b. _____

    c. _____

    d. _____

    e. _____

17. What is the significance of oligohydramnios?

CRITICAL THINKING EXERCISES

Test your knowledge of nonstress tests. Using Figure 15-9, A and B, in the text, answer the following questions about each strip:

Figure 15-9, A:

    a. Baseline fetal heart rate?

    b. Time duration of each strip?

    c. Number of accelerations?

    d. Number of decelerations?

    e. Beats per minute and duration of the accelerations?

    f. Reactive? Why or why not?

Figure 15-9, B:

    a. Baseline fetal heart rate?

    b. Time duration of each strip?

c. Number of accelerations?

d. Number of decelerations?

e. Beats per minute and duration of the accelerations?

f. Reactive? Why or why not?

CASE STUDIES

1. Joann is a primigravida with pregnancy-induced hypertension in her 35th week of pregnancy. She is scheduled for amniocentesis this morning.

   a. Why is she having the test?

   b. What preprocedure and postprocedure care are indicated?

2. Betty has type 1 diabetes and is in her 32nd week of pregnancy. She is scheduled for a nonstress test.

   a. Why is she having the test?

   b. What findings suggest that the fetus is healthy?

   c. How often is this test likely to be performed?

REVIEW QUESTIONS

Choose the correct answer.

1. The fetal heartbeat should be visible on ultrasound by the:
   a. 8th week following the last menstrual period.
   b. 12th week following the last menstrual period.
   c. 20th week following the last menstrual period.
   d. 22nd week following the last menstrual period.

2. Fewer fetal movements than expected suggest:
   a. intrauterine fetal growth retardation.
   b. inaccurate gestational age dating.
   c. rapid intrauterine fetal maturation.
   d. reduced placental perfusion with fetal hypoxia.

3. Choose the appropriate patient teaching related to maternal serum alpha-fetoprotein (MSAFP) analysis.
   a. Abnormal MSAFP levels should be followed by more specific tests.
   b. High MSAFP levels are usually associated with chromosome abnormalities.
   c. Having MSAFP testing will eliminate the need to perform an ultrasound examination.
   d. The initial MSAFP testing will be performed at 12 weeks of gestation.

4. Choose the correct patient teaching following amnio-centesis.
   a. Drink one to two quarts of clear fluid to replace fluid taken in the procedure.
   b. Resume all normal activities when desired.
   c. Report persistent contractions, vaginal bleeding, or fluid leakage.
   d. Eat a diet with increased iron content for two days after amniocentesis.

5. A woman who is assessing fetal movements each day should notify her health care provider if:
   a. more than six movements are felt during a 30- to 60-minute period.
   b. she perceives fewer than 10 fetal movements within 12 hours.
   c. the movement pattern changes very little from day to day.
   d. fetal movements are more frequent during the evening than in the morning.

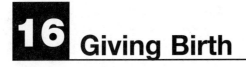

16 Giving Birth

MATCHING KEY TERMS

Match the term with the correct definition.

1. _____ Amniotomy
2. _____ Attitude
3. _____ Crowning
4. _____ EDD
5. _____ Engagement
6. _____ Molding
7. _____ Nuchal cord
8. _____ Station

a. Measurement of the descent of the fetal presenting part
b. Estimated date of delivery
c. Descent of widest fetal presenting part to zero station
d. Change in the shape of the fetal head during birth
e. Relationship of fetal body parts to one another
f. Umbilical cord around the fetal neck
g. Artificial rupture of the amniotic sac, or membranes
h. Appearance of the fetal presenting part at the vaginal opening

KEY CONCEPTS

1. Explain why each characteristic of uterine contractions is important during birth.

   a. Coordination

   b. Involuntary

   c. Intermittent

2. Describe the differences in how the upper and lower uterus contract during labor. Why is it important that the upper and lower parts of the uterus have different contraction characteristics?

3. Why should the nurse regularly check the woman's bladder during labor?

4. What maternal and fetal conditions may reduce fetal tolerance for the intermittent interruption in placental blood flow that occurs during contractions?

5. What are the changes in fetal lung fluid during pregnancy, during labor, and after birth?

6. What are the two powers of labor? When during labor do they come into play?

7. Why are the sutures and fontanels of the fetal head important during birth?

8. Describe the most common variations in:

   a. Fetal lie

   b. Fetal attitude

   c. Fetal presentation

9. Draw the three variations of a breech presentation. Which one is the most common?

10. What fetal anatomic reference point is used for each presentation or position?

   a. Vertex

   b. Face

   c. Breech

11. How can nursing measures help increase a woman's sense of control during labor?

12. How do each of these factors affect the onset of labor?

    a. Fetal hormone production

    b. Change in the maternal progesterone and estrogen relationship

13. Describe the common premonitory signs of labor. Are there differences between a nullipara and a parous woman?

14. Describe each mechanism of labor and its significance.

    a. Descent

    b. Engagement

    c. Flexion

    d. Internal rotation

    e. Extension

    f. External rotation

    g. Expulsion

15. Why must the fetal head and shoulders undergo rotation within the pelvis?

16. What are the three labor phases in stage one? What cervical dilation marks each phase?

17. How do the average durations of labor vary between nulliparas and multiparas for the first and second stages of labor?

18. List four signs that suggest that the placenta has separated.

    a. _____

    b. _____

    c. _____

    d. _____

19. Why is it important that the uterus remain firmly contracted after birth?

20. Complete the following chart regarding the characteristics of normal labor.

	First Stage	Second Stage	Third Stage	Fourth Stage
Duration Nullipara:				
Multipara:				
Cervical Dilation Latent phase:				
Active phase:				
Transition phase:				
Uterine Contractions Latent phase:				
Active phase:				
Transition phase:				
Discomfort				
Maternal Behaviors				

21. The two nursing priorities when a woman enters a birth center are to determine _____ and _____.

22. When should the nurse *not* perform a vaginal examination? Why?

23. List important nursing assessments after the membranes rupture. Describe normal and abnormal assessments, as appropriate.

24. Why is it important to place a small pillow under one hip if the mother must lie on her back?

25. What maternal vital signs may indicate problems?

    a. Blood pressure

    b. Temperature

26. Describe some basic comfort measures the nurse can provide during labor.

27. Immediate nursing care of the newborn includes supporting _____ and _____ functions and placing _____.

28. Nursing care of the mother during the fourth stage of labor focuses on observing for _____ and relieving _____.

29. Discuss the relationship between a full bladder and postpartum hemorrhage.

CRITICAL THINKING EXERCISES

1. Place a tennis ball in a sock. Slowly push it out of the cuff to get the idea of cervical effacement and dilation.

2. In performing a vaginal examination during labor, the nurse collects the following information:

   a. Cervix is open 4 cm and its length is approximately 0.5 cm.
   b. The presenting part is rounded and hard. A triangular depression on the presenting part has three linear depressions leading from it. Clear fluid flows from the vagina as the fetus moves during the examination.

   What is the correct interpretation of these findings?

3. During your clinical experience, note what effects fetal presentation and position have on the woman's comfort and the progress of labor.

4. Review the routine permits used in the intrapartal area at your birth facility.

5. During your clinical experience, use Leopold's maneuvers to identify the fetal presentation, position, and engagement.

CASE STUDY

Erin is an 18-year-old primigravida who calls the intrapartum unit because she thinks she may be in labor.

1. What information should the nurse obtain to help determine whether Erin is in true labor?

   The nurse decides that Erin may be in true labor and tells her to come to the birth center. On arrival, Erin says she thinks her "water broke."

2. What is the priority nursing care at this time?

3. What tests might the nurse use to verify that Erin's membranes have indeed ruptured?

   The nurse determines that Erin's contractions are every 5 minutes, of moderate intensity, and last 40 seconds. The fetal heart rate is 135 to 145 beats per minute (bpm), and it accelerates when the fetus moves. Amniotic fluid is light green with small white flecks in it. The vaginal examination reveals that the cervix is dilated 5 cm and is completely effaced. The fetal presenting part is hard and round, and a small triangular depression on the head can be felt in Erin's right posterior pelvis.

4. What stage (and phase, if applicable) of labor is Erin in?

5. How should the fetal heart rate be interpreted?

6. Is the amniotic fluid normal?

7. What is the fetal presentation and position?

Erin complains of back discomfort during each contraction.

8. What interventions might make this discomfort more tolerable?

After 4 hours of labor in the birth center, Erin's cervix is completely dilated and effaced, and the fetal station is +1. Erin feels the need to push during some contractions.

9. What is the safest way to advise Erin to push?

10. When should Erin be positioned for birth?

Erin gives birth to a boy. The nurse notes the following on the baby at 1 minute: heart rate is 138 bpm, loud vigorous crying, spontaneous movement and flexion of the extremities, and pink skin color except for a bluish color of the hands and feet.

11. What Apgar score will be assigned to the baby?

12. What are the priority nursing measures for the infant in relation to:

   a. Respiration

   b. Temperature regulation

Erin is now in the fourth stage of labor. She and her husband are getting acquainted with their baby, Derrick.

13. What time period does the fourth stage involve?

14. What nursing assessments are needed to observe for a hemorrhage?

15. What are appropriate pain relief methods during the fourth stage?

REVIEW QUESTIONS

Choose the correct answer.

1. When assessing a laboring woman's blood pressure, the nurse should:
   a. inflate the cuff at the beginning of a contraction.
   b. check the blood pressure between two contractions.
   c. expect a slight elevation in blood pressure.
   d. position the woman on her back with her knees bent.

2. A woman is admitted in active labor. Her leukocyte count is 14,500. Based on this information, the nurse should:
   a. assess the woman for other evidence of an infection.
   b. promptly inform the nurse-midwife of the results.
   c. use isolation techniques to limit the spread of infection.
   d. record the expected results in the woman's chart.

3. The most appropriate time for the nurse to encourage a laboring woman to push is during:
   a. the interval between contractions.
   b. first-stage labor.
   c. second-stage labor.
   d. whenever she feels the need.

4. The abbreviation LOA means that the fetal occiput is:
   a. on the examiner's left and in the front of the pelvis.
   b. in the left front part of the mother's pelvis.
   c. anterior to the fetal breech.
   d. lower than the fetal breech.

5. Choose the most reliable evidence that true labor has begun.
   a. Regular contractions that occur every 15 minutes
   b. Change in the amount of cervical thinning
   c. Increased ease of breathing with frequent urination
   d. A sudden urge to do household tasks

6. The nurse should note how long the interval between contractions lasts because:
   a. maternal cells restore their glucose levels during the interval.
   b. a very short interval requires earlier administration of analgesia.
   c. most exchange of fetal oxygen and waste products occurs.
   d. the interval becomes longer as cervical dilation increases.

7. What is the primary benefit of the stress of labor to the newborn?
   a. It stimulates breathing and eliminates lung fluid.
   b. It increases alertness and enhances parent–infant bonding.
   c. It speeds peristalsis to quickly eliminate meconium.
   d. It enhances the tolerance of microorganisms from others.

8. A station of +1 means that the:
   a. maternal cervix is open by 1 cm.
   b. mother's ischial spines project into her pelvis by 1 cm.
   c. fetus is unlikely to be born vaginally because the pelvis is small.
   d. fetal presenting part is 1 cm below the mother's ischial spine.

9. Bloody show differs from active vaginal bleeding in that bloody show:
   a. quickly clots on the perineal pad.
   b. is dark red and mixed with mucus.
   c. freely flows from the vagina during vaginal examination.
   d. decreases in quantity as labor progresses.

10. A laboring woman abruptly stops her previous breathing techniques during a contraction and makes low-pitched grunting sounds. The priority nursing action is to:
   a. ask her if she needs pain medication.
   b. turn her to her left side.
   c. Assess contraction duration.
   d. look at her perineum.

11. A woman's membranes rupture during a contraction. The priority nursing action is to:
   a. assess the fetal heart rate.
   b. note the color of the discharge.
   c. check the woman's vital signs.
   d. determine whether the fluid has a foul odor.

12. When palpating labor contractions, the nurse should:
   a. use the palm of one hand while palpating the lower uterus.
   b. avoid palpating during the period of maximum intensity.
   c. place the fingertips over the fundus of the uterus.
   d. limit palpations to three consecutive contractions.

13. When performing Leopold's maneuvers, the nurse palpates a hard round object in the uterine fundus. A smooth, rounded surface is on the mother's right side, and irregular, movable parts are felt on her left side. An irregularly shaped fetal part is felt in the suprapubic area and is easily moved upward. How should these findings be interpreted?
   a. The fetal presentation is cephalic, the position is ROA, and the presenting part is engaged.
   b. The fetal presentation is cephalic, the position is LOP, and the presenting part is not engaged.
   c. The fetal presentation is breech, the position is RST, and the presenting part is engaged.
   d. The fetal presentation is breech, the position is RSA, and the presenting part is not engaged.

14. When performing the fourth Leopold's maneuver, the nurse determines that the cephalic prominence is on the same side as the fetal back. How should this assessment be interpreted?
   a. The fetus is in a breech position with the head extended.
   b. The fetus is in a face presentation with the head extended.
   c. The fetus is in a transverse lie presentation with the face toward the mother's back.
   d. The fetus is in a cephalic presentation with the head well flexed.

15. The nurse notes the following contraction pattern:

Beginning of Contractions	End of Contractions
11:15:00	11:15:40
11:20:00	11:20:45
11:24:00	11:24:50
11:28:30	11:29:10
11:33:00	11:33:35

Choose the correct documentation for the pattern.
   a. Contractions every 4 to 5 minutes; duration 35 to 50 seconds
   b. Contractions every 5 minutes; duration 35 to 40 seconds
   c. Contractions every 3 to 5 minutes; duration 30 to 50 seconds
   d. Contractions every 3 to 4 minutes; duration 30 to 40 seconds

16. A woman who is having her third baby planned epidural analgesia for labor and birth. However, her labor was so rapid that she did not have the epidural. What is the best nursing approach in this case?
   a. Congratulate her on having a labor that was quicker than expected.
   b. Use open-ended questions to clarify her true feelings about the experience.
   c. Tactfully explain why a non-epidural labor and birth are actually better.
   d. Explain that it is often difficult to time epidural analgesia for labor.

17. A woman having her first baby has been observed for 2 hours for labor but is having false labor contractions. Choose the most appropriate teaching before she returns home.
   a. "It is unlikely that your labor will be fast, so you can stay home until your water breaks."
   b. "If your water breaks, you can wait until contractions are 5 minutes apart or closer."
   c. "As long as the baby is active, there is no hurry to return to the birth center."
   d. "Your contractions will usually be 5 minutes apart or closer for 1 hour if labor is real."

17 Intrapartum Fetal Surveillance

MATCHING KEY TERMS

Match the term with the correct definition.

1. _____ Amnioinfusion
2. _____ Hypoxia
3. _____ Nuchal cord
4. _____ Nadir
5. _____ Tocolytic
6. _____ Uterine resting tone
7. _____ Transducer

a. Translates fetal heart motion into electrical signals
b. Cord around the fetal neck
c. Reduced oxygen to the blood
d. Lowest point
e. Infusion of sterile isotonic solution into the uterus to reduce cord compression or to wash out meconium
f. Muscle tension of the uterus between contractions
g. Drug that reduces uterine muscle contractions

KEY CONCEPTS

1. List the five factors that affect fetal oxygenation.

   a. _____

   b. _____

   c. _____

   d. _____

   e. _____

2. Explain how each of these factors influences the fetal heart rate.

   a. Autonomic nervous system

   b. Baroreceptors

   c. Chemoreceptors

   d. Adrenal glands

   e. Central nervous system

3. Explain how each factor can reduce fetal oxygenation. How would you explain each in simple terms to a woman in labor?

   a. Maternal hypotension

   b. Maternal hypertension

   c. Maternal hypoxia

   d. Hypertonic uterine activity

   e. Placental disruptions

   f. Umbilical cord blood flow compression

   g. Fetal bradycardia or tachycardia

4. List the advantages and limitations of the two methods of an intrapartal fetal assessment: auscultation with the palpation of contractions and electronic fetal monitoring.

	Auscultation with Palpation	Electronic Fetal Monitoring
Advantages		
Limitations		

5. What must the nurse consider when evaluating intrauterine pressure from a solid catheter versus a fluid-filled catheter?

6. Define the following terms that describe the fetal heart rate.
   a. Normal

   b. Bradycardia

c. Tachycardia

d. Variability

7. List factors that may decrease variability.

8. Why is variability an important component of a fetal heart pattern evaluation?

9. Describe each fetal heart rate periodic change, list possible causes, and note whether the change is reassuring or nonreassuring and the basic actions to take if nonreassuring.

Periodic Change	Appearance on Strip	Possible Causes	Reassuring or Nonreassuring (with Nursing Actions)
Accelerations			
Early decelerations			
Late decelerations			
Variable decelerations			

10. Describe methods that may be used during labor to clarify the fetal condition.

11. The normal fetal scalp pH is _____ to _____. Use a medical–surgical nursing text to compare with the normal adult pH.

12. List possible nursing interventions to identify and/or correct the cause of a nonreassuring fetal monitor pattern.

a. Identifying the cause

b. Increasing placental perfusion

   c. Increasing maternal oxygen saturation

   d. Reducing umbilical cord compression

13. List two uses for amnioinfusion.

   a. _____

   b. _____

CRITICAL THINKING EXERCISES

1. Look at the fetal monitor strips in your clinical facility. Identify the following about each:

   a. Baseline rate

   b. Presence of variability (short and/or long term)

   c. Periodic changes

   d. Contraction frequency, duration, and intensity

   e. Nursing interventions for nonreassuring patterns

   f. Fetal responses to nursing interventions

2. Your friend is 7 months pregnant and is uncertain about whether she wants to have electronic fetal monitoring. Develop a plan to explain the pros and cons of each method of fetal surveillance during labor.

Choose the correct answer.

1. Firm contractions that occur every 3 minutes and last 100 seconds (1 minute, 40 seconds) may reduce fetal oxygen supply because they:
   a. cause fetal bradycardia and reduce oxygen concentration.
   b. activate the fetal sympathetic nervous system.
   c. limit the time for oxygen exchange in the placenta.
   d. suppress the normal variability of the fetal heart.

2. The expected response of the fetal heart rate to active fetal movement is:
   a. suppression of normal short-term variability for 15 seconds.
   b. acceleration of at least 15 beats per minute (bpm) for 15 seconds.
   c. increase in the long-term variability by 15 bpm.
   d. acceleration followed by a 15-second deceleration of the heart rate.

3. The nurse notes a pattern of variable decelerations to 75 bpm on the fetal monitor. The initial nursing action is to:
   a. reposition the woman.
   b. administer oxygen.
   c. increase the intravenous fluid infusion.
   d. stimulate the fetal scalp.

4. The tocotransducer should be placed:
   a. in the suprapubic area.
   b. in the fundal area.
   c. over the xiphoid process.
   d. in the uterus.

5. Choose an important precaution when a fluid-filled catheter is used to monitor the uterine contractions during labor.
   a. The tip of the catheter must be at the same level as the transducer.
   b. The fluid that fills the catheter must be warmed to room temperature.
   c. Understand that pressures within the fluid-filled catheter are higher than those in the solid catheter.
   d. Fluid-filled catheters cannot be used when a spiral electrode is applied.

6. The nurse notes a pattern of decelerations on the fetal monitor that begins shortly after the contraction and returns to baseline just before the contraction is over. The correct nursing response is to:
   a. give the woman oxygen by facemask at 8 to 10 L/min.
   b. position the woman on her opposite side.
   c. increase the rate of the woman's intravenous fluid.
   d. continue to observe and record the normal pattern.

18 Pain Management for Childbirth

MATCHING KEY TERMS

Match the term with the correct definition.

1. _____ Agonist

2. _____ Analgesia

3. _____ Anesthesia

4. _____ Antagonist

5. _____ Endorphin

6. _____ Pain tolerance

a. Blocking effect of a drug

b. Loss of sensation with or without the loss of consciousness

c. Maximum pain one is willing to endure

d. Relief of pain without the loss of consciousness

e. Causing a physiologic effect

f. Natural substance similar to morphine

KEY CONCEPTS

1. Explain how childbirth pain may differ from other pain.

2. How can excessive pain reduce fetal oxygenation?

3. How is labor affected when the fetus is in an occiput posterior (OP) position?

4. List four categories of nonpharmacologic techniques that can be used during labor.

5. Give an example of both direct and indirect effects of maternal drugs on the fetus.

6. What is the purpose of administering a test dose before doing an epidural block? What would be signs of problems after the test dose and what causes these signs?

7. What causes these adverse reactions to epidural block analgesia/anesthesia? What may be done to prevent or correct each?

a. Headache

b. Hypotension

c. Bladder distention

d. Prolonged second-stage labor

8. In which regional anesthesia method is it *desirable* to obtain cerebrospinal fluid (CSF)? Why?

9. Complete the following table on intrapartal pain relief methods.

Technique	Advantages	Disadvantages	Adverse Effects	Nursing Care
Systemic analgesics				
Epidural block				
Local infiltration				
Pudendal block				
Subarachnoid block				
General anesthesia				

10. List methods to relieve the pain of a postspinal headache.

11. Under what two circumstances should butorphanol (Stadol) or nalbuphine (Nubain) *not* be administered to a woman in labor?

CRITICAL THINKING EXERCISES

1. Make a plan to help a woman deal with the anxiety and fear that may accompany labor. Use the experience of a woman you have helped care for or that of a friend or relative or your own experience when making your plan.

2. Talk to an anesthesia clinician in your clinical facility about how the staff can compensate for the normal changes of pregnancy when giving anesthesia.

CASE STUDY

Alice is a 16-year-old primigravida in the latent phase of first-stage labor. She did not attend prepared childbirth classes. She is very anxious and tense, crying during each contraction. Her cervix is dilated to 3 cm, station 1, effacement 90%, and the membranes are ruptured (the fluid is clear). Her baseline vital signs are a pulse of 92 beats per minute (bpm), respirations of 24 breaths/min, and blood pressure of 120/70 mm Hg. The fetal heart rate is 126 to 136 bpm with average variability. Her 17-year-old husband is at her side but seems very frustrated and helpless. Her parents live out of town.

1. What assumptions must the nurse be careful to avoid when caring for Alice?

2. What initial nursing interventions are appropriate to help Alice cope with her contractions?

3. Can Alice be taught breathing techniques at this time? If so, how should the nurse approach such teaching?

4. Are analgesics desirable for Alice at this time? Why or why not?

Alice progresses to a 6-cm cervical dilation, effacement 100%, and fetal station 0. Maternal and fetal vital signs remain stable. Alice wants "something stronger" for the pain.

5. What pharmacologic options are possible for Alice, based on the information given?

Alice receives an epidural block analgesia.

6. What nursing care is essential related to the block? Why?

Alice gives birth to a 6-pound 2-ounce girl. Apgar scores are 7 at 1 minute and 9 at 5 minutes.

7. What are appropriate nursing measures are related to Alice's epidural while Alice is in the recovery area?

REVIEW QUESTIONS

Choose the correct answer.

1. Firm sacral pressure is likely to be most helpful in which situation?
   a. Rapid labor and birth
   b. Fetal occiput posterior position
   c. Oxytocin induction of labor
   d. If analgesics should be avoided

2. A woman receives meperidine (Demerol) during labor. Because this analgesic is being used, the nurse should have on hand:
   a. butorphanol (Stadol).
   b. lidocaine (Xylocaine).
   c. nalbuphine (Nubain).
   d. naloxone (Narcan).

3. When stocking a cart for epidural analgesia, the most important nursing action is to:
   a. add additional bags of intravenous (IV) normal saline.
   b. place anticoagulant drugs to allow rapid access.
   c. verify that no epidural drugs have preservatives.
   d. provide an indwelling catheterization tray.

4. The appropriate nursing action for a woman who has a postspinal headache is to:
   a. keep her bed in a semi-Fowler's position.
   b. encourage the intake of fluids that she enjoys.
   c. have her ambulate at least every 4 hours.
   d. restrict the intake of high-carbohydrate foods.

5. A woman having her first baby is trying to use breathing techniques during labor, but she has difficulty concentrating. She is 3-cm dilated, 80% effaced, and the station is 0. What nursing measure can best help her?
   a. Encourage her to change to a different breathing pattern.
   b. Have a family member other than her husband or coach her.
   c. Give her a very small dose of a narcotic that is ordered as needed (PRN).
   d. Help her find a specific point in the room on which she is to focus.

6. A woman must have general anesthesia for a planned cesarean birth because of a previous back surgery. Therefore, the nurse should expect to administer:
   a. naltrexone (Trexan).
   b. an oral barbiturate.
   c. ranitidine (Zantac).
   d. promethazine (Phenergan).

19 Nursing Care During Obstetric Procedures

MATCHING KEY TERMS

Match the term with the correct definition.

1. _____ Chignon
2. _____ Dystocia
3. _____ Iatrogenic
4. _____ Oligohydramnios

   a. Newborn scalp edema caused by a vacuum extractor
   b. Abnormally small amount of amniotic fluid
   c. Prolonged labor
   d. Adverse condition that results from a treatment

KEY CONCEPTS

1. List the potential complications of an amniotomy.

2. List the nursing considerations necessary before and after an amniotomy.

3. List two nursing measures following the use of prostaglandin E_2 to ripen the cervix and the rationale for each.

4. Describe the fetal and maternal nursing assessments associated with an oxytocin infusion. What are the signs of problems?

5. List the nursing interventions if the fetal or maternal assessments are not reassuring when the induction of oxytocin or augmentation of labor is being performed.

6. Explain the purpose of each aspect of care for the woman having an external version.

   a. Nonstress test

   b. Ultrasound

   c. Tocolytic drug

d. Rh immune globulin

e. Fetal heart rate (FHR) monitoring

f. Uterine activity monitoring

7. Describe the nursing care associated with a forceps or vacuum extractor–assisted birth. What is the rationale for each?

8. Describe techniques that may reduce the need for an episiotomy.

9. Explain why a cesarean birth is not necessarily easy for the newborn.

10. Explain the rationale for each intervention associated with a cesarean birth.

a. Medication, such as famotidine, is administered

b. Placing a wedge under one hip

c. Complete blood cell count, coagulation studies, blood type, and crossmatch

d. Antibiotics

e. Indwelling catheter

CRITICAL THINKING EXERCISES

1. Observe a cesarean birth and compare the sequence of events with those of a vaginal birth. What are the similarities and differences?

2. What measures do you see the nursing staff taking to keep the emphasis on the birth experience rather than on surgery when a woman has a cesarean birth?

3. Write a simply worded explanation that you might give to a woman immediately after birth about why you are placing a cold pack on her perineal area. How would you explain the change to warm packs the next day?

4. A woman gave birth to her first baby, a 9-pound boy. Low forceps with a mediolateral episiotomy were required. List three nursing diagnoses or collaborative problems that would be expected during the first 12 hours postpartum and appropriate nursing measures for each.

Nursing Diagnosis or Collaborative Problem	Nursing Interventions

CASE STUDY

Linda is a gravida 3, para 2, at 42 weeks of gestation. She is scheduled for an oxytocin induction of labor. Her first two pregnancies ended at 39 and 40 weeks, and the babies weighed 8 pounds 13 ounces and 9 pounds 11 ounces.

1. What is the probable reason for Linda's induction?

2. What tests might be performed before her induction?

Linda's initial assessments are normal, and the FHR is reassuring. She is having an occasional light contraction but no regular contractions.

3. How should the nurse set up the oxytocin infusion? What is the rationale for these precautions?

After 3 hours, Linda's cervix is dilated to 3 cm, the effacement is 80%, and the fetal station is +1. Contractions are every 4 to 5 minutes, lasting for 45 seconds, and are of moderate intensity. The FHR is 132 to 148 beats per minute (bpm). The physician decides to perform an amniotomy.

4. What nursing measures are appropriate before and after the amniotomy?

5. Should there be any change in the oxytocin infusion at this time? Why or why not?

Linda's labor progresses, and she is having contractions every 2 to 3 minutes, 75 to 90 seconds' duration, and firm. FHR is 130 to 140 bpm. She is dilated to 7 cm, the effacement is 90%, and the fetal station is −1.

6. Should there be any change in her oxytocin infusion at this time? Why or why not?

Despite adequate contractions, Linda's cervical dilation does not progress beyond 7 cm, and she will have a cesarean birth.

7. What nursing measures are appropriate for the planned birth?

Linda delivers a 10-pound 3-ounce girl via a low transverse cesarean birth.

8. What nursing care is appropriate for Linda during the recovery phase?

REVIEW QUESTIONS

Choose the correct answer.

1. After the physician performs an amniotomy, the fluid is dark green with a mild odor and the FHR is 130 to 140 bpm. The most appropriate nursing care is to:
   a. take the woman's temperature hourly until delivery.
   b. monitor the fetus more closely for nonreassuring signs.
   c. tell the woman that she cannot have anything by mouth.
   d. closely observe the woman for hypotension.

2. Choose the correct setup for an oxytocin induction of labor.
   a. Oxytocin is mixed with an electrolyte solution and delivered as a single infusion.
   b. Oxytocin is mixed with normal saline equal to 10 mL and administered by a slow intravenous (IV) push.
   c. Oxytocin is initiated at a rapid rate; its rate is decreased as labor progresses.
   d. Oxytocin is administered as a secondary infusion and is controlled by an infusion pump.

3. A method to prepare the cervix for the induction of labor the following day is:
   a. prostaglandin preparations.
   b. fetal fibronectin.
   c. oral oxytocin tablets.
   d. amniotomy.

4. Choose the nursing assessment finding that is most likely to occur with hypertonic uterine contractions.
   a. Foul-smelling amniotic fluid
   b. A contraction interval of 90 seconds
   c. A fetal heart rate of 80 to 100 bpm
   d. A maternal pulse of 80 to 90 bpm

5. A woman has external version to change her fetus' position from breech to cephalic. Choose the postprocedure nursing observation that would indicate that she should not be released to go home.
   a. The FHR is 135 to 145 bpm with average variability.
   b. Occasional mild, brief contractions occur.
   c. The maternal temperature is 99.2°F and pulse is 90 bpm.
   d. Vaginal discharge is a pale and watery fluid.

6. Parents of a newborn born with a forceps-assisted vaginal birth ask about small reddened areas on the infant's cheeks. The nurse should tell them that the areas:
   a. are temporary and will disappear.
   b. are typical of all vaginal births.
   c. will be reported to the physician.
   d. may lead to a serious infection.

7. A urinary catheter should be readily available when a woman has a forceps-assisted birth because:
   a. an emergency cesarean birth may be required.
   b. edema reduces the woman's sensation to void after birth.
   c. a full bladder reduces the available room in the pelvis.
   d. a large median or mediolateral episiotomy is likely.

8. During the recovery period after a low forceps birth with a median episiotomy, the nurse should:
   a. assess for purulent drainage from the episiotomy.
   b. promptly apply cold packs to the perineal area.
   c. expect a larger quantity of lochia rubra drainage.
   d. limit oral intake to ice chips until the transfer to a room.

9. Choose the correct preoperative teaching before a planned cesarean birth.
   a. Oral intake will be limited to clear fluids for 12 hours before surgery.
   b. IV fluids are usually continued for 2 days after birth.
   c. The woman will be asked to take deep breaths and cough regularly after birth.
   d. The nurse will help her ambulate to the restroom to urinate within 4 hours of birth.

10. The best method to prevent a hemorrhage after a cesarean birth is to:
    a. provide regular analgesia to enhance urination.
    b. reposition the woman from side to side.
    c. observe the vital signs for falling blood pressure.
    d. regularly assess the uterine fundus for firmness.

Chapter **19** **Nursing Care During Obstetric Procedures**

20 Postpartum Adaptations

MATCHING KEY TERMS

Match the term with the correct definition.

1. _____ Attachment
2. _____ Bonding
3. _____ Catabolism
4. _____ En face
5. _____ Engrossment
6. _____ Entrainment
7. _____ Fingertipping
8. _____ Fundus
9. _____ Involution
10. _____ Kegel exercises
11. _____ Puerperium
12. _____ REEDA
13. _____ Taking-in

a. Method to increase the tone of muscles in the vaginal and urinary meatal area

b. Part of the uterus above the openings of the fallopian tubes

c. Conversion of living cellular substances to simpler compounds

d. Acronym that helps assess wound healing (e.g., redness, edema, ecchymosis, discharge, approximation)

e. Period from childbirth until the return of the reproductive organs to their prepregnancy states

f. Retrogressive changes that return the reproductive organs to their prepregnancy states

g. First phase of maternal adaptation

h. Process by which an enduring bond between a parent and child is developed through pleasurable, satisfying interactions

i. Movement of the newborn in rhythm with the parent's voice

j. Position that facilitates eye-to-eye contact between the parent and newborn

k. Initial attraction felt by parents for their infants

l. Initial touch characteristics between the mother and newborn

m. Intense fascination between the father and newborn

KEY CONCEPTS

1. Describe postpartum changes in the:

   a. uterine muscle

   b. uterine muscle cells

   c. uterine lining

2. Describe the changes in lochia and when the aforementioned changes occur.

3. What is the significance of bradycardia during the early postpartum period?

4. What makes any pregnant and postpartum woman at risk for venous thrombosis? What factors increase this risk?

5. Explain how a full bladder at birth can lead to postpartum hemorrhage.

6. Describe the influence of these hormones on lactation.

   a. Estrogen

   b. Progesterone

   c. Prolactin

   d. Oxytocin

7. Discuss which postpartum mothers would be appropriate candidates for Rho(D) immune globulin and rubella vaccine.

8. Describe the proper techniques to massage a soft fundus. How should the nurse expel any clots?

9. Complete the following chart for postpartum assessments.

Assessment	What to Assess and Expected Findings	Deviations from Normal, Cause, and Nursing Actions
Fundus		
Lochia		

105

Bladder		
Perineum		
Vital signs		
Breasts		
Lower extremities		

10. Write out in simple terms how you would teach a woman about each of the following postpartum comfort measures:

    a. Cold packs

    b. Perineal care

    c. Topical medications

    d. How to sit

    e. Sitz baths

11. Describe additional nursing assessments and care for the woman who gave birth by cesarean.

    a. Respiratory

    b. Abdomen

    c. Intake and output

12. What teaching should you provide the postpartum woman to prevent constipation?

13. List the signs and symptoms that the postpartum woman should report to her physician or nurse-midwife.

14. Describe the processes of bonding and attachment. Note the similarities and differences in these processes.

15. Describe the progression of maternal touch.

16. Describe the progression of maternal verbal behaviors.

17. Complete the table by describing maternal behaviors in the three phases of maternal adaptation. How can nurses help these mothers meet their needs in each phase?

Phase	Maternal Behaviors	Nursing Considerations
Taking-in		
Taking-hold		
Letting-go		

18. Describe postpartum blues. What is the best response to them?

19. How can the nurse help the new father adapt to his role?

20. How should the nurse respond to the parent who is disappointed in the sex of the newborn?

21. What nursing measures can help the mother of twins attach to her babies?

22. New parents may not recognize signals from the infant that he or she has had enough stimulation and now needs to rest. What signals should the nurse teach parents to recognize?

CRITICAL THINKING EXERCISES

1. You may note that some postpartum women have a urine output that is greater than their oral fluid intake. Should you be concerned? Why or why not?

2. Ask a nurse on the gynecology surgery unit what the usual time is for a woman to first urinate after surgery (if a catheter is not used). How does this time interval compare with when a postpartum woman is expected to first urinate?

3. Write a narrative nurse's note to document the expected findings for a postpartum woman 12 hours after birth.

4. If you are a parent, did you or your partner experience separation grief because of the demands of employment? How did you deal with it?

5. During clinical practice, observe the reactions of siblings to a new infant. What steps do you see parents take to reassure the older child that he or she is still loved?

6. What cultural practices related to childbirth do you see in your clinical setting? Does the nursing staff support these? Discuss specific cultural practices with new parents of a different culture from your own.

CASE STUDY

Nita is a multipara who vaginally delivered twin boys 4 hours ago. One weighed 6 pounds and the other weighed 5 pounds 6 ounces. She is admitted to the mother–baby unit after an uneventful recovery. Your initial assessment reveals the following data: temperature 37.6°C (97.9°F), pulse 60 beats per minute (bpm), respirations 20 breaths/min, blood pressure 110/70 mm Hg; fundus slightly soft and located to the right of the umbilicus; lochia moderate; midline episiotomy intact with slight edema.

1. What is your interpretation of these data?

2. What is your first intervention? Why?

3. What should you immediately teach Nita?

Nita's vital signs 8 hours after birth are blood pressure 112/80 mm Hg, temperature 37.2°C (99°F), pulse 52 bpm, respirations 18 breaths/min.

4. Are any nursing interventions needed based on these vital signs? What is the rationale for your judgment?

Nita plans to breastfeed her twins. She successfully breastfed her other two children. However, she says, "I want to breastfeed, but I really have a lot of cramping when I nurse. I don't remember having that with the other two children."

5. What is the nurse's best response?

6. Why is Nita having more cramping than with her other two infants?

7. What intervention can help with this problem?

Nita is worried about constipation because she had this problem after her previous births and has been constipated during the last months of this pregnancy.

8. What interventions and teaching can help Nita avoid constipation?

Nita will receive the Rh immune globulin (RhoGAM) and rubella vaccine before discharge.

9. Under what circumstances are these drugs given?

10. What precautions should the nurse teach Nita?

On a home visit 2 days postpartum, the nurse assesses Nita's fundus as firm, midline, and −1.

11. Are these assessments normal? Why or why not? If they are not normal, is there an explanation?

12. What should the nurse expect to find in the lochia flow?

Nita's episiotomy is slightly reddened along the suture line, the edges are closely approximated, and there is no edema, bruising, or drainage.

13. Do these data support the supposition that the episiotomy is healing properly? Why or why not? What nursing actions are appropriate?

Choose the correct answer.

1. When checking a woman's fundus 24 hours after a cesarean birth of her third baby, the nurse finds her fundus at the level of her umbilicus, firm, and in the midline. The appropriate nursing action related to this assessment is to:
   a. document the normal assessment.
   b. determine when she last urinated.
   c. limit her intake of oral fluids.
   d. vigorously massage her fundus.

2. A woman who is 18 hours postpartum says she is having "hot flashes" and "sweats all the time." The appropriate nursing response is to:
   a. report her signs and symptoms of hypovolemic shock.
   b. tell her that her body is getting rid of unneeded fluid.
   c. notify her nurse-midwife that she may have an infection.
   d. limit her intake of caffeine-containing fluids.

3. A woman who is 3 hours postpartum has had difficulty urinating. She finally urinates 100 mL. The initial nursing action is to:
   a. insert an indwelling catheter.
   b. have her drink additional fluids.
   c. assess the height of her fundus.
   d. chart the urination amount.

4. When teaching the postpartum woman about peripads, the nurse should tell her that:
   a. she can change to tampons when the initial perineal soreness goes away.
   b. pads having cold packs within them usually hold more lochia than regular pads.
   c. blood-soaked pads must be returned in a plastic bag to the hospital after discharge.
   d. the pads should be applied and removed in a front-to-back direction.

5. A young mother is excited about her first baby. Choose the best teaching to help her obtain adequate rest after discharge.
   a. Plan to sleep or rest any time the infant sleeps.
   b. Do all housecleaning while the infant sleeps.
   c. Cook several meals at once and freeze for later use.
   d. Tell family and friends not to visit for the first month.

6. Choose the best independent nursing action to aid episiotomy healing in a woman who is 24 hours postpartum.
   a. Antibiotic cream application to the area
   b. Warm sitz baths taken four times per day
   c. Maintaining cold packs to the area at all times
   d. Checking the leukocyte level

7. To prevent breast engorgement, the nurse should teach the non-breastfeeding postpartum woman to:
   a. maintain loose-fitting clothing over her breasts.
   b. pump the breasts briefly if they become painful.
   c. limit fluid intake to suppress milk production.
   d. constantly wear a well-fitting bra or breast binder.

8. A woman who is 4 hours postpartum ambulates to the bathroom and suddenly has a large gush of lochia rubra. The nurse's first action should be to:
   a. determine whether the bleeding slows to normal or remains heavy.
   b. observe the vital signs for signs of hypovolemic shock.
   c. check to see what her previous lochia flow has been.
   d. identify the type of pain relief that was given when she was in labor.

9. To help the postpartum woman avoid constipation, the nurse should teach her to:
   a. avoid the intake of foods such as milk, cheese, or yogurt.
   b. take a laxative for the first 3 postpartum days.
   c. drink at least 2500 mL of non-caffeinated fluids daily.
   d. limit her walking until the episiotomy is fully healed.

10. Choose the sign or symptom that a new mother should be taught to report.
    a. Occasional uterine cramping when the infant nurses
    b. Oral temperature that is 37.2°C (99°F) in the morning
    c. Descent of the fundus one fingerbreadth each day
    d. Reappearance of red lochia after it changes to serous

11. Twelve hours after birth, a mother lies in bed resting. Although she will be discharged in another 12 hours, she does not ask about her baby or provide any care. What is the probable reason for her behavior?
    a. She is still in the taking-in phase of maternal adaptation.
    b. She shows behaviors that may lead to postpartum depression.
    c. She is still affected by medications given during labor.
    d. She may be dissatisfied with some aspect of the newborn.

12. A new father is reluctant to "spoil" his newborn when she cries by picking her up. The best nursing response is to:
    a. teach him that she will eventually stop crying if he waits.
    b. take the baby to the nursery to allow the parents to rest.
    c. pick the baby up and rock her until she sleeps again.
    d. tell the father that the baby cries to communicate a need.

13. A newborn is rooming in with his teenage mother, who is watching TV. The nurse notes that the baby is awake and quiet. The best nursing action is to:
    a. pick the baby up and point out his alert behaviors to the mother.
    b. tell the mother to pick up her baby and talk with him while he is awake.
    c. focus care on the mother, rather than the infant, so she can recuperate.
    d. encourage the mother to feed the infant before he begins crying.

14. The best nursing encouragement for parents to care for their infant is to:
    a. stay out of the room for as long as possible.
    b. have the grandmother nearby as a backup.
    c. give positive feedback when they provide care.
    d. correct their performance whenever they make a mistake.

21 The Normal Newborn: Adaptation and Assessment

MATCHING KEY TERMS

Match the term with the correct definition.

1. _____ Asphyxia

2. _____ Bilirubin

3. _____ Brown fat

4. _____ Jaundice

5. _____ Lanugo

6. _____ Neutral thermal environment

7. _____ Strabismus

8. _____ Surfactant

a. Slippery fluid that reduces the surface tension in lung alveoli

b. Tissue designed for newborn heat production

c. Surroundings in which the infant can maintain a stable temperature with minimal oxygen consumption and a low metabolic rate

d. Fine hair covering the fetus

e. Bilirubin staining of the skin and sclera

f. Low blood oxygen and high blood and tissue carbon dioxide

g. "Crossed" eyes

h. Unusable component of hemolyzed erythrocytes

Listed below are conditions that may be found when the newborn is assessed. Match the condition with the part(s) of the body where it would be observed. Note if it is found only in males or only in females. Mark a star by those that are abnormal variations.

9. _____ Candidiasis

10. _____ Pseudomenstruation

11. _____ Jaundice

12. _____ Engorgement

13. _____ Choanal atresia

14. _____ Cephalhematoma

15. _____ Syndactyly

16. _____ Preauricular sinus

17. _____ Hydrocele

18. _____ Subconjunctival hemorrhage

19. _____ Caput succedaneum

20. _____ Lanugo

21. _____ Epstein's pearls

22. _____ Hymenal tag

23. _____ Polydactyly

a. Head

b. Mouth

c. Skin

d. Genitalia

e. Spine

f. Ear

g. Eye

h. Nose

i. Breast

j. Hands and feet

k. Hip

24. _____ Developmental hip dysplasia

25. _____ Spina bifida

26. _____ Cataract

27. _____ Hypospadias

28. _____ Vernix caseosa

KEY CONCEPTS

1. Explain how each factor helps the newborn initiate respiration.

   a. Chemical

   b. Thermal

   c. Mechanical

   d. Sensory

2. Why is adequate functional residual capacity in the lungs important?

3. Number the following events in the correct order during fetal transition to extrauterine life.

   a. _____ Increased blood oxygen level

   b. _____ Respiration initiated

   c. _____ Closure of the ductus venosus

   d. _____ Increased pressure in the left side of the heart

   e. _____ Increased blood carbon dioxide level

   f. _____ Surfactant action keeps alveoli open

   g. _____ Foramen ovale closes

   h. _____ Ductus arteriosus constricts

4. List characteristics that predispose newborns to heat loss.

5. Describe each method by which the newborn can lose heat. Which ones can also be methods of heat gain?

Chapter **21** **The Normal Newborn: Adaptation and Assessment**

6. How does brown fat help the newborn maintain a near-constant temperature? Under what circumstances may newborns have inadequate brown fat and why?

7. Explain the relationship among oxygenation, body temperature, glucose stores, and bilirubin levels in the newborn.

8. Compare the normal values for fetal and adult erythrocytes, hemoglobin, and hematocrit.

9. How would you explain the prophylactic neonatal vitamin K injection to new parents?

10. Describe each newborn stool as you would explain it to a new parent. When should parents expect the first meconium stool? What differences in stools should parents expect if their infant is breastfed versus formula fed?

    a. Meconium stools

    b. Transitional stools

    c. Milk stools

11. What glucose level on a screening test requires further follow-up?

12. Which infants are at risk for hypoglycemia? Why?

13. Describe how each of the following factors can contribute to high newborn bilirubin levels. Which may be correctable with nursing intervention?

    a. Red blood cell quantity and life span

    b. Liver immaturity

    c. Intestinal factors

d. Time of first feeding

e. Birth trauma

f. Fatty acid production

g. Albumin-binding sites

h. Blood incompatibilities

i. Gestation

j. Family background

14. When does jaundice become pathologic rather than physiologic?

15. How does each of these problems result in jaundice? What is the usual treatment for each?
   a. Poor intake

   b. True breast milk jaundice

16. Compare extracellular water distribution in the newborn and adult.

17. What limitations does the newborn have in terms of:
   a. handling excess fluid

   b. compensating for inadequate fluid

18. What factors make the newborn vulnerable to infection that might not be a problem for an older infant or child?

19. Each of the following antibodies protects the newborn from which pathogens? Which one(s) are received from the mother?

a. IgG

b. IgM

c. IgA

20. Describe the two periods of reactivity. What are the nursing implications associated with each?

21. Describe the six behavioral states observed in the newborn.

22. What are the two immediate newborn assessments after birth?

23. Complete the following table.

Head Variation	Cause(s)	Characteristic Features	Parent Teaching
Caput succedaneum			
Cephalhematoma			

24. Explain the possible significance of each neonatal assessment.

a. Two-vessel umbilical cord

b. Simian line

c. Hair tuft on the lower spine

d. Ears below the level of the canthi of the eye

e. Drooping of one side of the mouth

25. Complete the following table on newborn measurements.

Measurement	Average for Full-Term Infant	Possible Causes for Deviations
Weight		
Length		
Head circumference		
Chest circumference		

26. List the normal ranges for each of the neonatal vital signs. Describe the correct assessment technique for each.

a. Pulse rate

b. Respiratory rate

c. Blood pressure

d. Temperature
- Rectal

- Axillary

27. List the signs that suggest neonatal respiratory distress.

Chapter **21** **The Normal Newborn: Adaptation and Assessment**

28. List the signs that suggest neonatal hypoglycemia.

29. Describe the normal assessments of female and male genitalia.

30. State the possible significance of each skin variance. Note if any special care is needed.

   a. Ruddiness

   b. Green-brown discoloration of the skin and vernix

   c. Red, blotchy areas with white or yellow papules in the center

   d. Blue-black marks over the sacral area

   e. Flat, purplish area that does not blanch with pressure

   f. Light-brown spots

31. What facial marks may be present if the infant had a nuchal cord?

CRITICAL THINKING EXERCISES

1. During clinical practice, note the steps taken to conserve the newborn's body heat. Identify which method of loss each is designed to interrupt.

2. Use a medical dictionary or laboratory manual to distinguish between indirect and direct bilirubin tests. How would each help identify possible causes of jaundice in the newborn?

3. What is the protocol for neonatal blood glucose screening at your clinical facility?

4. Find infants whose gestational age assessments were large for gestational age (LGA) or small for gestational age (SGA). Look at the mothers' charts to determine possible causes. Check the infants' charts to identify nursing assessments and care that were different (or more in depth) for these infants during the early hours after birth. Did any problems develop related to their being LGA or SGA?

5. Perform a gestational age assessment on an infant. Ask a classmate to assess the infant separately. Compare your scores and discuss reasons for any differences. Do the same with a staff nurse. Be careful not to stress the infant.

6. Identify different periods of reactivity in infants. Note the response of the mothers to the different periods. Determine their understanding of each period of reactivity and teach them as needed.

7. Identify habituation and self-consoling activities in infants. Determine what stimuli caused the habituation.

CASE STUDIES

You are admitting a newborn and performing a gestational age assessment. The infant weighs 6 pounds 10 ounces; her length is 19 inches, and her head circumference is 13 inches. You obtain the following information on assessment: fully flexed position; 0-degree wrist angle; 90- to 100-degree angle on arm recoil; 90-degree popliteal angle; the elbow reaches the sternum when extending the arm across the chest; lower leg at the 90-degree angle when flexing the thigh onto the abdomen. Skin is dry and cracking, and no blood vessels are visible through the skin. No lanugo is present. Sole creases cover the entire foot. Areola is 4 mm, and the ear cartilage is stiff. The clitoris and labia minora are completely covered by the labia majora.

1. Using Figure 21-23, circle the information given in the previous paragraph on the neuromuscular and physical maturity scale. What is your total score for both?

2. Determine the approximate weeks of gestation.

3. Using Figure 21-23, plot the infant's weight, length, and head circumference. (You will have to convert from English to metric measures.) Determine whether she is SGA, appropriate for gestational age (AGA), or LGA.

4. Based on your assessments, does the nurse need additional care for this infant? Why or why not?

119

REVIEW QUESTIONS

Choose the correct answer.

1. When performing an admission assessment on a term newborn, the nurse notes that the lung sounds are slightly moist. The skin color is pink except for acrocyanosis. Pulse is 156 beats/min (bpm), and respirations are 55 breaths/min and unlabored. The appropriate nursing action is to:
   a. notify the pediatrician regarding the abnormal lung sounds.
   b. continue to observe the infant's respiratory status.
   c. recheck the high respiratory and pulse rates in 30 minutes.
   d. keep the infant in the newborn nursery until stable.

2. A newborn has a hemoglobin level of 24 and a hematocrit value of 71%. The nurse should anticipate:
   a. temperature instability.
   b. high calcium levels.
   c. delayed breastfeeding.
   d. greater than normal jaundice.

3. Becoming cold can lead to respiratory distress, primarily because the infant:
   a. needs more oxygen than he or she can supply to generate heat.
   b. breathes more slowly and shallowly when hypothermic.
   c. reopens fetal shunts when the body temperature reaches 36.1°C (97°F).
   d. cannot supply enough glucose to provide fuel for respiration.

4. The primary purpose of surfactant is to:
   a. maintain normal blood glucose levels.
   b. keep lung alveoli partly open between breaths.
   c. inhibit excess erythrocyte production.
   d. stimulate the passage of the first meconium stool.

5. The foramen ovale closes because the:
   a. arterial pressure in the lungs is higher than that in the body.
   b. the presence of slight hypoxia and acidosis causes constriction.
   c. blood flow through it is redirected through the liver.
   d. pressure in the left atrium is higher than that in the right atrium.

6. Brown fat is used to:
   a. maintain temperature.
   b. facilitate digestion.
   c. metabolize glucose.
   d. conjugate bilirubin.

7. The infant of a diabetic mother is prone to hypoglycemia because:
   a. liver conversion of glycogen to glucose is sluggish.
   b. excess subcutaneous fat reduces blood flow to the tissues.
   c. high insulin production rapidly metabolizes glucose.
   d. vulnerability to infections increases metabolic stress.

8. The primary difference between physiologic and pathologic jaundice is the:
   a. number of fetal erythrocytes that are broken down.
   b. type of feeding method chosen by the mother.
   c. location of the yellow areas on the newborn's skin.
   d. time of onset and rate of increase in bilirubin levels.

9. The nurse can help prevent many cases of jaundice in the breastfed infant by:
   a. encouraging extra water intake between each nursing session.
   b. teaching the mother how to encourage regular and adequate breastfeeding.
   c. placing the infants under phototherapy prophylactically.
   d. advising mothers of suitable formulas to use if jaundice occurs.

10. Infection in the newborn often has subtle signs because:
    a. the body temperature slowly increases in response to pathogens.
    b. passive antibodies from the mother fight infection early.
    c. high urine output causes a lower body temperature.
    d. leukocyte responses and inflammatory signs are immature.

11. A hungry infant is vigorously crying. The best initial intervention is to:
    a. immediately give formula until the infant is satisfied.
    b. place the infant in a quiet, dark area, wrapped tightly.
    c. console the infant before the mother tries to feed it.
    d. encourage the parents to engage their infant in eye-to-eye contact.

12. A 9-pound 11-ounce infant was vaginally born. The labor nurse reports that there was shoulder dystocia at birth but that Apgar scores were 8 at 1 minute and 9 at 5 minutes. The nurse should do a focused assessment for:
    a. hip dysplasia.
    b. head molding.
    c. clavicle fracture.
    d. abnormal cord vessels.

13. The nurse notes that the infant's feet are turned inward. The appropriate nursing action is to:
    a. apply a splint to the feet and lower legs.
    b. notify the pediatrician or nurse practitioner.
    c. explain to the parents that this is typical for intrauterine position.
    d. determine whether the feet can be moved to a normal, straight position.

14. While performing an admission assessment on a term newborn, the nurse notes poor muscle tone and slight jitteriness. The appropriate nursing action is to:
    a. assess the infant's blood glucose level.
    b. stop the assessment and tightly wrap the infant in blankets.
    c. check the mother's chart for narcotics administered late in labor.
    d. give supplemental oxygen via a facemask.

15. While making a home visit to a mother and newborn on the second day after birth, the nurse notes that the infant's skin color is yellowish to the midsternal level. The most important action is to:
    a. teach the mother to breastfeed the infant at least every 2 to 3 hours.
    b. explain that jaundice after birth is common and will resolve without treatment.
    c. ask the mother whether she has been feeding the infant supplemental formula.
    d. notify the pediatrician or nurse practitioner of the early, intense jaundice.

16. Choose the nursing observation that is most important if the nurse notes a two-vessel umbilical cord.
    a. Urine output
    b. Onset of jaundice
    c. Respiratory rate
    d. Heart rhythm

17. An infant's gestational age assessment reveals that her weight is SGA. This means that:
    a. she was born before 37 completed weeks of gestation.
    b. her weight is between the 10th and 90th percentiles.
    c. she has a low birth weight in relation to her length.
    d. her weight is lower than expected for her gestation.

18. When weighing an infant, the nurse places a covering on the scale tray to:
    a. avoid causing multiple startle (Moro) reflexes when weighing.
    b. ensure that conductive heat loss from the infant is minimal.
    c. compensate for the negative weight balance to ensure the correct weight.
    d. avoid contaminating the nurse's hands with blood or other body substances.

19. Which newborn reflex can help the new mother learn to breastfeed?
    a. Tonic neck
    b. Rooting
    c. Palmar grasp
    d. Moro

20. The nurse notes a slight resistance when first inserting a rectal thermometer to take a newborn's first temperature. The best nursing action is to:
    a. notify the infant's pediatrician.
    b. rotate the thermometer to the left while inserting.
    c. listen for the presence of bowel sounds.
    d. check for rectal patency using the fifth digit.

21. The best location for an infant's glucose determination is the:
    a. great toe of either foot.
    b. nondominant heel.
    c. midline of the heel.
    d. lateral surface of the heel.

22 The Normal Newborn: Nursing Care

KEY CONCEPTS

1. What is the correct order for suctioning an infant's airway using a bulb syringe? Why?

2. Why is it particularly important that the infant's head be promptly dried?

3. What added assessments and interventions should the nurse perform if an infant has a subnormal temperature?

4. What type of heat loss can occur in each situation?

   a. Placing the newborn on a cold, unpadded scale

   b. Using a cold stethoscope to listen to breathing sounds

   c. Placing the infant's crib by a window on a snowy day

5. A newborn who is large for gestational age (LGA) has a low blood glucose on the first screening and will have repeat glucose screenings for approximately the next 8 hours. Explain in simple terms, as you would explain to the parents, the reason for promptly feeding the newborn and for repeat screenings.

6. When should the initial bath be given to a newborn?

7. What are the two primary nursing observations after circumcision?

8. What circumcision problems should parents be taught to report?

9. List the signs that suggest infection of the umbilical cord. What measures can prevent a cord infection?

10. What is the primary method of identifying the newborn and mother (or other support person)?

11. List five general signs of a newborn infection.

12. Explain why these medications are typically administered to newborns.

    a. Vitamin K

    b. Erythromycin eye ointment

    c. Hepatitis B immunization

13. Do infants of mothers who have hepatitis B need any additional medication? Why?

14. Compare the advantages and disadvantages of each type of postdischarge follow-up for mothers and infants.

	Advantages	Disadvantages
Home visits		
Telephone counseling		

CRITICAL THINKING EXERCISES

1. Newborn circumcision is a controversial topic. Consider common reasons for having the procedure performed on a newborn and refute each. Do the same for reasons for not performing circumcision.

2. What screening tests are routinely performed at your clinical facility? What information is given to parents regarding this testing?

123

3. Use a pediatric or clinical nursing skills text to compare the techniques for administering an intramuscular injection to an infant, a toddler, a preschool child, and a school-aged child. How do precautions differ? What needle sizes are appropriate for each age group? What are the maximum injection volumes for each?

4. What security measures are used at your clinical facility to prevent infant abduction? Ask several parents who have been previously taught security measures to restate these measures. How well do they recall them?

5. Does your clinical facility offer follow-up care, such as warm lines or home visits, for new parents? Ask staff members about its effectiveness.

REVIEW QUESTIONS

Choose the correct answer.

1. An infant's axillary temperature is 35.9°C (96.6°F). The priority nursing action is to:
   a. recheck the infant's temperature rectally.
   b. have the mother breastfeed the infant.
   c. place the infant in a radiant warmer.
   d. chart the normal axillary temperature.

2. To care for the uncircumcised penis, parents should be taught to:
   a. retract the foreskin with each diaper change.
   b. wash under the foreskin as far as it has separated.
   c. use an emollient cream to hasten foreskin separation.
   d. avoid putting soap on the foreskin before separation.

3. A nursing student has been caring for a woman and her newborn all morning. The student takes the infant to the nursery for screening tests before discharge. When the infant is returned to the mother, the correct procedure is to:
   a. have the mother read her printed band number and verify that it matches the infant's.
   b. ask the mother to state her name and the name of her infant.
   c. call out the mother's full name before leaving the infant with her.
   d. return the infant with no special procedure because the student knows both mother and infant.

4. A new mother should be taught to support her baby's head when holding the infant because:
   a. doing so will promote better eye contact and bonding.
   b. the baby's muscles are too weak to support the heavy head.
   c. it allows better guidance of the head toward the breast.
   d. less regurgitation of gastric contents will occur.

5. Choose the normal circumcision assessment.
   a. Slipping of the PlastiBell onto the shaft of the penis
   b. Oozing of blood from the site after a Gomco circumcision
   c. Delay in urination for 12 to 16 hours
   d. Development of a dry yellow crust on the site

6. Choose the correct parent teaching about cord care.
   a. Fold the diaper below the cord to speed drying.
   b. Expect the cord to detach in no more than 7 days.
   c. Tub baths are safe as soon as the cord detaches.
   d. Skin near the cord site may be red until it detaches.

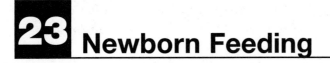

23 Newborn Feeding

MATCHING KEY TERMS

Match the term with the correct definition.

1. _____ Foremilk
2. _____ Hindmilk
3. _____ Mastitis
4. _____ Milk-ejection reflex

a. Release of milk from the alveoli into the ducts
b. Breast infection
c. Thirst-quenching milk
d. Higher fat milk

KEY CONCEPTS

1. Determine the number of calories per day needed by an infant weighing 8 pounds. Then calculate the number of ounces of breast milk or formula (each having 20 calories per ounce) the infant needs daily. What are the infant's daily fluid needs?

2. Describe changes in the composition and appearance of colostrum, transitional milk, and mature milk. When do these changes occur?

3. Complete the following table to contrast breast milk and cow's milk formula. What are the effects of these differences on newborns?

Component	Breast Milk	Cow's Milk Formula
Proteins		
Fats		
Vitamins		
Minerals		
Other substances, such as antibodies		

4. Describe the purposes of prolactin and oxytocin in breastfeeding. What can enhance or interfere with their secretion?

5. What care can help the mother who has flat or inverted nipples?

6. Describe the differences in breast fullness.

   a. Soft

   b. Filling

   c. Engorged

7. Describe each of these hand positions for breastfeeding. Which is preferred?

   a. "C" position

   b. V hold

8. Describe the differences between nutritive and nonnutritive suckling. How does an infant swallowing sound?

9. What should the mother be taught about removing the infant from the breast?

10. During the first few weeks, babies usually breastfeed approximately every _____ to _____ hours. They should eat approximately _____ times a day.

11. How does breastfeeding help resolve jaundice? Why should breastfeeding be frequent?

12. When is the best time to administer medications to a breastfeeding mother to decrease the amount of the drug being transferred to the baby?

13. Under which maternal conditions is breastfeeding not advised?

14. What should the mother be taught about storage of breast milk?

    a. Containers

    b. Temperature

    c. Thawing frozen milk

15. Describe the use and precautions associated with each type of formula.

    a. Ready-to-use

    b. Concentrated liquid

    c. Powdered

16. Explain what a new mother should be taught about each of these aspects of formula feeding.

    a. Frequency

    b. Propping the bottle

    c. Microwaving formula

    d. Discarding formula

CRITICAL THINKING QUESTIONS

1. Ask women you care for during clinical practice what their reasons were for choosing their method of feeding. Were any of their reasons based on cultural influences?

2. Make a teaching plan to help mothers with these breastfeeding problems.

   a. Engorgement

   b. Sore nipples

   c. Flat or inverted nipples

   d. Sleepy baby or one who falls asleep soon after nursing begins

3. A mother tells you that she does not think she has enough milk for her baby. How can you guide her?

4. If your clinical experience includes postpartum clinics or home visits, ask breastfeeding mothers whether they have encountered problems since they were discharged. If they have stopped breastfeeding, why? Have any of the women forgotten information that was taught when they were in the birth center?

CASE STUDY

Margaret is breastfeeding for the first time. She seems awkward in handling her baby and says that the baby is not feeding well. The baby frequently cries while Margaret tries to feed her.

1. What is the first nursing action to take in this situation?

2. What additional nursing actions can help Margaret?

   After your nursing actions, the infant latches on to the breast and begins vigorously suckling. Margaret begins to relax. She says, "I thought this would be easy, but it isn't."

3. What basic teaching is appropriate for Margaret?

   After approximately 3 minutes, Margaret asks, "Shouldn't I change breasts now? I don't want to have sore nipples."

4. What teaching is appropriate about nursing duration and frequency?

5. What should you tell Margaret about caring for her breasts?

Margaret successfully completes her first breastfeeding. She asks, "The baby seemed to suck a lot, but how do I know she is getting enough to eat?"

6. What infant signs or behaviors can you teach Margaret to look for that indicate adequate milk intake?

REVIEW QUESTIONS

Choose the correct answer.

1. A new mother wants to nurse her infant for only 5 minutes at each breast to avoid sore nipples. Choose the appropriate teaching.
   a. Limiting the time during early days can lessen the trauma to the nipples and allow them time to toughen.
   b. Limiting time can cause frequent infant hunger because the baby does not receive richer milk.
   c. Limiting time at the breast does not reduce sore nipples but does reduce engorgement.
   d. Limiting time at the breast delays the transition from colostrum to transitional and true milk.

2. A new mother wants to breastfeed but also to feed her infant formula occasionally. The nurse should teach her to:
   a. avoid using any bottles in the first month to establish her milk supply.
   b. make a clear choice to feed by one method or the other to avoid nipple confusion.
   c. limit formula feeding to once each day until her milk supply is well established.
   d. alternate formula and nursing to allow the infant to become accustomed to both.

3. A woman has had a baby at 29 weeks of gestation. She tells the nurse that she cannot breastfeed because the baby is so small and early. The nurse should tell her that:
   a. she will be able to establish lactation when the baby is strong enough to nurse.
   b. special formulas are actually better for preterm infants than her breast milk.
   c. infections are more likely to occur if the infant takes stored breast milk.
   d. she can use a breast pump to maintain lactation until nursing is possible.

4. A breastfeeding mother is reluctant to take a prescribed analgesic because she does not want to pass it to the baby. The nurse should teach her that:
   a. less medication will reach the baby if she takes it after a feeding.
   b. limiting the duration of feedings when she needs medication will reduce the transfer to the baby.
   c. it is best to avoid all medications during nursing, including analgesics.
   d. formula feeding while she needs analgesics may be best for the baby.

5. The maximum length of time formula should be kept after preparation is:
   a. 12 to 18 hours.
   b. 18 to 24 hours.
   c. 24 to 48 hours.
   d. 48 to 72 hours.

6. A new mother is worried because her 1-day-old baby is taking only 3/4 ounces of formula at most feedings. The nurse should teach her that:
   a. her baby should be taking 2 to 3 ounces at each feeding by the next day.
   b. the amount the baby is taking at each feeding is normal at this time.
   c. the baby might take more if a different formula is used.
   d. the nipple may be too firm for the baby to easily suck.

24 The Childbearing Family with Special Needs

MATCHING KEY TERMS

Match the term with the correct definition.

1. _____ Crack
2. _____ Egocentrism
3. _____ Fetal alcohol syndrome
4. _____ Methadone
5. _____ Opiate
6. _____ Abstinence syndrome

a. Interest centered on self rather than on others
b. Symptoms observed when an individual who is addicted to a specific drug abstains
c. Fetal disorders associated with maternal alcohol use
d. CNS depressant that produces mental dullness, drowsiness, and stupor
e. Highly addictive form of cocaine
f. Long-acting drug to substitute heroin or morphine

KEY CONCEPTS

1. Explain how pregnancy affects the adolescent's:

    a. development of independence

    b. education

    c. employment opportunities

2. What pregnancy risks are higher for adolescents than for adults?

3. List complications the mature pregnant woman is more likely to encounter.

    a. Genetic

    b. Pre-existing disorders

    c. Obstetric complications

4. What problems is the mature mother likely to encounter in terms of the following?

   a. Fatigue

   b. Support of friends or family

5. Why do substances ingested by the mother tend to have a more pronounced effect on her fetus than on her?

6. Complete the following chart related to the fetal and neonatal effects of maternal substance use.

	Fetal Effects	Neonatal Effects
Tobacco		
Alcohol		
Cocaine		
Marijuana		
Opioids		
Amphetamines and methamphetamine		
Antidepressants		

7. Why might the birth center staff screen a woman for cocaine if she is admitted in preterm labor and having intense contractions?

8. What therapeutic management is necessary for a pregnant woman who desires to discontinue her use of heroin during pregnancy?

9. List the antepartal signs associated with drug abuse.

   a. Behaviors

   b. Physical appearance

   c. Obstetric history

   d. Emotional reaction to pregnancy

10. What signs might the woman have during the intrapartum period if she has recently ingested these drugs?

    a. Cocaine

    b. Heroin

11. What special concerns exist if the infant has facial or genital anomalies?

12. Why is grief an essential aspect of attachment to an infant with an anomaly?

13. Why is it important that both fathers and mothers be supported in the grief aspects of having a baby with an anomaly or of perinatal loss?

14. Describe the risks to an abused pregnant woman and her fetus.

15. Describe each phase of the violence cycle.

CRITICAL THINKING EXERCISES

1. If you care for a teenage mother, discuss the involvement of the infant's father and the grandmother in infant care. What evidence of the "honeymoon phase" did you observe? What are the future plans of the young mother (and father, if involved)? Are their plans realistic? Why or why not?

2. What does your state require if either the mother or infant shows evidence of drug abuse in toxicology screenings?

3. Discuss with your hospital's emergency department about their experience with battered women. Do they note any differences in abuse when a woman is pregnant?

REVIEW QUESTIONS

Choose the correct answer.

1. The best way for the nurse to evaluate the quality of a pregnant adolescent's diet is to:
   a. ask her how well she eats in a nonthreatening manner.
   b. assume it is inadequate and give her advice.
   c. ask her to describe what she ate the previous day.
   d. have her record everything she eats for 1 week.

2. Correct advice for women who ask about using alcohol during pregnancy is that it is:
   a. safest if taken during the last trimester.
   b. best to avoid consumption during the first 12 weeks.
   c. unknown if there is any fetal harm from its use.
   d. important to avoid it entirely throughout pregnancy.

3. When first presenting an infant with an anomaly to parents, the nurse should:
   a. have the physician initially discuss the causes of the anomaly, if known.
   b. emphasize the most normal aspects of the infant before showing them the anomaly.
   c. wait until the mother has had time to recuperate from the stress of labor.
   d. limit their time with the infant the first time they see him or her.

4. A woman who had a stillborn infant at 37 weeks of gestation angrily asks the nurse why her physician did not "take the baby early." The nurse should understand that the mother's behavior:
   a. is unusual when stillbirth occurs this late in gestation.
   b. suggests a discord between the woman and her partner.
   c. should be expected as part of the normal grieving process.
   d. reflects intense guilt about her own self-care during pregnancy.

5. The main goal when caring for battered women is to:
   a. emphasize that they have the right not to be hurt.
   b. help them to better identify their role in the family.
   c. encourage them to ask their partners about counseling.
   d. limit their ability to return to the abusive partner.

Chapter **24** The Childbearing Family with Special Needs

25 Pregnancy-Related Complications

MATCHING KEY TERMS

Match the term with the correct definition.

1. _____ Cerclage

2. _____ Kernicterus

3. _____ Maceration

a. Bilirubin accumulation within the brain that may cause damage

b. Degeneration of a fetus retained in the uterus after its death

c. Encircling the cervix with sutures

KEY CONCEPTS

1. Define spontaneous abortion.

2. Complete the table on the types of spontaneous abortions.

	Clinical Manifestations	Therapeutic Management
Threatened		
Inevitable		
Incomplete		
Complete		
Missed		
Recurrent		

3. Describe altered laboratory studies seen in disseminated intravascular coagulopathy (DIC).

4. Write a simply worded response that you might use if a woman expresses the feeling that she did something to cause her spontaneous abortion.

5. What is the possible significance of sudden shoulder pain during early pregnancy?

6. What teaching is needed for the woman receiving methotrexate therapy for an early ectopic pregnancy?

7. List the typical signs and symptoms of a hydatidiform mole.

8. What is the relationship between a hydatidiform mole and cancer? What precautions related to cancer detection are taken after the evacuation of the mole?

9. List foods that should be emphasized for a woman who experienced bleeding complications with pregnancy (at any gestation). How would you explain simply the need for these foods?

10. Complete the following chart to compare placenta previa with abruptio placentae.

	Placenta Previa	Abruptio Placentae
Placenta location		
Character of bleeding		
Presence of pain		
Uterine activity		
Diagnosis		
Therapeutic management		

11. List the nursing teaching associated with home care when a woman has placenta previa.

12. What is the relationship between cocaine use and abruptio placentae?

13. Why is the amount of external bleeding in abruptio placentae not a reliable indicator of the true amount of blood loss?

14. List the early and late signs of hypovolemic shock.

15. List the nursing measures and their rationales to promote maternal and fetal oxygenation in hemorrhagic disorders.

16. Describe how generalized vasospasm of preeclampsia affects each organ and how these effects are manifested.
    a. Kidneys

    b. Liver

    c. Brain

    d. Lungs

    e. Placenta

17. What is the primary difference between the expected edema of pregnancy and that of preeclampsia?

18. What is the significance of epigastric pain in a woman with preeclampsia?

19. List the signs of magnesium toxicity.

20. What is the antidote for magnesium toxicity?

21. What feature distinguishes chronic hypertension from pregnancy-induced hypertension?

22. What conditions are necessary for the woman to receive the anti-Rh$_O$(D) immunoglobulin? What does each mean?

    a. Rh of the woman

    b. Rh of the fetus or newborn

    c. Indirect Coombs test (woman)

    d. Direct Coombs test (newborn)

23. How can ABO incompatibility occur?

CRITICAL THINKING EXERCISES

1. Examine your own feelings about induced abortion. Are your feelings different for early and later abortions? Can you care for a woman who is having an induced abortion?

2. Ask the staff nurses at your clinical facility about their experiences with women who have hyperemesis gravidarum. Do you detect any preset beliefs about the disorder among the nurses?

CASE STUDY

Patricia is a 17-year-old gravida 1, para 0 at 34 weeks of gestation who is visiting her doctor for a routine prenatal visit. When weighing Patricia, the nurse finds that she has gained 8 pounds in the past month.

1. What is the main objective after this initial assessment?

2. What is the most important question or problem that must be solved during Patricia's prenatal visit?

3. What are the nurse's priority assessments? Why?

The nurse obtains a clean catch urine specimen from Patricia and takes her vital signs (temperature: 37°C [98.6°F], pulse: 82 beats/min (bpm), respiration: 20 breaths/min, blood pressure: 146/90 mm Hg) and fetal heart rate (FHR: 144 to 150 bpm). The deep tendon reflexes are normal (2+), with no clonus.

4. What testing would you expect to be performed on this urine specimen? Why?

5. What information might the nurse need from previous prenatal visits and why?

6. What questions should the nurse ask Patricia while assessing her?

Patricia's physician diagnoses her with mild preeclampsia and will initially manage Patricia at home.

7. What findings would lead the physician to the diagnosis of mild preeclampsia?

8. Why do you think the physician is recommending home management at this time?

9. What teaching is essential regarding Patricia's home care?

REVIEW QUESTIONS

Choose the correct answer.

1. Choose the primary distinction between a threatened and inevitable abortion.
   a. Presence of cramping
   b. Rupture of membranes
   c. Vaginal bleeding
   d. Pelvic pressure

2. A woman is admitted to the emergency department with a possible ectopic pregnancy. Choose the signs and symptoms that should be immediately reported to her physician.
   a. Low levels of β-human chorionic gonadotropin (β-hCG)
   b. Hemoglobin level of 11.5; hematocrit value of 34%
   c. Light vaginal bleeding
   d. Pulse increases from 78 to 100 bpm

3. When caring for a woman who had a hydatidiform mole evacuated, the clinic nurse should primarily:
   a. reinforce the need to delay a new pregnancy for 1 year.
   b. ask the woman whether she has any cramping or bleeding.
   c. observe the return of her blood pressure to normal.
   d. palpate the uterus for the return to its normal size.

4. The woman who is receiving methotrexate for an ectopic pregnancy should be cautioned to avoid:
   a. driving or operating machinery.
   b. eating raw vegetables or fruits.
   c. using latex condoms for intercourse.
   d. taking vitamins with folic acid.

5. A woman who is 34 weeks pregnant is admitted with contractions every 2 minutes, lasting 60 seconds, and a high uterine resting tone. She says she had some vaginal bleeding at home, and there is a small amount of blood on her perineal pad. The priority action of the nurse is to:
   a. establish whether she is in labor by performing a vaginal examination.
   b. ask her whether she has had recent intercourse or a vaginal examination.
   c. evaluate the maternal and fetal circulation and oxygenation.
   d. determine whether this is the first episode of pain she has had.

6. Nursing teaching for the woman who has hyperemesis gravidarum should include:
   a. adding favorite seasonings to foods while cooking.
   b. eating simple foods such as breads and fruits.
   c. lying down on the right side after eating.
   d. eating creamed soup with every meal.

7. The nurse makes the following assessments on a woman who is receiving intravenous magnesium sulfate: FHR: 148 to 158 bpm, pulse: 88 bpm, respiration: 10 breaths/min, and blood pressure: 158/96 mm Hg. The priority nursing action is to:
   a. increase the rate of the magnesium infusion.
   b. maintain the magnesium infusion at the current rate.
   c. slow the rate of the magnesium infusion.
   d. discontinue the magnesium infusion.

8. When providing intrapartal care for a woman with severe preeclampsia, priority nursing care is to:
   a. maintain the ordered rate of anticonvulsant medications.
   b. promote placental blood flow and prevent maternal injury.
   c. administer intravenous fluids and observe the urine output.
   d. reduce maternal blood pressure to the prepregnancy level.

9. Clonus indicates that the:
   a. central nervous system is very irritable.
   b. renal blood flow is severely reduced.
   c. lungs are filling with interstitial fluid.
   d. muscles of the foot are inflamed.

10. The feature that distinguishes preeclampsia from eclampsia is the:
    a. amount of blood pressure elevation.
    b. edema of the face and fingers.
    c. presence of proteinuria.
    d. onset of generalized seizures.

11. Which woman should receive $Rh_O(D)$ immunoglobulin after birth?
    a. Rh-negative mother; Rh-positive infant; positive direct Coombs test
    b. Rh-positive mother; Rh-negative infant; negative direct Coombs test
    c. Rh-negative mother; Rh-positive infant; negative direct Coombs test
    d. Rh-positive mother; Rh-positive infant; positive direct Coombs test

26 Concurrent Disorders During Pregnancy

MATCHING KEY TERMS

Match the term with the correct definition.

1. _____ Dystocia

2. _____ Euglycemia

3. _____ Seroconversion

4. _____ Gluconeogenesis

a. Development of antibodies in response to infection or immunization

b. Difficult or prolonged labor

c. Formation of glycogen from noncarbohydrate sources such as proteins and fats

d. Normal blood glucose levels

KEY CONCEPTS

1. List the four classic signs of diabetes.

   a. _____

   b. _____

   c. _____

   d. _____

2. Why is the maintenance of a normal blood glucose level before and during early pregnancy particularly important?

3. What are the effects of maternal vascular involvement on the fetus/newborn of a diabetic mother?

4. Do insulin requirements increase, decrease, or remain stable during the following periods? Why?

   a. First trimester

   b. Second and third trimesters

   c. Labor

   d. Postpartum

5. When would the physician want a pregnant woman to have an oral glucose tolerance test?

6. Why is it important to give a pregnant woman who has diabetes as many choices as possible?

7. What steps minimize insulin leakage from the injection site?

8. Why is it recommended that a woman who has hypoglycemia avoid sucrose or unrefined sugar, such as candy?

9. List the early signs and symptoms of congestive heart failure.

10. Janet is a 26-year-old woman who is 30 weeks pregnant with her first baby. She has rheumatic heart disease. She had to stop working at her desk job at 20 weeks of pregnancy because of fatigue. She has no problems when sitting quietly, but tasks, such as making her bed or gathering laundry to wash, cause slight chest pain and a rapid heartbeat. She complains that she always feels tired. What class of heart disease do her symptoms suggest?

11. What anticoagulant is recommended if one is needed during pregnancy? Why?

12. Why are labor and the immediate postpartum period especially dangerous for a woman who has a heart disease?

13. A woman who is 32 weeks pregnant and has class II heart disease visits the antepartal clinic for a routine visit. You find that she has gained 7 pounds since her last visit. Is her weight gain normal? What possibilities should you consider?

14. Why is it important to take folic acid before and during pregnancy?

15. Why does maternal sickle cell crisis make fetal death more likely?

16. Describe the signs of sickle cell crisis.

17. List the pregnancy-associated risks for a woman who has systemic lupus erythematosus.

18. Why is the drug management of a woman who has epilepsy difficult during pregnancy?

19. Describe the four stages of the course of an human immunodeficiency virus (HIV) infection.

20. Complete the table to learn more about viral infections during pregnancy.

Infection	Maternal Effects	Fetal and Neonatal Effects	Prevention	Treatment
Cytomegalovirus				
Rubella				
Varicella zoster				
Herpes viruses				
Parvovirus B19				
Hepatitis B				

21. At what point is a person said to have acquired immunodeficiency syndrome (AIDS)?

22. Which drug is recommended for HIV-infected pregnant women to prevent viral transmission to the fetus?

23. What nursing care is appropriate for the HIV-infected pregnant woman?

24. Complete the table to learn more about non-viral infections during pregnancy.

Infection	Maternal Effects	Fetal and Neonatal Effects	Prevention	Treatment
Toxoplasmosis				
Group B streptococci				
Tuberculosis				

CRITICAL THINKING EXERCISES

1. Review patients' charts to determine whether they had a glucose challenge test and their response to it. What follow-up was performed if their blood level was 140 mg/dL or higher?

2. Examine your attitudes toward people with HIV. Are you fearful of them? Did you have to confront this fear before entering nursing school? How do you feel about pregnant women who have HIV? Are your feelings for "innocent" victims, such as infants, different from feelings for those who acquired the infection through unsafe sexual intercourse or intravenous drug use?

CASE STUDY

Debra is a 22-year-old gravida 1, para 0, who has had type 1 diabetes for 6 years. Her last menstrual period was 12 weeks ago.

1. How will Debra's diabetes be affected by her pregnancy?

2. What changes will she most likely have to make in her diabetes management because she is pregnant?

3. What routine assessments will be made at each prenatal visit?

4. What additional tests will Debra need as her pregnancy progresses?

5. How may Debra's fetus be affected by her diabetes?

6. What nursing management during labor should be expected?

7. What newborn problems should the nurse anticipate?

8. What added care will Debra's infant need?

REVIEW QUESTIONS

Choose the correct answer.

1. The test used to screen for gestational diabetes is the:
   a. glycosylated hemoglobin test.
   b. glucose challenge test.
   c. oral glucose tolerance test.
   d. postprandial glucose test.

2. The best evaluation for the patient goal of accurate insulin administration is that she will:
   a. repeat the instructed steps of the technique.
   b. accurately withdraw, mix, and inject the insulin.
   c. have normal fasting and postprandial glucose levels.
   d. state that she understands the teaching provided.

3. Rheumatic heart disease is usually preceded by which infection?
   a. Streptococcal pharyngitis
   b. Syphilis
   c. Pneumococcal pneumonia
   d. Chlamydial vaginitis

4. The primary fetal risk when a mother has any type of anemia is:
   a. neonatal anemia.
   b. elevated bilirubin.
   c. limited infection defenses.
   d. reduced oxygen delivery.

5. Intrapartum nursing care for a woman who has sickle cell disease focuses on:
   a. maintaining oxygenation and preventing dehydration.
   b. controlling pain and avoiding unnecessary movement.
   c. preventing excess exertion and limiting visitors.
   d. increasing calorie intake and avoiding internal monitoring.

6. When caring for a pregnant woman with systemic lupus erythematosus, the clinic nurse must especially observe for the development of:
   a. urinary tract infections.
   b. excessive weight gain.
   c. elevated blood pressure.
   d. reduced blood glucose level.

7. Choose the appropriate infant care teaching for the woman who gave birth by cesarean because of active herpes.
   a. Do not breastfeed the infant until all the lesions are healed.
   b. Thoroughly wash your hands before handling the infant.
   c. Wear a mask when breastfeeding or holding the infant close.
   d. No special precautions are needed when caring for the infant.

8. The nurse should expect the HIV-infected pregnant woman to receive:
   a. antibiotics.
   b. protease inhibitors.
   c. zidovudine.
   d. acyclovir.

9. Expected drug treatment for a pregnant woman who has tuberculosis is:
   a. acyclovir and zidovudine.
   b. isoniazid and rifampin.
   c. cefotaxime and vancomycin.
   d. ampicillin and gentamicin.

27 The Woman with an Intrapartum Complication

MATCHING KEY TERMS

Match the term with the correct definition.

1. _____ Abruptio placentae
2. _____ Hydramnios
3. _____ Placenta accreta
4. _____ Shoulder dystocia
5. _____ Tocolytic

a. Delayed or difficult birth of the shoulders after the head has emerged
b. Premature separation of a normally implanted placenta
c. Excessive volume of amniotic fluid
d. Placenta that is abnormally adherent to the uterine muscle
e. Medication to stop preterm or hypertonic labor contractions

KEY CONCEPTS

1. What are three characteristics of effective uterine activity?

   a. _____

   b. _____

   c. _____

2. Complete the following table to compare the characteristics of hypotonic and hypertonic labor dysfunction.

	Hypotonic Dysfunction	Hypertonic Dysfunction
Contraction characteristics		
Uterine resting tone		
Phase of labor when it is most common		
Therapeutic management		

3. What two measures may be used to stimulate labor that slows down after it is established?

   a. _____

   b. _____

4. What is the central principle of nursing actions when dysfunctional labor is a result of ineffective maternal pushing?

5. Why are upright positions good for women who have ineffective second-stage pushing?

6. List the nursing measures to promote normal labor when maternal pushing is ineffective for each reason listed.

   a. Fear of injury

   b. Exhaustion

7. Why are upright maternal positions best to relieve persistent occiput posterior positions?

8. List four intrapartal problems that are more likely to occur if the woman has a multifetal pregnancy.

   a. _____

   b. _____

   c. _____

   d. _____

9. What are the expected rates for dilation and fetal descent for the following?

   a. Nulliparas

   b. Parous women

10. List the nursing measures for the woman having prolonged labor and for her fetus.

11. List the nursing measures that may be used when the woman has precipitate labor.

   a. Promoting fetal oxygenation

   b. Promoting maternal comfort

12. What factors may make the woman think her membranes have ruptured when they have not?

13. A patient will be discharged with ruptured membranes at 32 weeks of gestation. Write a summary of patient teaching in simple terms that you might use.

14. List the side effects that may occur with β-adrenergic drugs such as terbutaline. What drug should be available to reverse the serious adverse effects of β-adrenergic drugs, and what is its classification?

15. How do these drugs stop preterm labor? Give an example of each.

    a. Prostaglandin synthesis inhibitors

    b. Calcium antagonists

16. What are the primary nursing assessments related to each of these tocolytic drugs?

    a. Terbutaline

    b. Magnesium sulfate

    c. Indomethacin

    d. Nifedipine

    e. Corticosteroids

17. What are the two variations of a prolapsed cord?

    a. _____

    b. _____

18. What are the two objectives if an umbilical cord prolapse occurs or is suspected?

    a. _____

    b. _____

147

19. Describe the three variations of a uterine rupture.

    a. _____

    b. _____

    c. _____

20. Why might amniotic fluid embolism result in disseminated intravascular coagulation?

21. If the pregnant woman suffers trauma, why should medical and nursing care focus on her stabilization before fetal stabilization?

22. The woman at 32 weeks of gestation has had a car accident. Her vital signs are stable, and the fetal heart rate is 150 to 160 beats/min (bpm). What should the nurse suspect if the woman's uterus seems to be enlarging? What is the correct action?

CRITICAL THINKING EXERCISES

1. During clinical practice, observe and discuss with the nurses what measures they use for women having back labor.

2. Practice the positions listed for back labor so that you will be familiar with them during clinical practice.

3. If you had to be on bed rest for preterm labor, possibly for 6 weeks, what adjustments would you and your family have to make to achieve that recommendation? What would be the single most important obstacle to adhering to bed rest in your life? What type of quiet activities could you do while maintaining bed rest?

CASE STUDIES

Ann Craig is admitted at 33 weeks of gestation saying that she thinks her "water broke." This is her fourth pregnancy. Two of her infants were preterm, born at 32 and 27 weeks of gestation, and she has had one elective abortion. She has had regular prenatal care since 6 weeks of gestation.

1. What are the most important additional assessments that the nurse should make?

   The nurse notes that a small amount of cloudy fluid is draining from Ann's vagina. A nitrazine paper turns blue-black in color, and a fern test is positive. The maternal vital signs are a temperature of 37.2°C (99°F), pulse of 86 bpm, respiration of 22 breaths/min, and blood pressure of 132/80 mm Hg. The fetal heart rate is 162 to 170 bpm and has average variability. Ann occasionally has a contraction that lasts for 20 to 30 seconds.

2. What data from the aforementioned assessments are the most relevant?

3. What is the main judgment you would make from these data? What is the basis for that judgment?

4. Would you perform a vaginal examination at this point? Why or why not?

Shawna is an 18-year-old primigravida admitted to the birth center at 27 weeks of gestation in probable preterm labor. Her membranes are intact. The physician writes these orders:

- NPO except ice chips
- Complete blood count
- Catheterize urine for routine analysis, culture, and sensitivity
- IV fluids: Ringer's lactate at 200 mL/hr for 1 hour, then 125 mL/hr
- Routine fetal monitoring and maternal vital signs

5. Which of these orders has priority? Why?

6. What position is appropriate for Shawna? Why?

Shawna will receive magnesium sulfate for tocolysis.

7. What nursing observations are essential with respect to magnesium sulfate? Why?

The contractions stop, and Shawna will begin taking oral terbutaline before she is discharged.

8. What teaching is appropriate related to the home use of this drug?

9. What additional teaching is important before Shawna is discharged?

REVIEW QUESTIONS

Choose the correct answer.

1. The woman is having hypotonic labor and is very frustrated because this is her third trip to the birth center. What nursing measure is most appropriate for her?
    a. Do not allow any oral intake.
    b. Initiate oxytocin at a low rate.
    c. Offer her a warm shower or bath.
    d. Reassure her that her problem is common.

2. The woman has shoulder dystocia when giving birth. The nurse should expect:
    a. an immediate forceps delivery.
    b. the application of suprapubic pressure.
    c. oxytocin for labor augmentation.
    d. turning to a hands-and-knees position.

3. While in bed, a good position for the woman laboring with a twin pregnancy is:
   a. supine.
   b. hands and knees.
   c. knee–chest.
   d. side-lying or lateral.

4. Choose the primary nursing measure to promote fetal descent.
   a. Remind the woman to empty her bladder every 1 to 2 hours.
   b. Assist fetal head rotation while performing a vaginal examination.
   c. Have the woman push at least three times with each contraction.
   d. Promote the intake of glucose-containing fluids during labor.

5. An infant weighing 8 pounds 10 ounces is vaginally born. Shoulder dystocia occurred at birth. Because of this problem, the nurse should assess the infant for:
   a. head swelling that does not extend beyond the skull bone.
   b. inward turning of the feet and/or legs.
   c. creaking sensation when the clavicles are palpated.
   d. limited abduction of one or both hips.

6. The woman is fully dilated, and the fetal station is 0. The fetus is in a right occiput posterior position. Choose the optimal maternal position for pushing.
   a. Squatting
   b. Left side-lying
   c. Hands and knees
   d. Semi-sitting

7. The woman is having very rapid labor with her fourth child. What nursing measure is most appropriate to help her manage the pain?
   a. Offer meperidine (Demerol) when she reaches a 5-cm cervical dilation.
   b. Keep her in an upright position until full cervical dilation.
   c. Avoid vaginal examinations during the peak of a contraction.
   d. Coach her to use breathing techniques with each contraction as it occurs.

8. Choose the nursing assessment that most clearly suggests an intrauterine infection.
   a. Fetal heart rate of 145 to 155 bpm
   b. Cloudy amniotic fluid
   c. Maternal temperature of 37.8°C (100°F)
   d. Increased bloody show

9. The woman telephones the labor unit and says she has been having back discomfort all day. She is at 32 weeks of gestation. The nurse should tell the woman that she:
   a. is experiencing discomfort that is typical of a late pregnancy.
   b. should come to the hospital if she has increased vaginal drainage.
   c. can increase her fluid intake to reduce the Braxton Hicks contractions.
   d. should come to the hospital for further evaluation.

10. The woman is receiving magnesium sulfate to stop preterm labor. The essential nursing assessment related to this drug is:
    a. for the frequency and duration of uterine contractions.
    b. hourly vital signs, heart sounds, and lung sounds.
    c. for the presence of fetal movements with contractions.
    d. vaginal examination for cervical dilation, effacement, and station.

11. A few minutes after the woman's membranes rupture during labor, the fetal heart rate decreases from an average of 140 bpm to 75 to 80 bpm. The nurse should immediately:
    a. call the physician via the telephone and report the decreased fetal heart rate.
    b. assess for other signs that indicate chorioamnionitis.
    c. perform a vaginal examination and palpate for a prolapsed cord.
    d. insert an indwelling catheter to keep the bladder empty.

12. The woman telephones the labor unit saying that she has recent onset of pain between her shoulder blades that is worse when she breathes in. The nurse should:
    a. ask her whether she has had a recent upper respiratory infection.
    b. explain that the growing fetus reduces space for breathing.
    c. have her palpate her uterus for frequent contractions.
    d. tell her that she should promptly come to the hospital.

13. Choose the nursing assessment that most clearly suggests hypovolemia.
    a. A urine output of 20 to 25 mL/hr
    b. Fetal heart rate of 155 to 165 bpm
    c. Blood pressure of 108/84 mm Hg
    d. Maternal heart rate of 90 to 100 bpm

28 The Woman with a Postpartum Complication

MATCHING KEY TERMS

Match the term with the correct definition.

1. _____ Atony

2. _____ Embolus

3. _____ Hematoma

4. _____ Hypovolemia

5. _____ Psychosis

6. _____ Thrombus

a. Blood clot within a vessel

b. A clot, usually a thrombus, forced into smaller vessels by the blood circulation

c. Lack of muscle tone

d. Decreased volume of circulating fluid

e. Localized collection of blood

f. Mental state in which a person's ability to recognize reality is impaired

KEY CONCEPTS

1. What is the time difference between an early and late postpartum hemorrhage? What quantity of blood loss constitutes a postpartum hemorrhage?

2. What is the most common cause of an early postpartum hemorrhage? Describe the pathophysiology of this cause of a hemorrhage.

3. How will the nurse recognize uterine atony?

4. What are the correct nursing actions if uterine atony is discovered?

5. What signs typically distinguish a postpartum hemorrhage caused by uterine atony from that caused by lacerations of the birth canal?

6. How do the signs and symptoms of a hematoma differ from those of uterine atony or a bleeding laceration?

7. Describe the body's reaction to hypovolemia and the clinical signs that the nurse might detect.

   a. Compensatory

   b. Failure of compensatory mechanisms

8. What discharge teaching related to a late postpartum hemorrhage is essential?

9. Why are pregnant and postpartum women prone to developing venous thrombosis?

10. Complete the following chart on venous thrombosis. Include the preventive measures.

	Signs and Symptoms	Medical and Nursing Management
Superficial venous thrombosis		
Deep vein thrombosis		

11. What laboratory studies should the nurse expect if the woman is administered heparin anticoagulation or if she is administered warfarin anticoagulation?

12. List the patient teaching related to long-term anticoagulation.

13. What are the signs and symptoms of a pulmonary embolism?

14. Define *puerperal infection.*

15. What anatomic features of the woman's reproductive tract make an infection in this location potentially serious?

16. What changes in uncomplicated childbirth further increase the woman's risk for a reproductive tract infection? What are her protective factors?

17. What is the significance of a distended, painful abdomen in the woman who has endometritis? Are other assessments needed? What action should the nurse take?

18. List the signs and symptoms of a wound infection.

19. What liquids can help acidify urine? Why is this helpful in preventing or treating a urinary tract infection?

20. Why is it important that the breastfeeding mother with mastitis empty her breasts completely?

21. How does septic pelvic thrombophlebitis differ from thrombophlebitis?

22. What is the key difference between postpartum "blues" and postpartum depression?

23. Describe the characteristics of each category of postpartum psychosis.

CRITICAL THINKING EXERCISES

1. During clinical practice, review the charts of postpartum women. List all the factors that put them at a higher risk for infection and the type of infection that would probably occur based on these factors. How should your nursing care change according to their risk for infection and/or the site of the infection?

2. Use the information in Chapter 14 to plan a diet for a breastfeeding woman who had a postpartum hemorrhage without blood replacement.

CASE STUDY

Jana is a gravida 1, para 1, who had a vaginal birth of a 9-pound baby 1.5 hours ago. Her fundus has remained firm, midline, and one fingerbreadth below the umbilicus. She has not yet voided. Her vital signs are stable, and she is afebrile. She received two tablets of hydrocodone with acetaminophen (Vicodin) for perineal pain 30 minutes after the birth. She now requests "something stronger" for the pain because the previous analgesic has been ineffective.

1. What are some possible explanations for the ineffectiveness of the analgesic?

2. Does the nurse need more information? If so, what?

The nurse checks Jana's vital signs 30 minutes later. Her blood pressure is near its previous levels, but her pulse is slightly higher. Her fundal height, firmness, and amount of lochia are unchanged. Her perineum is intact and has a small amount of edema. The nurse replaces the ice pack on the perineum that has been in place since Jana's recovery period began.

3. Are any other interventions warranted? If so, what are they and why are they appropriate?

REVIEW QUESTIONS

Choose the correct answer.

1. The nurse notes that the woman has excess lochia at 2 hours after the vaginal birth of an 8-pound baby. The priority nursing action is to:
   a. catheterize her to check the urine output.
   b. check her blood pressure, pulse, and respiration.
   c. assess the firmness of her uterus.
   d. notify her physician or nurse-midwife.

2. Choose the signs and symptoms that suggest a concealed postpartum hemorrhage.
   a. Rectal pain accompanied by an increasing pulse
   b. Cramping accompanied by a steady trickle of blood
   c. Soft uterine fundus and a decreasing blood pressure
   d. Heavy lochia accompanied by tachypnea and dyspnea

3. One hour after the woman gives birth vaginally, the nurse notes that her fundus is firm, two fingerbreadths above the umbilicus, and deviated to the right. The lochia rubra is moderate. Her perineum is slightly edematous, with no bruising; an ice pack is in place. The priority nursing action is to:
   a. chart the expected assessments.
   b. have the woman empty her bladder in the bathroom.
   c. change the perineal ice pack to a warm pack.
   d. increase the rate of the oxytocin infusion.

4. What drug should be readily available when the woman is receiving heparin therapy?
   a. Vitamin K
   b. Methylergonovine
   c. Ferrous sulfate
   d. Protamine sulfate

5. The nurse's initial response to a suspected pulmonary embolism should be to:
   a. initiate a second intravenous (IV) line of a hypotonic solution.
   b. raise the head of the bed and administer oxygen.
   c. insert a catheter to monitor urine output.
   d. lower the head of the bed and elevate the legs.

6. The woman has an 8-pound 9-ounce baby after an 18-hour labor that required a low-forceps delivery. Her membranes were ruptured for 15 hours. Based on these facts, patient teaching should emphasize:
   a. reporting foul-smelling lochia.
   b. delaying intercourse for at least 6 weeks.
   c. eating a diet that is high in iron.
   d. losing weight over at least a 6-month period.

7. Postpartum teaching related to urinary health should emphasize:
   a. drinking any type of fluid whenever thirsty.
   b. allowing the bladder to fill to promote emptying.
   c. cleansing the perineum in a front-to-back direction.
   d. eating two servings of acidic fruits or vegetables each day.

8. The best position for the woman who has postpartum endometritis is:
   a. left lateral.
   b. Trendelenburg.
   c. supine.
   d. Fowler's.

9. A breastfeeding woman develops mastitis. She tells the nurse that she will just feed her baby formula instead of breastfeeding. The best nursing response is that:
   a. emptying the breast is important to prevent an abscess.
   b. a tight breast binder or bra will help reduce engorgement.
   c. she should continue to drink extra fluids while weaning.
   d. breastfeeding can continue when her temperature is normal.

10. The woman who has a postpartum bipolar psychosis is most likely to demonstrate:
   a. intermittent feelings of letdown or frustration with the baby and her life.
   b. gradual reduction of interest in her surroundings and family.
   c. hyperactivity and poor judgment alternating with tearfulness and guilt.
   d. delusions that her baby is dead or will be kidnapped by a stranger.

29 The High-Risk Newborn: Problems Related to Gestational Age and Development

MATCHING KEY TERMS

Match the term with the correct definition.

1. _____ Bronchopulmonary dysplasia

2. _____ Containment

3. _____ Necrotizing enterocolitis

4. _____ Pulse oximetry

5. _____ Retinopathy of prematurity

a. Damage to blood vessels by oxygen use that may cause blindness

b. Method to determine blood oxygen saturation level

c. Inflammatory condition of the intestines

d. Chronic lung disease

e. Method to increase comfort in infants by tucking

Classify each of these newborn physical characteristics as (a) preterm, (b) term, or (c) postterm. Some letters may be used more than once.

6. _____ Underdeveloped flexor muscles

7. _____ Abundant hair on the head

8. _____ Loose skin

9. _____ Little or no lanugo

10. _____ Poor muscle tone

11. _____ Long fingernails

12. _____ Visible blood vessels on the abdomen

13. _____ Thin body

14. _____ Creases cover the entire sole

15. _____ May have an apprehensive look

16. _____ No subcutaneous fat

17. _____ Dry and peeling skin

18. _____ "Frog-leg" position

19. _____ Meconium staining

20. _____ Abundant vernix caseosa

21. _____ Thick ear cartilage

22. _____ Soft, flexible ears

23. _____ Labia majora covers the clitoris and labia minora

1. Explain the newborn classifications of gestational age and birth weight.

   a. Preterm

   b. Low birth weight

   c. Very low birth weight

   d. Extremely low birth weight

   e. Intrauterine growth restricted

2. Distinguish periodic breathing from apneic spells.

3. Why is the prone position not advised for normal newborns but good for the preterm infant?

4. Why is proper hydration important to maintain a good respiratory status?

5. Describe the four major disadvantages the preterm infant has in regulating temperature.

   a. _____

   b. _____

   c. _____

   d. _____

6. List the common measures used to help the preterm infant maintain thermoregulation.

7. What factors make fluid and electrolyte balance difficult in the preterm infant?

8. Describe the measures used to evaluate the fluid status in the preterm infant.

9. List the signs of dehydration and overhydration.

10. What factors typically increase a preterm infant's risk for an infection?

11. What are the possible reasons why a preterm infant will need intravenous or gavage feedings?

12. List four methods to identify intestinal complications.

a. _____

b. _____

c. _____

d. _____

13. What is the purpose of giving an infant a pacifier when gavage feeding?

14. What advantages do nursing and breast milk have for the preterm infant?

15. What signs suggest the development of respiratory distress syndrome?

16. What are the two complications of oxygen therapy that may be manifested in preterm infants?

a. _____

b. _____

17. What are the two possible consequences for a postterm fetus?

a. _____

b. _____

18. Why is the postterm infant likely to have problems with the following?

a. Hypoglycemia

b. Thermoregulation

c. Hyperbilirubinemia

19. What is the difference between symmetric and asymmetric growth restriction (GR)?

20. What are some possible complications of birth for a large-for-gestational-age (LGA) infant?

CRITICAL THINKING EXERCISES

1. During clinical practice, assess the gestational age of infants you care for and plot their weight, length, and head circumferences on a chart to classify them as a small for gestational age (SGA), appropriate for gestational age (AGA), or LGA. Identify those who have GR and what type of GR exists (symmetric or asymmetric).

2. Note sources of environmental stress in the newborn nursery (for either normal or sick infants). How might these stresses be reduced while supervising the babies?

CASE STUDY

Kaylee was born 2 weeks ago at 30 weeks of gestation. Her mother had placenta previa. Because of continued bleeding along with persistent contractions, a cesarean birth was performed. Kaylee weighed 3 pounds 10 ounces (1642 g) at birth. She had surfactant therapy and mild respiratory distress but did not require mechanical ventilation. She is no longer receiving supplemental oxygen. Her present weight is 3 pounds 7 ounces (1558 g), after a low weight of 3 pounds 4 ounces (1474 g). She is being fed breast milk by a combination of gavage with bottle or breastfeeding.

1. What are the three priority nursing diagnoses likely in this scenario? What factors support the nursing diagnoses?

   a. _____

   b. _____

   c. _____

2. What nursing interventions can help Kaylee's parents feel that she is indeed *their* baby?

REVIEW QUESTIONS

Choose the correct answer.

1. To promote the drainage of lung secretions in the preterm infant, the nurse should:
   a. position the infant in a head-down position.
   b. frequently change the infant's position.
   c. keep the infant in the supine position with the head elevated.
   d. place a small roll under the infant's neck and shoulders.

2. After discharge teaching to the parents of a preterm infant, the nurse recognizes that further teaching is required when the parent states:
   a. "My baby may have problems with breastfeeding."
   b. "Our other children can immediately play with this baby."
   c. "My baby will need to be closely watched for breathing problems."
   d. "My baby will take less care than my other children when they were newborns."

3. The purpose of containment in care of the preterm infant is to:
   a. simulate the enclosed uterine environment when stressful procedures must be performed.
   b. gradually reduce the percentage of supplemental oxygen needed to prevent hypoxia.
   c. recover fluid lost by insensible means and return it to the infant.
   d. limit the formula administered by gavage feedings as the infant starts nipple feeding.

4. Discharge teaching for the parents of an infant with bronchopulmonary dysplasia should emphasize:
   a. that recurrent grunting and retractions are common.
   b. the importance of providing enzyme formula supplements.
   c. careful handling to prevent a pulmonary hemorrhage.
   d. managing equipment for oxygen supplementation.

5. Nursing care that reduces the risk for periventricular or intraventricular hemorrhage includes:
   a. assessing for abnormal heart rhythms or murmurs.
   b. minimal and gentle handling of the infant.
   c. limiting the duration of parental visits.
   d. examining the eyes at 4 weeks and 8 weeks.

6. What intervention should be expected for the late preterm infant during the first 24 hours after birth?
   a. Blood glucose determinations
   b. Placement under phototherapy
   c. Surfactant replacement
   d. Blood transfusions

7. The mother of a preterm infant weighing 1200 g is worried because her baby does not seem to respond to her. The nurse's best response is that:
   a. she should stroke her baby as well as talk to him.
   b. infants this young cannot sense the presence of others.
   c. her baby is too immature to tolerate too much stimulation.
   d. the baby will respond to her better just before feeding.

30   The High-Risk Newborn: Acquired and Congenital Conditions

MATCHING KEY TERMS

Match the term with the correct definition.

1. _____ Asphyxia

2. _____ Bilirubin encephalopathy

3. _____ Neonatal abstinence syndrome

4. _____ Persistent pulmonary hypertension

5. _____ Transient tachypnea of the newborn

a. Brain damage that results from bilirubin toxicity

b. Vasoconstriction of the infant's pulmonary vessels after birth

c. Insufficient oxygen and excess carbon dioxide in the blood

d. Condition of rapid respiration caused by inadequate absorption of the fetal lung fluid

e. Signs exhibited by the newborn exposed *in utero* to maternal substance abuse

KEY CONCEPTS

1. What is the difference between primary and secondary apnea? Which is more ominous? Why?

2. Compare these newborn respiratory complications.

	Transient Tachypnea of the Newborn	Meconium Aspiration Syndrome	Persistent Pulmonary Hypertension
Cause(s)			
Manifestations			
Therapeutic management			
Nursing considerations			

3. What is the relationship among bilirubin, jaundice, kernicterus, and bilirubin encephalopathy?

4. Why is phototherapy initiated at lower bilirubin levels if the infant is preterm rather than full-term?

5. Formulate a simple explanation about phototherapy to provide to the parents of a jaundiced newborn. Include in your explanation why the treatment is needed, how it works, and what precautions are needed to prevent injury.

6. What is the purpose of an exchange transfusion?

7. Determine which neonatal infection(s) each of these statements refers to (see Table 30-1, Common Infections in the Newborn).

   a. Infection is preventable through immunization.

   b. This is typically manifested by white patches in the mouth that resemble milk curds.

   c. Intellectual disability is associated with the infection.

   d. Antibiotics may be administered to high-risk mothers in labor or to an infant after birth.

   e. Antibiotic prophylaxis administered soon after birth can prevent blindness.

   f. Maternal antiviral treatment during pregnancy can reduce transmission to the infant.

8. List the factors that make newborns more vulnerable to sepsis neonatorum.

9. Compare early and late-onset sepsis.

10. How does the newborn manifest an infection compared with an older child? Why is it particularly important to identify newborn sepsis early?

11. Why are tests for drug levels often needed for antibiotics?

12. How can diabetes cause both intrauterine growth restriction and large-for-gestational-age infants?

13. Explain these complications that may occur in the infant of a diabetic mother.

    a. Respiratory distress syndrome

    b. Hypoglycemia

    c. Hypocalcemia

    d. Polycythemia

14. Describe the typical appearance of a macrosomic infant of a diabetic mother (IDM).

15. List signs of neonatal hypoglycemia.

16. Why does the IDM with polycythemia require adequate hydration?

17. List infant behaviors that should cause a nurse to suspect prenatal drug exposure.

18. Why are gavage feedings sometimes required for a drug-exposed infant, even if born at term?

19. Early screening and treatment for phenylketonuria (PKU) are necessary to prevent _____.

CRITICAL THINKING EXERCISES

1. Imagine that you are the nurse caring for an infant who requires resuscitation at birth. List the things you would want to have readily available. Write out your actions and what you think the actions of other team members will be from the time the infant is brought to the warmer until he or she is adequately breathing.

2. How might the actions in the previous scenario change if there were thick meconium in the amniotic fluid?

3. Compare an IDM with other newborns. What similarities and differences do you note? Can any of these be explained by how well the woman's diabetes was controlled during pregnancy?

4. Observe the reception that a mother of an infant exposed to drugs prenatally receives when she visits the nursery. Are the nurses' reactions positive or negative? If they are not positive, what nursing actions might better benefit the mother?

CASE STUDY

Steven is 12 hours old. He was vaginally born with forceps following a 16-hour labor. He has bilateral cephalhematomas. His mother is Rh negative, while Steven is Rh positive. His bilirubin level was 7.5, and his Coombs test was positive on a cord blood sample.

1. Which information in the previous scenario indicates a pathologic condition?

2. What other assessments should be performed?

Twenty-four hours after birth, Steven's bilirubin level is 13.5 and his skin is jaundiced.

3. What treatment does Steven require at this time? How does the treatment affect his bilirubin level?

4. Identify the required nursing interventions for Steven once treatment for jaundice has begun.

5. What are the possible side effects of this treatment?

Steven's bilirubin level continues to increase and becomes dangerously high.

6. What complication can occur with dangerously high bilirubin levels?

7. What treatment should Steven receive at this time to lower his bilirubin levels?

8. What blood type should be used for Steven's treatment and why?

9. How is an exchange transfusion performed?

10. What are the expected results of the transfusion?

11. What are some possible complications of an exchange transfusion?

12. What is the nurse's role in an exchange transfusion?

REVIEW QUESTIONS

Choose the correct answer.

1. Naloxone for neonatal use is supplied in 1 mg/mL vials. The correct volume of naloxone for a neonate weighing 5 pounds 2 ounces is approximately:
   a. 0.1 mL
   b. 0.2 mL
   c. 0.3 mL
   d. 0.4 mL

2. If meconium is present in the amniotic fluid, the infant's mouth and pharynx should be suctioned after the head is born but before the rest of the body. The primary reason for this action is to:
   a. limit the transfer of infectious substances to the lower airways.
   b. reduce the likelihood that secondary apnea will occur.
   c. prevent the persistence of abnormal cardiac shunts.
   d. avoid drawing meconium into the lower airways with the first breath.

3. Infants receiving phototherapy should be fed every 2 to 3 hours to:
   a. promote the excretion of bilirubin from the bowel.
   b. prevent the development of hypothermia.
   c. increase the life span of fetal erythrocytes in the blood.
   d. increase renal and liver perfusions.

4. The nurse notes that a 24-hour-old infant is lethargic and her temperature is below normal, a change from an earlier assessment that was normal. Her mother states that she did not breastfeed well and that the infant spit up the small amount she had ingested. The nurse's next action should be to:
   a. reassure the mother that infants are often sluggish this soon after birth.
   b. feed the infant formula to accurately determine how much intake she is getting.
   c. determine whether there is jaundice over the thoracic and abdominal areas.
   d. assess for signs of sepsis and report these assessments to the physician.

Chapter **30** The High-Risk Newborn: Acquired and Congenital Conditions

5. A mother who has diabetes is concerned because her 36-hour-old baby is "so yellow." She tells the nurse that she thought her baby's problems were over when his blood glucose stabilized, although he was smaller than expected. The best nursing response is that:
   a. her baby's liver is also less mature than expected and cannot handle normal red blood cell breakdown.
   b. her baby lived in a lower-than-normal oxygen environment during pregnancy and must eliminate more red blood cells.
   c. the baby's high blood glucose levels immediately after birth caused a slight dehydration that increases jaundice.
   d. early feedings slowed the elimination of meconium that would have also eliminated excess bilirubin.

6. The nurse notes that a 12-hour-old infant is jittery, but his blood glucose level is normal. The infant appears hungry but takes only ¼ ounce of formula with difficulty. The nurse's next action should be to:
   a. recheck the glucose levels at 30 minutes after the feeding.
   b. apply a bag to collect the next sample of urine.
   c. limit infant contact with the mother for the next 12 hours.
   d. swaddle the infant tightly and try to feed more formula.

7. Choose the caregiver teaching that is most appropriate for the infant who was prenatally exposed to cocaine.
   a. Breastfeeding is especially important to the infant's recovery from prenatal drug exposure.
   b. Align the infant's face with yours to allow prolonged eye contact that better facilitates bonding.
   c. Do not burp your baby until at least 1 ounce of formula has been taken.
   d. Swaddle your baby with arms and legs flexed to reduce startling.

31 | Management of Fertility and Infertility

HELPFUL HINT

HELPFUL HINT

A fundamentals-of-nursing textbook can provide additional information on many of the topics covered in the chapter as they relate to the nursing profession.

MATCHING KEY TERMS

Match the term with the correct definition.

1. _____ Basal body temperature
2. _____ Endometriosis
3. _____ Gestational surrogate
4. _____ Infertility
5. _____ Oligospermia
6. _____ Spermicide
7. _____ Tubal ligation

a. A chemical that kills sperm
b. Cutting the fallopian tubes to prevent fertilization
c. Growth of the uterine lining tissue outside the uterine cavity
d. Body temperature at rest
e. Inability to conceive after 1 year
f. A woman who carries the embryo of an infertile couple and relinquishes the child
g. Decreased number of sperm in the semen

KEY CONCEPTS

1. Why is the typical or actual failure rate of a contraceptive more useful than the theoretical failure rate?

2. What are the major side effects of Depo-Provera?

3. When may a perimenopausal woman discontinue contraception?

4. Why should a man have his semen analyzed following a vasectomy?

5. How do hormone injections prevent pregnancy?

6. How do estrogen–progestin oral contraceptives prevent conception?

7. How do progestin-only oral contraceptives prevent conception?

8. What teaching is appropriate in each area related to oral contraceptive use?

   a. Back-up contraception

   b. Time of day

   c. Possible pregnancy

   d. Use during lactation

   e. Other medications

9. What annual examinations should the woman have if she takes oral contraceptives?

10. List some types of emergency contraception.

11. Why should women using an intrauterine device (IUD) be in a mutually monogamous relationship?

12. What teaching is important related to IUD use?

13. What are the two main advantages of barrier methods of contraception?

14. Why is the use of a spermicide with condoms advisable?

15. What should the woman who uses spermicides be taught about douching?

16. Why is it essential to help the man or woman understand the difference between natural membrane condoms and latex condoms?

17. What are the major problems associated with the female condom?

18. At what times should the woman who uses a diaphragm for contraception have the fit checked?

19. What is the major problem associated with using natural family planning methods?

20. Complete the following table to describe the advantages and disadvantages of each contraceptive method.

Contraceptive Methods	Advantages	Disadvantages
Sterilization		
Hormone injection		
Oral contraception		
Intrauterine device		
Chemical barriers		
Male condom		
Female condom		
Diaphragm		
Natural family planning		

169

21. List the factors that may impair the ability of sperm to fertilize the ovum.

22. List the factors that may impair normal erections.

23. List the causes of abnormal ejaculation.

24. List the factors that may impair the function of seminal fluid.

25. List the factors that may disrupt the hormonal secretions a woman requires to achieve pregnancy.

26. List the factors that may impair normal ovulation.

27. List the factors that may impair the structure and function of the fallopian tubes.

28. List the factors that may obstruct or impair the function of the woman's cervix.

29. List the factors that may be associated with repeated pregnancy loss.

30. Describe the nursing care associated with each of the more common diagnostic tests for infertility.
    a. Semen analysis

    b. Postcoital test

    c. Hysterosalpingogram

31. Describe two complications associated with medications that are administered to induce ovulation.

a. _____

b. _____

32. What are some reasons for choosing therapeutic insemination?

33. What precautions decrease the risk that a man will transmit an infection or genetic disorders when he donates his sperm?

34. Complete the following table comparing *in vitro* fertilization (IVF), gamete intrafallopian transfer (GIFT), and tubal embryo transfer (TET).

Procedure	Description	Advantages	Disadvantages
IVF			
GIFT			
TET			

CRITICAL THINKING EXERCISES

1. Have you known adolescents who have some of the erroneous beliefs discussed in your textbook? Did you have any of these beliefs when you were an adolescent? How might you use age-appropriate counseling to correct the misinformation listed? How would you address the issue of confidentiality?

2. Practice how you might tactfully introduce the subject of contraception to an adolescent, a postpartum woman, and a woman in her mid-40s.

3. You are asked for contraceptive information by a 16-year-old girl, a 28-year-old woman with three children, and a 45-year-old woman with one child. If you could ask only two questions of each woman to help find the best method for her, what questions would be most important? If you had to choose only two types of contraception to offer each, what would they be?

a. 16-year-old

b. 28-year-old

c. 45-year-old

4. If you could design the perfect contraceptive method, what qualities would it have? Who would use it? How would it be obtained?

5. Oral contraceptives are available without prescription in many countries and may be available over-the-counter in the United States in the near future. What are the advantages and disadvantages of this?

6. What is your opinion about monetary compensation for a woman who is a surrogate mother and contributes her ovum to the child? What if she is a gestational surrogate and carries the fetus to term but does not contribute a gamete?

7. Should compensation be different for male sperm donors and females who donate their ovum and carry the fetus? Why?

8. What are your feelings regarding the use of blastomere analysis to identify genetic defects before the implantation of an embryo that results from an assisted reproductive technology procedure? Should an embryo that has an identified defect be implanted? If it is discarded, do you view it as abortion?

9. Should health insurance cover all infertility diagnostic studies and therapy? If not, which ones should not be covered?

10. Should public assistance funds, such as Medicaid, cover infertility therapy? Why or why not?

REVIEW QUESTIONS

Choose the correct answer.

1. A woman is considering having a tubal ligation after she gives birth to her second child. The nurse should counsel her that:
   a. she should wait until several months after birth to be certain that the infant is healthy.
   b. the procedure should be considered permanent and irreversible.
   c. sterilization is an easier procedure to perform after the postpartum period.
   d. she must provide signed informed consent by the sixth month of pregnancy.

2. Postprocedural teaching for a man who has had a vasectomy should include the discussion that:
   a. urinating may be difficult for several times after the procedure.
   b. a catheterized urine specimen should be obtained in 1 week.
   c. testosterone levels may fluctuate for the first few months.
   d. another form of contraception should be used until the semen is free of sperm.

3. Which woman would be a good candidate for hormone contraception?
   a. A 30-year-old woman who thinks she has completed her family
   b. A 22-year-old breastfeeding woman who just gave birth
   c. A 29-year-old woman who has type 2 diabetes secondary to obesity
   d. A 25-year-old woman who takes an anticonvulsant

4. A woman decides to change from the diaphragm to Depo-Provera. Her last menstrual period ended 1 week ago. She should be taught that she should:
   a. take the oral contraceptive during this cycle only.
   b. return in 1 week to have the hormone injection.
   c. continue to use the diaphragm for the rest of her cycle.
   d. expect heavier periods than she had when using the diaphragm.

5. How should a woman take oral contraceptives?
   a. On an empty stomach, with a full glass of water
   b. At approximately the same time each day
   c. Before every episode of intercourse
   d. In the morning and at bedtime

6. Choose the safety teaching related to oral contraceptives.
   a. A barrier method should also be used to protect from infection.
   b. Nausea suggests that stroke is imminent.
   c. Toxic shock syndrome is more likely to occur when the pill is used.
   d. Increase fluids if urinary frequency or urgency occurs.

7. The IUD is an appropriate contraceptive for the woman who:
   a. has unplanned intercourse with several partners.
   b. was recently hospitalized for the treatment of a pelvic infection.
   c. is in a mutually monogamous relationship.
   d. has had two ectopic pregnancies.

8. If the IUD strings are longer than usual, the woman should:
   a. know that this is expected when the IUD is first inserted.
   b. immediately have a Pap smear to rule out cervical cancer.
   c. take her temperature twice a day for 1 week.
   d. visit her physician and use another method of contraception.

9. The major advantage of using a condom for contraception is that it:
   a. requires a visit to the health care provider yearly.
   b. reduces transmission of infections.
   c. can be placed several hours before intercourse.
   d. may be incorporated as a part of foreplay.

10. When teaching a woman fertility awareness, the nurse should emphasize that the basal body temperature:
    a. is the average temperature taken each morning.
    b. should be recorded each morning before any activity.
    c. has a higher degree of accuracy in predicting ovulation than the cervical mucus test.
    d. can be taken with a mercury thermometer but not a digital one.

11. At ovulation, the basal body temperature usually:
    a. abruptly increases and then decreases after 1 or 2 days.
    b. decreases and remains low for the last half of the cycle.
    c. is higher during the first half of the cycle than in the latter half.
    d. slightly decreases at ovulation and is higher during the last half of the cycle.

12. Cervical mucus at ovulation should be:
    a. clear, thin, and slippery and should stretch to at least 6 cm.
    b. cloudy, with a mild odor, and should stretch to at least 6 cm.
    c. thick, clear, and of a large quantity.
    d. thin and tinged with a small amount of blood.

13. Choose the correct instructions for a man who must provide a semen sample.
    a. After collecting the sample in a condom, refrigerate it until it is transported to the laboratory.
    b. Masturbation is the only way a good sample can be obtained.
    c. Keep the sample near the body, and transport it to the laboratory within 1 hour.
    d. Do not take any regularly scheduled drugs for 3 days before obtaining the sample.

14. A woman who is taking clomiphene citrate (Clomid) calls the infertility clinic and says that she has some nausea each morning and frequency of urination. She suspects that she may be pregnant. The correct nursing response is to:
    a. tell her that pregnancy cannot be determined until she misses her next period.
    b. have her promptly come to the clinic for a sensitive pregnancy test.
    c. have her continue taking the drug until she completes this cycle and then have a pregnancy test.
    d. reassure her that her symptoms are commonly seen in women who take this drug.

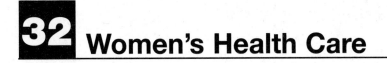

32 Women's Health Care

MATCHING KEY TERMS

Match the term with the correct definition.

1. _____ Climacteric
2. _____ Condyloma
3. _____ Dysmenorrhea
4. _____ Dyspareunia
5. _____ Dysplasia
6. _____ Menarche

a. Wart-like growth on genitalia
b. Painful menstruation
c. Onset of menstruation
d. Abnormal tissue development
e. Painful intercourse in women
f. Menopause

KEY CONCEPTS

1. What are the three major preventable problems in women?

   a. _____

   b. _____

   c. _____

2. When should a breast self-examination be performed?

3. What are the current recommendations for screening mammography?

4. What is the recommendation for a vulvar self-examination?

5. What preparation should a woman make for a pelvic examination with Pap test?

6. Describe the signs, symptoms, and treatment for each benign breast disorder.

   a. Fibroadenoma

   b. Fibrocystic breast changes

   c. Ductal ectasia

   d. Intraductal papilloma

7. Describe the major management methods for breast cancer.

8. Define each type of amenorrhea and state common causes for each.

   a. Primary

   b. Secondary

9. List the common causes of abnormal uterine bleeding.

10. What is the nurse's role when caring for women who have abnormal uterine bleeding?

11. What treatment is typical for each type of menstrual cycle pain?

    a. Mittelschmerz

    b. Primary dysmenorrhea

    c. Endometriosis

12. What nursing measures are appropriate when a woman has premenstrual syndrome (PMS)?

13. Explain the purpose for each technique that may be used in elective termination of a pregnancy and state any side or adverse effects, if applicable.

	Purpose	Side/Adverse Effects
Mifepristone		
Dilation and aspiration with curettage		
Laminaria		
Prostaglandin E_2		

14. Why should a woman promptly report unexpected uterine bleeding after menopause?

15. What is the purpose of giving estrogen with progestin to relieve the symptoms of menopause?

16. List the risks of estrogen–progesterone replacement therapy.

17. What signs occur when a woman has osteoporosis?

18. What screening tests may be used to identify female reproductive tract cancers early?

19. Complete the following table on sexually transmitted diseases as you read your text.

	Signs and Symptoms	Treatment	Teaching
Candidiasis			
Trichomoniasis			
Bacterial vaginosis			

177

Chlamydia			
Gonorrhea			
Syphilis			
Herpes genitalis			
Condylomata acuminata			
AIDS			

20. How does pelvic inflammatory disease occur? What are the symptoms?

CRITICAL THINKING EXERCISES

1. Talk with a woman who has had breast cancer about her feelings upon learning the diagnosis and during the wait between diagnosis and treatment.

2. When caring for people who have experienced age-related fractures, such as a hip fracture, note how many of them are older and female. Do you note any other adverse effects of osteoporosis?

REVIEW QUESTIONS

Choose the correct answer.

1. A breast self-examination should be performed using the:
   a. palm of the left hand to palpate the right breast in a wedge pattern.
   b. horizontal pattern to palpate across both breasts at one pass.
   c. middle three fingertips of the left hand to palpate the right breast.
   d. thumb of the opposite hand to palpate each breast in a circular pattern.

2. Your friend calls to tell you that she noticed a small amount of nipple retraction in her right nipple when she was showering. As a nurse, you should advise her to:
   a. perform a complete breast self-examination to determine if any lumps are present.
   b. wait until 1 week after her next menstrual period and then perform a breast self-examination.
   c. note whether there is any change in the amount of nipple retraction for 2 weeks.
   d. see her primary health care provider for a professional examination.

3. A woman will have screening for fecal occult blood. Choose the correct instructions.
   a. Do not take nonsteroidal anti-inflammatory drugs for 48 hours before collecting the sample.
   b. Eat two servings of red meat each day for 3 days before obtaining the specimen.
   c. Collect a small sample of stool from the first stool expelled each morning for 3 days.
   d. Refrigerate the samples until they can be returned to the laboratory for testing.

4. Preoperative nursing care for the woman anticipating a modified radical mastectomy for breast cancer includes preparation for:
   a. restricted arm movement on the operative side for 2 weeks after surgery.
   b. a small dressing applied to the operative site.
   c. drainage tubes that will remove fluid that accumulates under the operative area.
   d. a hospital stay of 3 to 4 days.

5. To relieve her menstrual cramps, a woman should be taught to take ibuprofen:
   a. within 8 hours of the onset of menstruation.
   b. before onset of menstruation and cramps.
   c. every 4 hours during the 2 days preceding menstruation.
   d. on an empty stomach before the pain becomes severe.

6. Your friend is having hot flashes as she enters menopause. She is interested in hormone replacement to improve these symptoms but is fearful of breast cancer. As a nurse, you should tell her that:
   a. her physician or nurse practitioner can evaluate her actual risk and help her make a better decision.
   b. the risk for breast cancer is very small for women who are younger than 60 years when menstrual periods stop.
   c. taking the estrogen with progestin will reduce the risk for estrogen-induced breast cancer.
   d. the benefits of estrogen replacement therapy far outweigh any risks associated with it.

7. A woman who has age-associated urinary incontinence should be taught to:
   a. avoid alcohol and caffeinated drinks.
   b. reduce fluid intake before special events.
   c. limit ingestion of foods that acidify urine.
   d. urinate at least every 2 hours while awake.

8. To reduce the risk for toxic shock syndrome, women should be taught to:
   a. avoid changing tampons until they are thoroughly saturated.
   b. use a diaphragm with spermicidal jelly during the menstrual period.
   c. wash hands thoroughly before inserting a tampon or diaphragm into the vagina.
   d. limit the use of superabsorbent tampons to the times when flow is heavy.

33 Physical Assessment of Children

HELPFUL HINT

Review the physical assessment of the infant and child in a nursing health assessment textbook.

MATCHING KEY TERMS

Match the term with the correct definition.

1. _____ Auscultation

2. _____ Circumduction

3. _____ Crepitation

4. _____ Development

5. _____ Fasciculation

6. _____ Fremitus

7. _____ Growth

8. _____ History

9. _____ Inspection

10. _____ Obtund

11. _____ Palpation

12. _____ Percussion

13. _____ Systematic assessment

a. Vibration perceptible on palpation or auscultation

b. Organized method of collecting data

c. Use of touch to determine temperature, moisture, and organ placement

d. Circular movement of a limb or an eye

e. Aggregate of subjective data that describes the past and present health status

f. Tapping of the body to determine density, location, and size of organs

g. Elicitation and evaluation of sounds produced by the body

h. Observations to identify physical findings

i. Dry, crackling sound or sensation

j. Small, local, involuntary muscle contraction visible under the skin

k. To render dull or blunt

l. Change that occurs over time in functional, psychosocial, and cognitive behavior

m. Measurable physical and physiologic changes that occur over time

GENERAL APPROACHES TO PHYSICAL ASSESSMENT

Answer as either true (T) or false (F).

1. _____ It is appropriate to auscultate the heart, lungs, and abdomen while an infant is sleeping.

2. _____ Stranger anxiety makes the physical examination of an older infant more difficult.

3. _____ Parents should not be present during a young child's physical examination.

4. _____ In all age groups, uncomfortable procedures should be saved until the end of the examination.

5. _____ Adolescents should be allowed to participate in deciding who will be present during the physical examination.

6. _____ For adolescents, the physical examination proceeds from head to toe.

TECHNIQUES FOR PHYSICAL EXAMINATION

Fill in the blanks.

1. Using an ophthalmoscope is an example of _____ inspection.

2. In palpating the lymph nodes for general assessment, the nurse uses the _____.

3. In palpating the lymph nodes specifically for heat, the nurse uses the _____.

4. When percussing the liver, the nurse would expect to hear _____ sounds.

5. The _____ of the stethoscope is most effective in auscultating low-pitched sounds.

Match each type of history with its description.

6. _____ Complete history

7. _____ Episodic history

8. _____ Well-interim history

a. Information about a specific problem is added to an existing database.

b. Information about a child from conception to the present

c. Information gathered from last well visit to current visit

Answer as either true (T) or false (F).

9. _____ Axillary temperatures are preferable to rectal temperatures because they are less invasive.

10. _____ The apical impulse is palpated to determine the position of the heart.

11. _____ All irregular heart rhythms in children require immediate attention.

12. _____ The respiratory rate in infants can be counted by observing the movement of the abdomen.

13. _____ An adolescent with a blood pressure of 120/80 mm Hg is considered to be pre-hypertensive.

14. Give two ways of measuring the length of an infant.

   a. _____

   b. _____

15. Why is the head circumference measured at every visit until the child is 3 years old?

Fill in the blanks.

16. All scales must be _____ before use.

17. Chest circumference is measured at the _____.

18. Midarm circumference is a measure of _____ and _____.

19. An adolescent who is 62 inches tall and weighs 120.5 lb has a body mass index (BMI) of:

   _____.

20. To complete a growth chart on a child's height, the nurse should do the following:

   a. Use a chart appropriate for the child's _____ and _____.

   b. Find the child's age on the _____ axis.

   c. Find the child's height on the _____ axis.

   d. Mark the location of the two lines. _____

   e. Note the _____.

21. Increased thickness and pigmentation of the skin on the posterior neck, on the armpits, and behind the knees and elbows can indicate that a child might have: _____.

22. On a child, the nurse assesses skin turgor on the _____ or _____.

23. Unusual hair loss is called _____; excessive hair growth is called _____.

24. When a child has head lice, nits are found on the _____.

25. Capillary refill should be within _____ seconds.

26. When assessing a child's face, the nurse examines the cranial nerves _____ and _____.

27. Frequent wiping of the nose indicates that the child probably has _____.

28. The philtrum is the _____.

29. How does the nurse examine cranial nerve XII (hypoglossal nerve)? _____

30. When eliciting the gag reflex with a tongue blade, the nurse is evaluating cranial nerve _____.

Match each test or chart with its description.

31. _____ Lea chart

32. _____ Sweep test

33. _____ Ishihara cards

34. _____ Weber test

35. _____ Snellen chart

36. _____ Pure tone test

a. Tests ability to hear via bone conduction

b. Tests visual acuity in a 30-month-old child

c. Test used to determine the extent of hearing loss

d. Tests color vision

e. Tests for hearing loss

f. Tests visual acuity in a 12-year-old child

Answer as either true (T) or false (F).

37. _____ Breathing is more diaphragmatic in a school-age child than in a toddler.

38. _____ Before auscultation of breath sounds, have a toddler sit upright on the parent's lap.

39. _____ Normal breath sounds are called adventitious.

40. _____ The apical pulse is also called the point of maximal impulse (PMI).

41. _____ Auscultation of the heart is best done by listening with the bell of the stethoscope only.

42. _____ A pause between the closing of the pulmonic and aortic valves is a normal finding in children.

43. _____ Functional heart murmurs require immediate intervention.

44. When should adolescent females start performing monthly breast self-examinations?

45. To ascertain the absence of bowel sounds, the nurse listens to the area for up to _____ minutes.

46. Describe how to test for rebound tenderness.

47. How can the nurse decrease adolescent anxiety during a genital examination?

48. Why are adolescent males taught to do monthly testicular examinations?

Match each term with its description.

49. _____ Lordosis   a. Performed until the child is 1 year old

50. _____ Ortolani maneuver   b. Common in young children

51. _____ Genu varum   c. Related to poor posture

52. _____ Scoliosis   d. Bowleg

53. _____ Kyphosis   e. Lateral non-painful curvature of the spine

Answer as either true (T) or false (F).

54. _____ To evaluate neurologic functioning in a child younger than 5 years, use the Denver Developmental Screening Test II (DDST-II).

55. _____ The nurse should test all of the cranial nerves at the beginning of the physical examination.

56. _____ *Obtunded* is a term used to describe one of the altered levels of consciousness.

57. _____ As part of the neurologic examination, it is important to assess a toddler's orientation to person, place, and time.

58. _____ Depression may alter a child's ability to solve problems.

59. _____ Assessing a child's ability to balance evaluates cerebellar function.

60. _____ Responses to eliciting the Babinski reflex depend on the child's ability to walk.

61. _____ Neurologic "soft" signs are normal variants and require no further assessment.

STUDENT LEARNING ACTIVITY

1. Perform a complete history and physical assessment on an infant, a child, and an adolescent. Describe your findings clearly and coherently in writing.

STUDENT LEARNING APPLICATIONS

Enhance your learning by discussing your answers with other students.

During a physical assessment on an infant, child, or adolescent, many variables can alter either the process or the findings. Describe how you would handle a physical assessment in each of the following situations.

1. A toddler's parents are not present during the examination.

2. A school-age child's level of cognitive functioning is far below average.

3. An adolescent is experiencing moderately severe abdominal pain.

4. A 9-month-old infant is exhibiting a high degree of stranger anxiety.

5. A preschooler believes that undergoing the physical examination is punishment for being bad.

REVIEW QUESTIONS

Choose the correct answer.

1. A 1-year-old child is at the pediatrician's office for a well-interim visit. When interviewing the parents, the nurse should:
   a. obtain a complete history from conception to the present.
   b. record information about the child's chief complaint.
   c. obtain a family history.
   d. gather data about what has occurred since the last visit.

2. Before auscultating a toddler's lungs, the nurse should:
   a. examine the child's ears and throat.
   b. ask the parent(s) to leave the room.
   c. allow the child to examine the stethoscope.
   d. do none of the above.

3. The nurse begins auscultation of the abdomen in the:
   a. RUQ.
   b. RLQ.
   c. LUQ.
   d. LLQ.

4. Which is an abnormal finding?
   a. Posterior fontanel is flat and soft in an 8-month-old infant.
   b. A 7-month-old sits using hands for support.
   c. Breathing is abdominal in a 3-month-old child.
   d. A 5-year-old's pupils dilate when focusing on a distant object.

5. Which is a normal finding in a school-age child?
   a. Bone conduction is greater than air conduction.
   b. Cerumen is found in the external auditory meatus.
   c. Discharge is present in the ear canal.
   d. The tympanic membrane is stationary.

6. An assessment technique of the chest and lungs normally reserved for the advanced nursing practitioner is:
   a. inspection.
   b. auscultation.
   c. palpation.
   d. percussion.

7. The PMI is located at the fifth intercostal space in the midclavicular line after approximately age:
   a. 2 months.
   b. 18 months.
   c. 4 years.
   d. 7 years.

8. An example of a "soft" neurologic sign is:
   a. a short attention span.
   b. left handedness.
   c. non-mirroring movement of the extremities.
   d. none of the above.

9. Which sound occurs when parts of the lungs lose their lubricating fluid?
   a. High-pitched wheezing
   b. Pleural friction rub
   c. Rales
   d. Sonorous rhonchi

10. Which reflex is elicited by suddenly and briskly dorsiflexing the child's foot and applying moderate pressure?
    a. Clonus
    b. Babinski
    c. Cremasteric
    d. Patellar

34 Emergency Care of the Child

HELPFUL HINT

Review the anatomy and physiology of the cardiac and respiratory systems.

MATCHING KEY TERMS

Match the term with the correct definition.

1. _____ ABCDEs

2. _____ Cardiopulmonary resuscitation (CPR)

3. _____ Dental emergency

4. _____ Envenomation

5. _____ Extracorporeal membrane oxygenation

6. _____ Hypothermia

7. _____ Ingestion

8. _____ Shock

9. _____ Submersion injury

10. _____ Trauma

11. _____ Trauma score

12. _____ Traumatic brain injury

13. _____ Triage

a. Injury from an external cause

b. Protocol performed when an individual's respiratory and cardiovascular systems require support to maintain vital functions

c. Temporary method of providing cardiovascular, respiratory, and circulatory support for children for whom other methods of treatment are not effective

d. Cooling of the body temperature to subnormal levels

e. Injury or infection of a tooth in which prompt medical attention is critical for the survival of the tooth or to alleviate pain

f. Swallowing of a potentially toxic substance

g. Sorting process used to decide the urgency of an individual's illness or injury and to allocate appropriate resources effectively

h. Injuries resulting from a near-drowning incident

i. Injection of venom by an animal

j. Critical components of the primary assessment of a critically ill or injured child: airway, breathing, circulation, disability, and exposure

k. Numeric score assessed by health care providers to determine the extent of the trauma

l. A leading cause of death or permanent disability

m. Inadequate tissue perfusion that results in cardiovascular or respiratory compromise

Chapter 34 Emergency Care of the Child

Copyright © 2018, Elsevier Inc. All rights reserved.

GENERAL GUIDELINES FOR EMERGENCY NURSING CARE

1. List five interventions that can facilitate a more positive and comfortable emergency experience for a child and family.

    a. _____

    b. _____

    c. _____

    d. _____

    e. _____

2. List three strategies that the nurse could use when dealing with a family experiencing great emotional distress because they have been told that their child's injuries are life-threatening.

    a. _____

    b. _____

    c. _____

Match each medication with its use in pediatric emergency care.

3. _____ Activated charcoal   a. Reverses the effects of some narcotics

4. _____ Atropine sulfate   b. Treats symptomatic bradycardia

5. _____ Amiodarone   c. Treats bradycardia or asystolic arrest

6. _____ Dextrose   d. Treats ventricular tachycardia

7. _____ Epinephrine   e. Treats severe acidosis

8. _____ Naloxone hydrochloride   f. Reduces drug absorption in toxic ingestions

9. _____ Sodium bicarbonate   g. Treats hypoglycemia

GROWTH AND DEVELOPMENT ISSUES IN EMERGENCY CARE

Match each age group with the appropriate nursing interventions.

1. Infant   a. Ascertain the child's level of understanding and allow time for questions.

2. Toddler   b. Allow the child to have familiar objects to help him or her feel safe.

3. Preschooler   c. Use a soothing voice and touch, rock, or cuddle the child.

4. School-age child   d. Carefully explain the procedures and allow choices.

5. Adolescent   e. Talk to the child throughout the procedure explaining how he or she can help.

The Family of a Child in Emergency Care

Fill in the blanks.

1. _____ and _____ are the two most common emotions experienced by parents of children cared for in emergencies.

2. The underlying cause of the anger that some parents express toward health care providers in the emergency setting is often _____.

Emergency Assessment of Infants and Children

1. Describe the role of the triage nurse.

2. Name three essential factors in an initial pediatric triage assessment.

   a. _____

   b. _____

   c. _____

3. List the components of the *primary assessment*.

   A:

   B:

   C:

   D:

   E:

Answer as either true (T) or false (F).

4. _____ A respiratory rate of more than 60 breaths/min is considered abnormal for a child of any age.

5. _____ Tachycardia and decreased peripheral perfusion are early signs of cardiovascular compromise in a child.

6. _____ Infants and young children have a higher percentage of fluid located in the intracellular compartment.

7. _____ For the first several months of life, the presence of nasal secretions can cause respiratory compromise in infants.

8. _____ Abdominal breathing is an abnormal finding in infants and young children.

9. What are the four components of the *secondary assessment?*

    F:

    G:

    H:

    I:

10. Give the suggested order for measuring vital signs in children.

11. Identify the elements of a **SAMPLE** history.

    S: _____

    A: _____

    M: _____

    P: _____

    L: _____

    E: _____

12. Which laboratory tests are considered standard protocol in an emergency setting?

13. Why is determining the child's weight essential during emergency care?

Cardiopulmonary Resuscitation of the Child

1. What are the two most common causes of cardiopulmonary arrest in children?

2. Ventilations should be given at a rate of _____ or approximately one breath every _____ seconds.

3. What is the emergency intervention for an obstructed airway in a conscious child?

4. What is the emergency intervention for an obstructed airway in an unconscious child?

5. What is the rationale for *not* performing blind finger sweeps for infants and children?

6. What is the emergency intervention for removal of a foreign object from an infant?

7. Before and during cardiac compressions, the nurse feels for a pulse in the infant at the _____;

   for a child older than 1 year, at the _____.

8. According to the American Heart Association, chest compressions are performed at a rate of

   _____.

9. In the community setting, an automatic external defibrillator (AED) should be used on a child who has had a cardiac arrest after _____ cycles of CPR have been performed.

THE CHILD IN SHOCK

Indicate whether each statement refers to hypovolemic (H), cardiogenic (C), or distributive (D) shock.

1. _____ This is the most common type of shock seen in children.

2. _____ This occurs when a myocardial function is unable to produce cardiac output that meets the metabolic demands of the body.

3. _____ This occurs when microbial toxins are in the bloodstream.

4. _____ Early signs include warm extremities and purpuric skin lesions.

5. _____ Diuretics are often prescribed when there is an excess of increased intravascular volume.

6. _____ Periorbital edema, crackles, and diaphoresis are clinical manifestations.

7. _____ Initial treatment involves administration of normal saline or Ringer's lactate solution.

Answer as either true (T) or false (F).

8. _____ Hypotension is an early sign of shock in children.

9. _____ Septic shock is the most common cause of hypovolemic shock.

10. _____ Early signs of cardiogenic shock include hypothermia or hyperthermia.

11. _____ Dopamine and milrinone are the initial drugs of choice for treating distributive shock.

PEDIATRIC TRAUMA

Answer as either true (T) or false (F).

1. _____ Injury is the leading cause of death for children older than 1 year.

2. _____ Injuries from blunt trauma are seen after falls and motor vehicle collisions.

3. _____ Children weighing more than 40 lb can safely sit in the front passenger seat of a car if they are restrained with lap belts and shoulder harnesses.

4. _____ Acceleration-deceleration force is known as Waddell's triad.

5. _____ An example of a penetrating injury is a gunshot wound.

6. _____ State the goals of the *primary survey* in pediatric trauma.

7. Identify the four elements of the *primary survey* used in the management of pediatric trauma.

   A:

   B:

   C:

   D:

8. What is included in the *secondary survey?*

9. For each of the following types of injury, write two questions that the nurse should ask when obtaining a history of the injury.

   Motor vehicle accident

   Fall

   Penetrating injury

10. List five indicators or physical findings that should raise suspicion of child maltreatment.

11. What is the most critical aspect of nursing care of the pediatric trauma patient?

INGESTIONS AND POISONINGS

1. Most poisonings occur as a result of _____.

2. List the five methods used to treat toxic exposure or ingestion.

   a.

   b.

   c.

   d.

   e.

3. Why does the American Academy of Pediatrics no longer recommend the use of syrup of ipecac in the home setting?

Answer as either true (T) or false (F).

4. _____ Respiratory acidosis is an early manifestation of aspirin toxicity.

5. _____ Hydrocarbon ingestion is associated with chemical pneumonitis.

6. _____ Milk or water is recommended to dilute ingested acids.

7. _____ Activated charcoal has become the recommended treatment for acute poisoning in the pediatric population.

8. _____ Gastric lavage is used to empty the stomach of the toxic substance in the first 1 to 2 hours after an ingestion.

9. _____ The dosage of activated charcoal usually administered is 3 to 4 g/kg.

10. _____ The antidote for acetaminophen ingestion is naloxone.

11. _____ Emesis should be induced following ingestion of corrosive substances.

12. _____ A serum lead level that is greater than 10 mcg/dL is considered harmful.

13. List three questions that should be asked when a child has ingested a poisonous substance.

   a.

   b.

   c.

Environmental Emergencies

1. List four local signs and symptoms of a snake bite.

   a.

   b.

   c.

   d.

2. Describe the nursing care of an injury from a dog bite.

SUBMERSION INJURIES

1. The injury to organ systems that occurs in drowning is the result of _____.

2. Briefly explain the diving reflex. _____

3. Most long-term sequelae of near-drowning incidents affect the _____ system.

HEAT-RELATED EMERGENCIES

1. What is the first priority in the management of all pediatric heat-related illnesses?

2. Describe the treatment for heat exhaustion.

3. What are the clinical manifestations of heat stroke?

DENTAL EMERGENCIES

Answer as either true (T) or false (F).

1. _____ In subluxation, the socket of the injured tooth is damaged.

2. _____ An avulsed tooth can be placed in saline or milk for transport to emergency care.

SUGGESTED LEARNING ACTIVITY

1. Arrange to observe in an emergency department that handles pediatric patients. Ask the nurses about the kinds of pediatric problems that are seen most often.

STUDENT LEARNING APPLICATION

Enhance your learning by discussing your answers with other students.

You are observing in the emergency department when the paramedics bring in a 6-year-old girl who ingested many aspirins while visiting with her grandmother while her father was at work. The nurse is performing a primary survey on the child when she goes into cardiac arrest. Her father arrives at the emergency department while the trauma team is performing CPR on his child. When the father is told about his daughter's condition, he begins sobbing and keeps repeating, "Please don't let her die." The nurse says, "Don't worry now. We won't. Everything will be fine."

1. While the child is being stabilized, what questions should be directed at the child's grandmother?

2. How would the nurse explain the rationale behind gastric lavage and the administration of activated charcoal after the child has been stabilized?

3. What do you think about the nurse's response to the child's father? Offer an alternative response.

4. How can the nurse be supportive of the father and grandmother during this emergency situation?

REVIEW QUESTIONS

Choose the correct answer.

1. A 2-year-old boy is brought to the emergency department after swallowing over-the-counter antihistamine tablets approximately 30 minutes earlier. He is now irritable and lethargic. What is the best approach for gastric emptying in this situation?
   a. Dilute the toxic substance with water or milk.
   b. Administer an antidote such as naloxone.
   c. Perform gastric lavage.
   d. Administer syrup of ipecac.

2. Which medication is used to treat severe acidosis associated with cardiac arrest?
   a. Epinephrine
   b. Calcium chloride
   c. Sodium bicarbonate
   d. Atropine sulfate

3. Which nursing action might help the toddler feel more secure in the emergency department?
   a. Perform the most distressing procedures first.
   b. Distract the child by counting numbers.
   c. Give the child a reward for cooperative behavior.
   d. Allow the child to hold his favorite toy.

4. What is assessed first in an initial triage assessment?
   a. Respiratory rate and effort
   b. Skin color and temperature
   c. Response to environment
   d. Heart rate and rhythm

5. When a child's breathing makes a high-pitched sound on inspiration, what term should the nurse use to identify this breath sound?
   a. Snoring
   b. Stridor
   c. Wheezing
   d. Crackles

6. What is one reason that a small child is at a greater risk for airway problems than an adult?
   a. The child's thicker, inflexible trachea can more easily obstruct the airway.
   b. Children younger than 3 years are obligate nose breathers.
   c. The child's airway is narrower and more easily obstructed by small amounts of mucus.
   d. The child's smaller tongue creates more space for foreign body obstruction.

7. Which vitals sign indicates that a 5-year-old child requires immediate attention?
   a. Systolic blood pressure of 80 mm Hg
   b. Bulging, pulsatile posterior fontanel
   c. Heart rate of 94 beats/min (bpm)
   d. Respiratory rate of 68 breaths/min

8. Which finding in a 1-year-old child with hypovolemic shock should be reported immediately?
   a. Flat anterior fontanel
   b. Palpable peripheral pulses
   c. Moist mucous membranes
   d. Less responsive to painful stimuli

9. What is the most common form of distributive shock?
   a. Septic
   b. Hypovolemic
   c. Cardiogenic
   d. Anaphylactic

10. The primary focus of assessment of cardiovascular status in a child with multiple traumas is to identify:
    a. hypovolemia.
    b. septic shock.
    c. cardiac arrest.
    d. electrolyte imbalance.

11. An indicator of hypovolemic shock in a 2-month-old infant is:
    a. bulging anterior fontanel.
    b. capillary refill of less than 2 seconds.
    c. parental report of two wet diapers in past 24 hours.
    d. extremities warm to the touch.

12. When near-drowning occurs, injury to organ systems is the result of:
    a. hypoxia.
    b. respiratory acidosis.
    c. hypokalemia.
    d. hypoglycemia.

13. After a 10-year-old child falls on his face, his mother notices that the upper central incisors are loose. What should she do?
    a. Remove the loose teeth and put them in a container of milk.
    b. Call the dentist and schedule an appointment within the week.
    c. Leave the teeth alone and call the dentist for an immediate appointment.
    d. Ask the child to wiggle the teeth loose while driving to the nearest emergency department.

14. Which vital sign is measured first in children?
    a. Temperature
    b. Pulse
    c. Respiratory rate
    d. Blood pressure

15. The first compensatory mechanism for decreased cardiac output in children is:
    a. tachycardia.
    b. hypotension.
    c. cyanosis.
    d. diminished breath sounds.

35 The Ill Child in the Hospital and Other Care Settings

HELPFUL HINT

In your textbook, review Chapter 4, "Communicating with Children and Families"; Chapters 5 through 9 on growth and development; Chapter 36, "The Child with a Chronic Condition or Terminal Illness"; and Chapter 39, "Pain Management for Children."

MATCHING KEY TERMS

Match the term with the correct definition.

1. _____ Denial

2. _____ Egocentrism

3. _____ Regression

4. _____ Separation anxiety

5. _____ Situational crisis

6. _____ Therapeutic play

a. An unanticipated event that poses a threat to an individual's well-being

b. Guided play that promotes the child's psychosocial or psychologic well-being

c. Distress and apprehension caused by being removed from the parents, home, or familiar surroundings

d. Preoccupation with one's own interests and needs

e. Defense mechanism in which unpleasant realities are kept out of conscious awareness

f. Defense mechanism in which a conflict or frustration is resolved by returning to a behavior that was successful in earlier years

SETTINGS OF CARE

1. List four settings where the pediatric nurse can provide health or illness care to children.

   a. _____

   b. _____

   c. _____

   d. _____

Answer as either true (T) or false (F).

2. _____ One role of the pediatric nurse in a hospital setting is that of a tour guide.

3. _____ A child having an asthma episode may be admitted to the hospital for a 24-hour observation.

4. _____ Because of time constraints in an emergency setting, preparing a child for a procedure is not an important nursing action.

5. _____ Teaching the child and family is less of a concern in an outpatient facility than it is in an acute care setting.

6. _____ In a rehabilitative setting, nurses must balance nurturing the child with setting limits as the child learns to be more self-sufficient.

7. _____ The nurse working in a school-based clinic needs to be sensitive to parental concerns regarding sexuality issues.

8. _____ In a community clinic, the nurse integrates health promotion and primary prevention into acute care.

9. _____ In home care, the nurse serves as case manager and care coordinator.

STRESSORS ASSOCIATED WITH ILLNESS AND HOSPITALIZATION

1. Identify four factors that influence a child's reaction to illness.

   a. _____

   b. _____

   c. _____

   d. _____

2. Separation anxiety is most significant in the _____ and _____ age groups.

3. Describe the behaviors associated with the three stages of separation anxiety.

   Protest

   Despair

   Detachment

4. How can nurses help parents cope with their child's regression in the hospital?

5. How can nurses minimize disruption in a toddler's usual routines during hospitalization?

6. How can hospitalization intensify a preschooler's fear of injury?

7. What can the nurse do to promote a sense of control during hospitalization for the school-age child?

8. Why is it important to provide hospitalized adolescents the opportunity to meet and interact with each other?

9. Give two examples of regressive behavior the nurse might observe in a child who is hospitalized.

   a. _____

   b. _____

197

FACTORS AFFECTING A CHILD'S RESPONSE TO ILLNESS AND HOSPITALIZATION

1. Identify three factors that affect how a child copes with illness or hospitalization.

   a. _____

   b. _____

   c. _____

2. Provide two strategies that might facilitate a child's ability to cope with illness and hospitalization.

   a. _____

   b. _____

3. Identify two potential psychologic benefits of hospitalization.

   a. _____

   b. _____

PLAYROOMS IN HEALTH CARE SETTINGS

1. What makes therapeutic play different from normal play?

2. What is emotional outlet play?

3. How can the nurse maintain the hospital playroom as a "safe place" for the child?

4. Give an example of how a child's cooperation with a treatment plan can be enhanced through play.

ADMITTING THE CHILD TO A HOSPITAL SETTING

1. How can the nurse set a positive tone for the child and family on admission?

2. What should take precedence over completing the admission "paperwork" when a child is admitted to the hospital?

THE ILL CHILD'S FAMILY

1. How does the parental role change as a result of hospitalization?

2. Identify three common reactions that a child might have to a sibling being hospitalized.

   a.

   b.

   c.

DEVELOPMENTAL APPROACHES TO THE HOSPITALIZED CHILD

Match each intervention with the appropriate age group. (Age groups may be used more than once.)

1. _____ Be particularly careful to follow home routines and rituals.

2. _____ Provide a special area for activities with this age-group.

3. _____ Provide safe outlets for acting out aggression, such as painting and using play dough.

4. _____ Reassure the child that he or she did not cause the illness.

5. _____ Assist the child in contacting friends.

6. _____ Limit the number of caregivers assigned to the child.

7. _____ Provide opportunities for nonnutritive sucking and oral stimulation.

a. Neonates

b. Infants

c. Toddlers

d. Preschoolers

e. School-age children

f. Adolescents

SUGGESTED LEARNING ACTIVITIES

1. Arrange for clinical observations in a school or community clinic, pediatrician's office, home care setting, or some other non-acute care setting. Compare the role of the pediatric nurse in these settings with that of the pediatric nurse in the hospital.

2. Develop a plan for a toddler experiencing separation anxiety during hospitalization.

STUDENT LEARNING APPLICATIONS

Enhance your learning by discussing your answers with other students.

David is a 3-year-old child who had an emergency appendectomy late last night. David has not been hospitalized before. His mother is with him now. His father left for work after David came out of anesthesia; he is planning to visit this evening after work. The family lives approximately 1 hour's distance from the hospital. David has a 7-year-old sister, Sara, who is in the second grade. The grandmother is taking care of Sara after school today.

1. What stressors do you think the family might be experiencing at this time?

2. When you get a report on David, you learn that he clings to his mother every time a hospital staff person comes into his room. How can you help David cope with his fears?

3. David's mother tells you that she will be going home tonight with her husband because she needs to make arrangements for Sara's care. She expresses how guilty she feels about leaving David. How can you be supportive of her and her decision?

4. When you ask David whether he wants to have his blood pressure taken, he says, "No." What would you do now?

5. David has cried inconsolably for 2 hours since his parents left. When you go to check on him, you find that he has wet his pajamas. What is your interpretation of these behaviors? How would you explain them to David's mother when she calls to check on him?

6. What would be important to convey in your report to the nurse replacing you on the following shift?

REVIEW QUESTIONS

Choose the correct answer.

1. Which child is most likely to have difficulty with separation during hospitalization?
   a. A 3-month-old
   b. An 18-month-old
   c. A 4-year-old
   d. A 7-year-old

2. Which type of behavior would be expected when a child is in the despair stage of separation?
   a. Agitated
   b. Playful
   c. Withdrawn
   d. Anxious

3. A young child cries, kicks, and clings to his mother when she tries to leave. What is the nurse's best comment to the mother about this behavior?
   a. "This child is experiencing ineffective coping."
   b. "Parents should not leave their children when they are hospitalized."
   c. "Wait until the child falls asleep to leave."
   d. "This behavior actually shows a healthy attachment between you and your child."

4. Which action is not developmentally appropriate for a hospitalized adolescent?
   a. Allow the adolescent to wear her own clothing.
   b. Provide privacy when giving treatments.
   c. Suggest that her parents bring in her favorite foods.
   d. Discourage visits from school friends.

5. Which nursing intervention might help the hospitalized toddler feel a sense of security and control?
   a. Follow the child's usual bedtime routine.
   b. Place the child in a crib with a cover over it.
   c. Tell the child what needs to be done and do not offer choices.
   d. Suggest to the parents that they bring new toys to the child.

6. What is the best nursing response to a father who is concerned because his 4-year-old daughter has been using the bathroom independently for more than a year now but has had a few "accidents" since she has been hospitalized?
   a. Suggest that he take his daughter to the bathroom more often.
   b. Assure him that this behavior will disappear immediately after the discharge.
   c. Explain that children often exhibit regressive behaviors because of the stress of hospitalization.
   d. Set up a reward system to motivate the child to use the bathroom.

7. A 7-year-old child, who is going to have a lumbar puncture later today, tells the nurse, "I'm really nervous about this test." What is the best way to minimize the child's anxiety until time for the procedure?
   a. Review the lumbar puncture procedure with him.
   b. Give him a relaxation tape to practice.
   c. Read a book to him about being in the hospital.
   d. Distract him by playing his favorite board game with him.

8. Ten-year-old Meg told the school nurse that she is worried about her twin sister, Mary, who is in the hospital. What might increase Meg's stress about this situation?
   a. Meg's grandparents are helping to care for her at home.
   b. Meg's parents have explained Mary's illness to her.
   c. Meg wonders whether she will get sick too.
   d. Meg plans to call her sister on the phone after school.

9. Emotional outlet play would be appropriate for which child?
   a. A child who does not feel well enough to play
   b. A child who is having a hip spica cast applied in the morning
   c. A child who is scheduled for surgery next week
   d. A child who has been physically abused

10. Why might a 4-year-old child think that she caused her younger sibling's illness, which necessitated hospitalization?
    a. Preschool-age children have a beginning understanding of disease transmission.
    b. The child feels insecure since the birth of the sibling.
    c. The feeling of closeness to her sibling makes her feel responsible for the illness.
    d. Children are magical thinkers at this age.

Chapter **35**   The Ill Child in the Hospital and Other Care Settings

36 The Child with a Chronic Condition or Terminal Illness

HELPFUL HINT

Review Elizabeth Kübler-Ross's work on death and dying.

MATCHING KEY TERMS

Match the term with the correct definition.

1. _____ Anticipatory grief

2. _____ Chronic condition

3. _____ Chronic grief

4. _____ Chronic sorrow

5. _____ Hospice care

6. _____ Illness trajectory

7. _____ Normalization

8. _____ Palliative care

a. The course of an illness, including its effect on those involved

b. Responses used to counteract an illness or abnormal behavior in order to maintain appropriate and valued social roles

c. A system of comprehensive care that provides support and assistance to patients and families affected by terminal illness

d. Recurrent feelings of grief, loss, and fear related to the child's illness and the loss of the ideal, healthy child

e. The processes of mourning, coping, interacting, planning, and psychosocial reorganization that occur as part of the response to the impending death of a loved one

f. Treatments or procedures that promote comfort and quality of life, rather than those that aim to cure the underlying disease

g. An illness that is long term and either without a cure or with residual effects that limit activities of daily living

h. Excessively long mourning that interferes with resuming normal activities

9. In what ways has the experience of childhood chronic illness changed?

10. What is meant by the term *children with special healthcare needs?*

THE FAMILY OF THE CHILD WITH SPECIAL HEALTH CARE NEEDS

1. What does the term *situational crisis* mean?

2. The predominant trait exhibited by resilient families is _____.

3. List four processes that enhance a family's resilience.

a. _____

b. _____

c. _____

d. _____

Answer as either true (T) or false (F).

4. _____ In resilient families, the child's condition-related needs become the focus around which family activities revolve.

5. _____ For resilient families, coping is an active process that involves learning about their child's condition and available resources.

THE GRIEVING PROCESS

1. The nurse caring for a child with a chronic illness must keep in mind that the most important aspect of a chronic illness

   is that it affects _____.

2. Identify the five stages of the grieving process delineated by Kübler-Ross.

a. _____

b. _____

c. _____

d. _____

e. _____

Answer as either true (T) or false (F).

3. _____ Children move through the five stages of the grieving process sequentially.

4. _____ Children with chronic conditions may use denial more often than adults.

THE CHILD WITH SPECIAL HEALTH CARE NEEDS

1. Children's responses to chronic illness are influenced by their _____ and their

   _____.

2. Nurses caring for children with chronic conditions must understand issues concerning _____

   and _____ in relation to each stage of growth and development.

Answer as either true (T) or false (F).

3. _____ Temporary regression may be observed in children of all ages.

4. _____ Rearing a child with a chronic illness necessitates that parents learn a different set of child-rearing techniques.

THE CHILD WITH A CHRONIC ILLNESS

1. The goal for a child with a chronic illness is _____.

2. List three goals for the family of a child with a chronic illness.

a. _____

b. _____

c. _____

3. What is the first factor the nurse must consider when planning care for a child with a chronic illness?

4. List five ways health care professionals can support the parents of children with a chronic condition.

a. _____

b. _____

c. _____

d. _____

e. _____

Answer as either true (T) or false (F).

5. _____ The nurse should convince the parents that it is always better to express emotions than to hold them inside.

6. _____ Honesty and trust must be maintained at all times when caring for a child with a chronic condition.

7. _____ Siblings of a chronically ill child may also experience a developmental regression.

8. _____ Siblings should not participate in the ill child's physical care.

THE TERMINALLY ILL OR DYING CHILD

Match each age group with the corresponding concept of death.

1. _____ Infants/toddlers

2. _____ Preschoolers

3. _____ School-age children

4. _____ Adolescents

a. Death is temporary and reversible.

b. Death is a sad and irreversible event.

c. Death is viewed as the loss of a caretaker.

d. Death is inevitable and irreversible.

Answer as either true (T) or false (F).

5. _____ One of the primary concerns of dying children is the fear of being alone.

6. _____ The health care team must uphold the family's decisions about continuing curative care for their child.

7. _____ An important aspect of supporting the sibling of a child who has died is to acknowledge that the loss is significant.

CARING FOR THE DYING CHILD

1. Identify three self-care measures that can assist nurses caring for terminally ill children.

a. _____

b. _____

c. _____

2. The most common issue for families surrounding a child's impending death is _____.

Answer as either true (T) or false (F).

3. _____ Pain control is a primary concern for dying children, their families, and the nursing staff.

4. _____ Many hospice organizations offer palliative care for families after their child dies.

5. _____ The nurse should make every effort to provide privacy for the dying child and family.

6. _____ Adequate oral intake is crucial to the dying child's comfort.

7. _____ Hearing is the last sense to shut down before death.

8. _____ The young child is usually not aware of the presence of parents during the dying process.

9. _____ Respiratory changes are always the earliest indicators of imminent death.

10. _____ Hypercapnia has a sedative effect.

11. _____ The nurse's response to caring for a dying child correlates to a certain degree with the Kübler-Ross stages of grieving.

12. _____ Nurses with many years of experience in caring for dying children will typically not experience grief when a child dies.

SUGGESTED LEARNING ACTIVITIES

1. Investigate the availability of pediatric hospice care in your area.

2. Arrange to make a home visit to the family of a child with a chronic illness. How does home care compare with hospital care?

STUDENT LEARNING APPLICATIONS

Enhance your learning by discussing your answers with other students.

1. What are your fears or concerns about caring for a child who is dying? Talk with other students about your thoughts. Are your fears or concerns similar to or different from those of the other students?

2. Talk to a nurse who has worked with dying children and their families. What has been the most rewarding aspect of this work? The most difficult? Share what you learned with other students.

REVIEW QUESTIONS

Choose the correct answer.

1. The most significant concern of the parents of a dying child is the child's:
   a. pain.
   b. hydration.
   c. safety.
   d. privacy.

2. A preschooler understands death as:
   a. the loss of a caretaker.
   b. a temporary separation.
   c. sad and permanent.
   d. something that happens to everyone.

3. Although an individual may move back and forth among the various stages of the grieving process, the first stage is usually:
   a. denial.
   b. resentment.
   c. bargaining.
   d. depression.

4. Chronic illness with frequent hospitalizations can affect the psychosocial development of a school-age child by:
   a. leading to feelings of inferiority.
   b. preventing a sense of initiative.
   c. interfering with parental attachment.
   d. blocking the development of identity.

5. What is the best response to an adolescent who asks whether he should talk to his dying brother?
   a. "You might want to hold his hand instead because he cannot hear you."
   b. "Although he may not answer you, your brother can still hear what you are saying."
   c. "He can't hear you, but he can feel your presence nearby."
   d. "Talk about happy things because you don't want to upset him."

6. Which action represents the predominant trait of resilient families?
   a. Disengaging the family from the community
   b. Maintaining rigid family roles
   c. Engaging in efforts to keep the family intact
   d. Focusing on the child's condition-related needs

7. Which intervention is appropriate when caring for a chronically ill toddler?
   a. Prepare for procedures days in advance.
   b. Arrange for friends to visit in the hospital.
   c. Limit parental participation in the child's care.
   d. Keep security objects nearby.

8. What is the nurse's first consideration when planning care for the child with a chronic illness?
   a. Child's physiologic condition
   b. Child's development
   c. Family's coping mechanisms
   d. Family's understanding of the prognosis

37 Principles and Procedures for Nursing Care of Children

HELPFUL HINT

Review Chapter 4, "Communicating with Children and Families," and Chapter 35, "The Ill Child in the Hospital and Other Care Settings."

MATCHING KEY TERMS

Match the term with the correct definition.

1. _____ Informed consent
2. _____ Apical pulse rate
3. _____ Enteral
4. _____ Antipyretic
5. _____ Pyrogen
6. _____ Lavage

a. Substance that produces a fever

b. By way of the digestive system

c. Requirement that both the child and the parent/guardian completely understand the proposed procedures or treatments

d. Agent that reduces or relieves fever

e. Process of washing out or irrigating an organ

f. Heart rate determined by placing the stethoscope over the point of maximum impulse (PMI) and counting for 1 minute

PREPARING CHILDREN FOR PROCEDURES

1. List five assessments the nurse should make in preparing a child and family for an invasive procedure.

a. _____

b. _____

c. _____

d. _____

e. _____

Answer as either true (T) or false (F).

2. _____ Children need to be prepared before any procedure that is performed.

3. _____ Parents need to be prepared before a procedure is performed on their child.

4. _____ It is preferable to perform painful or invasive procedures in the treatment room.

5. _____ The nurse should praise children only when they have been cooperative during a procedure.

6. _____ Parents should be asked to step out of the room before an invasive procedure is started.

7. _____ Informed consent is obtained from the parent before any surgical or diagnostic invasive procedures.

8. _____ Children older than 7 years can give informed consent for procedures.

TRANSPORTING INFANTS AND CHILDREN

1. Name four factors that must be considered when choosing the method of transportation for a hospitalized child.

   a. _____

   b. _____

   c. _____

   d. _____

USING RESTRAINTS

Answer as either true (T) or false (F).

1. _____ Restraints are applied only as a last resort and not for the staff's convenience.

2. _____ The physician's order for restraints should indicate why the restraints are necessary and how long they should be in place.

3. _____ When restraints are applied, the distal extremity is assessed for temperature, pulses, capillary refill, sensation, and movement.

4. _____ Restraints should be removed every 4 hours for range of motion and repositioning.

INFECTION CONTROL

1. List the four body components to which Standard Precautions apply.

   a. _____

   b. _____

   c. _____

   d. _____

2. Second-tier precautions are also called _____.

3. Describe the Centers for Disease Control and Prevention (CDC) recommendations for *hand hygiene*.

BATHING INFANTS AND CHILDREN

1. The temperature of water used to bathe a child should not exceed _____.

2. If a thermometer is not accessible, the nurse can determine whether the water temperature is comfortable by _____.

3. When bathing an infant in the tub, the nurse makes sure that the water level does not exceed _____ inches.

4. What is the rationale for avoiding talcum powder after a child's bath?

ORAL HYGIENE

Answer as either true (T) or false (F).

1. _____ Wipe the infants' gums with a wet cloth after each feeding.

2. _____ A quarter-sized amount of toothpaste should be placed on the toothbrush each time the child brushes his or her teeth.

3. _____ Cleaning teeth is avoided when the child is at risk for gingival bleeding.

FEEDING

1. What is the rationale for not propping a bottle when feeding an infant?

2. Name three strategies that might make hospital meals more desirable for young children.

   a. _____

   b. _____

   c. _____

VITAL SIGNS

1. What are the indications for measuring axillary temperatures in children?

2. What factors might cause an inaccurate measurement of oral temperature?

Answer as either true (T) or false (F).

3. _____ Mercury thermometers are recommended for use only in the acute-care setting.

4. _____ Tympanic temperature measurements have been demonstrated to be accurate for measuring core body temperature.

5. _____ Radial pulse measurements are appropriate for children older than 2 years.

6. _____ When measuring an apical pulse, the nurse counts the heart rate for 1 full minute.

7. _____ When measuring respirations in a 6-month-old, the nurse auscultates breath sounds for 30 seconds and then multiplies the result by two to record the respiratory rate.

8. _____ The nurse measuring blood pressure on a child hears a systolic pressure at 86 mm Hg and continues to hear it down to a measurement of 0 mm Hg. This blood pressure would be recorded as 86/0 mm Hg.

9. _____ Blood pressure can be measured in the upper or lower arm, the thigh, the calf, and the ankle.

FEVER-REDUCING MEASURES

1. List two environmental measures that can be taken to reduce a child's fever.

   a. _____

   b. _____

2. The drugs (generic names) used to treat fever in children are _____ and _____.

SPECIMEN COLLECTION

1. Regardless of the type of specimen to be obtained, the nurse should use _____ Precautions.

2. The technique used for collecting a sample of an infant's nasopharyngeal secretions is _____.

3. Children who undergo frequent catheterizations are at high risk for developing _____ sensitivity.

4. The most common site for bone marrow aspiration in the child is the _____.

Chapter **37**   **Principles and Procedures for Nursing Care of Children**

GAVAGE AND GASTROSTOMY

1. When and how often should the nurse check the placement of a nasogastric tube?

2. How can the nurse determine the placement of a nasogastric tube before a bolus feeding?

Answer as either true (T) or false (F).

3. _____ A reliable method for determining nasogastric tube placement is an auscultation of the air entering the stomach.

4. _____ Tube placement and residual volumes should be checked every 24 hours when continuous enteral feedings are infusing.

5. _____ The only definitive method of determining the correct position of a feeding tube is by getting X-ray confirmation.

6. _____ When a bolus feeding is completed, the child is placed on the left side with the head of the bed elevated for at least 30 minutes.

ENEMAS

1. When giving an enema to a 7-year-old child, the nurse should use a volume of _____ and insert the tube into the rectum no farther than _____.

CARE OF OSTOMIES

Answer as either true (T) or false (F).

1. _____ The consistency of the stool through an ostomy is determined by the anatomic location of the stoma.

2. _____ The nursing care of a child with an ostomy differs very little from that of an adult.

OXYGEN THERAPY

1. List five ways that oxygen therapy can be delivered to infants and children.

    a. _____

    b. _____

    c. _____

    d. _____

    e. _____

ASSESSING OXYGENATION

1. The nurse measures a child's pulse oximetry to be 98%. What does this finding indicate?

2. What action should the nurse take if this child's pulse oximetry drops to 89%?

CHEST PHYSIOTHERAPY

1. Define *percussion*.

2. Define *postural drainage*.

3. When should chest physiotherapy be performed in relation to meals?

TRACHEOSTOMY CARE

1. What are the five elements of routine tracheostomy care?

    a. _____

    b. _____

    c. _____

    d. _____

    e. _____

2. How often should the nurse perform tracheostomy care?

3. Catheter insertion and suctioning time should be limited to _____.

4. The suction catheter is inserted with the suction _____.

SURGICAL PROCEDURES

1. At what point preoperatively should clear liquids be stopped?

2. List five nursing interventions that are appropriate for preventing atelectasis postoperatively.

    a. _____

    b. _____

    c. _____

    d. _____

    e. _____

3. Identify five stressors that may be experienced by a child undergoing surgery.

    a. _____

    b. _____

    c. _____

    d. _____

    e. _____

SUGGESTED LEARNING ACTIVITIES

1. Follow a child through a surgical experience. Take note of preoperative procedures and teaching, as well as postanesthesia care. When the child returns to the unit, provide immediate postoperative care. How is this nursing care similar to or different from preoperative and postoperative care of an adult?

STUDENT LEARNING APPLICATIONS

Enhance your learning by discussing your answers with other students.

Betsy is a 3-year-old child who is going to have a bilateral ureteral reimplantation to correct vesicoureteral reflux. She is scheduled for surgery in the morning. She and her parents have just arrived at her assigned room, and you are assigned to admit Betsy to the unit. Betsy's admission orders include routine urinalysis and complete blood count (CBC).

1. How are you going to measure Betsy's vital signs?

2. Betsy is not toilet trained yet. How would you collect a urine specimen from her?

3. Her mother tells you that she wants to stay with Betsy when you take blood for the CBC. What is your response? Where are you planning to do this procedure?

4. How would you explain the procedure for venipuncture to Betsy?

5. Betsy's father wants to know when she has to stop eating before surgery. What would you tell him?

6. What do you want to know from Betsy and her parents before you do any preoperative teaching?

REVIEW QUESTIONS

Choose the correct answer.

1. A parent wants to wait outside until a procedure is completed on his child. The nurse's best response is:
   a. "It would be better for your child if you were by his side."
   b. "That is fine. I will stay with your child during the procedure."
   c. "It is hospital policy for parents to step out of the room during procedures."
   d. "This test will only take a few minutes. Why don't you stay?"

2. Which core body temperature should be reported?
   a. 96.5°F
   b. 36.5°C
   c. 37.2°C
   d. 100°F

3. What advice should the nurse offer a parent about reducing a child's fever?
   a. Give the child an alcohol bath.
   b. Offer the child additional oral fluids.
   c. Administer baby aspirin.
   d. Dress the child in heavy-weight clothing.

4. What indicates that the nurse is correctly measuring vital signs on an infant?
   a. Measuring oral temperature for 5 minutes
   b. Counting apical pulse for 60 seconds
   c. Recording the respiratory rate from the cardiorespiratory monitor
   d. Recording blood pressure as P/46

5. A 9-year-old child asks the nurse where the doctor is going to put the needle for his bone marrow test. The nurse describes the location as the:
   a. lower middle part of his back.
   b. middle part of his chest.
   c. right or left side of his hip.
   d. top bone in his leg.

6. When an extremity is restrained, it is essential for the nurse to assess the affected area for:
   a. clubbing.
   b. pallor.
   c. spasm.
   d. crepitus.

7. Nasogastric tube placement should be checked:
   a. before initiating a bolus feeding.
   b. when the feeding is completed.
   c. every 12 hours during continuous feedings.
   d. when residual volumes are excessive.

8. The nurse should discontinue a bolus gavage feeding if what occurs?
   a. Fatigue
   b. Crying
   c. Phlebitis
   d. Vomiting

9. Which statement about ostomies is correct?
   a. The lower the stoma along the intestinal tract, the more liquid is the stool.
   b. Urinary stomas do not begin to drain until the second postoperative day.
   c. A minimal amount of drainage from colostomies is normal up to 4 days after surgery.
   d. Children usually do not require appliances on their stomas.

10. What should the nurse teach parents about chest physiotherapy?
    a. Give treatments before meals.
    b. Schedule treatments approximately 30 minutes after meals.
    c. Treatments should last approximately 45 minutes to 1 hour.
    d. Children must be placed in all of the postural drainage positions with each treatment.

11. A 2-year-old is scheduled for surgery tomorrow. The parents have been told to arrive at the short procedure unit at 8:00 A.M. The nurse should expect preoperative feeding instructions to include:
    a. clear liquids until midnight tonight, then nothing by mouth.
    b. stopping solid food at 5:00 A.M., then clear liquids until 7:00 A.M.
    c. fluids including milk and orange juice until arrival at the hospital.
    d. clear liquids until 6:00 A.M., then nothing to eat or drink.

12. A nursing student is caring for a 3-year-old with asthma who has been placed on a cardiorespiratory monitor. Just as the student enters the room, the monitor alarm sounds. According to the monitor, the child's heart rate is 32 beats/min (bpm) and decreasing. What should the nursing student do first?
    a. Find the nurse who is assigned to the child.
    b. Assess the child's ABCs.
    c. Call a rapid response.
    d. Initiate cardiopulmonary resuscitation (CPR).

38 Medication Administration and Safety for Infants and Children

HELPFUL HINT

Review pharmacodynamics and pharmacokinetics in a pharmacology or fundamentals of nursing textbook.

MATCHING KEY TERMS

Match the term with the correct definition.

1. _____ EMLA

2. _____ Metered-dose inhaler

3. _____ Pharmacodynamics

4. _____ Pharmacokinetics

5. _____ Central venous access device

6. _____ Peripherally inserted central catheter (PICC) line

a. Central line inserted via the antecubital vein into the superior vena cava

b. Hand-held device that delivers "puffs" of medication for inhalation

c. Cream used to numb skin at a depth of 0.5 mm

d. Behavior of medications at the cellular level

e. Venous access device placed in the superior vena cava or jugular vein

f. Time and movement relationships of medications

PHARMACOKINETICS IN CHILDREN

1. Name four factors that influence the absorption of medications orally administered.

   a. _____

   b. _____

   c. _____

   d. _____

Answer as either true (T) or false (F).

2. _____ Infants have a larger body surface area-to-weight ratio than adults.

3. _____ Compared with an adult, a child requires a lower dose per kilogram of a water-soluble medication to achieve its desired effect.

4. _____ The immaturity of the blood–brain barrier in a child results in a decreased distribution of medications to the brain.

5. What factors affect drug excretion in the infant?

6. Why would a medication's peak and trough serum levels be measured?

7. The level at which the serum concentration is lowest is referred to as the medication _____.

PSYCHOLOGIC AND DEVELOPMENTAL DIFFERENCES

1. Name three ways parents can assist the nurse with administering medications to children.

   a. _____

   b. _____

   c. _____

2. Describe two strategies to elicit cooperation from each age group of children.

   Toddler

   a. _____

   b. _____

   Preschooler

   a. _____

   b. _____

   School-age child

   a. _____

   b. _____

CALCULATING DOSAGES

Answer as either true (T) or false (F).

1. _____ Standard doses exist for pediatric medications.

2. _____ Pediatric doses are usually calculated based on the child's weight in pounds.

3. _____ The most reliable method for determining pediatric medication dosages is to use the body surface area (BSA) formula.

MEDICATION ADMINISTRATION PROCEDURES

1. List three procedures that should be followed to avoid medication errors when giving medications to children.

   a. _____

   b. _____

   c. _____

2. What is meant by *medication reconciliation?*

3. What should a nurse do if a child cannot swallow tablets or capsules?

Chapter **38** **Medication Administration and Safety for Infants and Children**

4. Why should the nurse mix a powdered or crushed medication with a "nonessential" food?

Answer as either true (T) or (F) false.

5. _____ Medications can be mixed with small amounts of natural honey and administered to infants.

6. _____ A sustained-release tablet can be crushed if the child cannot swallow it.

7. _____ Liquid medications should be placed in the infant's mouth along the side of the cheek using an oral syringe.

8. _____ Oral medications should be administered with the child in an upright position.

9. How can the nurse position a 3-year-old child who does not want to take oral medication?

10. What nursing action should be taken if the child vomits a medication 15 minutes after it was administered?

11. What procedures should be followed when administering medications via a feeding tube?

ADMINISTERING INJECTIONS

1. What are the guidelines for giving an explanation to a child before administering an injection?

2. What can the nurse do to make injections less painful?

Match each injection site with its indication for use.

3. _____ Vastus lateralis

4. _____ Ventrogluteal

5. _____ Deltoid

a. Not used for young children because muscle cannot hold the volume of medication

b. Usually used for children younger than 3 years

c. Safe for children older than 18 months

Answer as either true (T) or false (F).

6. _____ The nurse documents the amount of medication injected and the site used.

7. _____ The air bubble technique is used when preparing pediatric injections.

8. _____ Preschoolers can safely receive up to 1.5 mL of a drug in the ventrogluteal site.

9. _____ Viscous medication is less painful when injected through a smaller-gauge needle.

ADMINISTERING SUBCUTANEOUS INJECTIONS

1. A subcutaneous injection should not be used if the child's _____ is impaired.

2. Name four areas of the body that are preferred subcutaneous injection sites.

    a. _____

    b. _____

    c. _____

    d. _____

Answer as either true (T) or false (F).

3. _____ Subcutaneous injection sites need to be rotated to prevent the development of abscesses.

4. _____ The angle of needle insertion for a subcutaneous injection is usually 90 degrees.

5. _____ Volumes for subcutaneous injections can be as large as 3 mL.

INTRADERMAL INJECTIONS

1. The intradermal route is most often used for _____.

2. What sites are used for intradermal injections?

3. Describe the procedure for administering an intradermal injection.

RECTAL AND VAGINAL ADMINISTRATION

Answer as either true (T) or false (F).

1. _____ The vaginal route is used to treat candidal infections.

2. _____ The child should be placed in a prone position for administration of a rectal suppository.

3. _____ The nurse should direct the child to take a deep breath as medication is inserted into the rectum.

OPHTHALMIC AND OTIC ADMINISTRATION

Answer as either true (T) or false (F).

1. _____ Instillation of ophthalmic drops is a sterile procedure.

2. _____ Otic solutions should be warmed to room temperature before being administered.

3. _____ To administer eardrops to a 5-year-old child, pull the pinna of the ear down and back.

INHALATION THERAPY

1. A _____ used with a metered-dose inhaler increases the effectiveness of the medication.

2. If a child inhales too quickly when using a metered-dose inhaler with a spacer, he or she will hear a

    _____.

3. How long should a child hold the breath after inhaling a "puff" of medication from a metered-dose inhaler?

INTRAVENOUS THERAPY

1. What factors should be considered when selecting a site for an intravenous (IV) line?

2. Name a nonpharmacologic technique for helping a child cope with the discomfort of intravenous catheter insertion.

3. What are the guidelines for using EMLA [eutectic mixture of local anesthetic(s)] cream before inserting an IV catheter?

4. Why should a volumetric infusion pump be used when administering IV fluids?

5. How frequently should an IV site be assessed?

6. What assessments of the site should be made?

7. Give the formula for calculating maintenance fluid needs.

8. Calculate the maintenance fluid requirements for children of the following weights:

   35 kg: _____

   16 kg: _____

9. What is meant by IV push medications?

10. How does the nurse administer medication via the IV retrograde route?

11. Why is it important to flush the IV tubing after administering an IV piggyback (IVPB) medication?

12. How frequently should an intermittent infusion port or heparin lock be flushed?

13. In what types of situations are central venous access devices used?

14. What is an implanted venous access device?

15. The major complications of PICC lines are _____.

ADMINISTERING BLOOD OR BLOOD PRODUCTS

Answer as either true (T) or false (F).

1. _____ Blood should be infused with a dextrose solution on a piggyback setup.

2. _____ Packed red blood cells are administered to infants and children to prevent circulatory hypovolemia.

3. _____ Blood products should be used within 30 minutes of arrival from the blood bank.

4. _____ An important nursing action is to take the child's vital signs before initiating a blood transfusion.

5. _____ When a transfusion reaction is suspected, the nurse immediately discontinues the blood infusion and removes the IV.

CHILD AND FAMILY EDUCATION

1. List six points that need to be addressed when teaching parents about administering medications to a child at home.

a. _____

b. _____

c. _____

d. _____

e. _____

f. _____

SUGGESTED LEARNING ACTIVITIES

1. Review a child's medication administration record. Calculate dosages for prescribed medications. Determine whether the prescribed dosage is safe for the child. Observe the medication administration. What techniques were helpful to the child and nurse?

STUDENT LEARNING APPLICATIONS

Enhance your learning by discussing your answers with other students.

Kelly is a 9-year-old girl with cystic fibrosis (CF). Kelly is in the hospital because of a CF exacerbation. Her cough has worsened, she has lost weight, and she is mildly dehydrated. She weighs 55 lb. Kelly's admission orders include IV fluids and medications.

1. Kelly needs to have an IV line placed for fluids and medications. What could you do to minimize her discomfort before and during the venipuncture?

2. There is an order to administer Kelly D_5 .225 NS at 65 mL/hr. Calculate her maintenance fluid requirements. How does this order compare with your calculation?

3. There is an order to administer tobramycin 40 mg IVPB every 8 hours. The dosage range for children is 6 to 7.5 mg/kg/day divided every 8 hours. Is Kelly's dose within that range?

Chapter **38** Medication Administration and Safety for Infants and Children

4. Two days later, Kelly's maintenance IV line is converted to a heparin lock. How does the care of a heparin lock differ from that of a continuous IV?

5. Kelly's IV line has infiltrated, and a PICC line is discussed. What is a PICC line? What are the advantages of having a PICC line instead of a heparin lock?

6. When you approach Kelly to administer her oral medications, she turns her head away and puts her hand over her mouth. What would you do to get Kelly to take her medications? What would you do if Kelly's mother were present?

REVIEW QUESTIONS

Choose the correct answer.

1. Physiologic differences in the gastrointestinal system between children and adults affect which component of a drug's action?
   a. Absorption
   b. Distribution
   c. Metabolism
   d. Excretion

2. Drug toxicity may occur more rapidly in the infant for which reason?
   a. Larger surface area requires a larger dosage.
   b. Fewer enzymes are available to bind with the drug.
   c. Renal immaturity may delay drug excretion.
   d. The blood–brain barrier becomes less selective with maturity.

3. The pediatric maintenance dosage for Dilantin (phenytoin) is 4 to 8 mg/kg/day in three equal doses. A safe morning dose for a child weighing 15 kg is:
   a. 30 mg.
   b. 60 mg.
   c. 90 mg.
   d. any of these dosages.

4. Which food is the best choice for mixing with a medication to be administered to an infant?
   a. Honey
   b. Rice cereal
   c. Similac with iron
   d. Pudding

5. When administering insulin subcutaneously, the nurse should:
   a. use a 1- to 1½-inch needle.
   b. rotate injection sites.
   c. administer a very small volume such as 0.1 mL.
   d. inject the needle at a 30-degree angle.

6. Which action is appropriate for the administration of a rectal suppository?
   a. Position the child on his abdomen.
   b. Insert the suppository 1 to 2 inches.
   c. Direct the child to take a deep breath.
   d. Ask the child to get up and walk around after insertion.

7. Which statement about the administration of IVPB medications is correct?
   a. The undiluted medication is pushed directly into the IV catheter through the port closest to the patient.
   b. The medication is injected into the port nearest the child and flushed through the tubing slowly.
   c. The IV catheter is used intermittently when medication is infused over a 1- to 2-hour period.
   d. The medication is diluted in at least 20 mL of IV fluid and infused over at least 15 minutes.

39 Pain Management for Children

HELPFUL HINT

Review pain management in a medical-surgical nursing textbook.

MATCHING KEY TERMS

Match the term with the correct definition.

1. _____ Addiction

2. _____ Adjuvant

3. _____ Epidural

4. _____ Neuropathic pain

5. _____ Nociceptive

6. _____ Pain

7. _____ Pain threshold

8. _____ Opioid

9. _____ Tolerance

a. Pain resulting from trauma to or malfunction of the nervous system

b. Natural or synthetic opium derivative used for analgesia

c. Impulse giving rise to the sensation of pain

d. Psychologic or neurologic state of the need for and compulsive use of illegal and legal drugs

e. Unpleasant sensory and emotional experience associated with actual or potential tissue damage

f. Situated within the spinal canal, on or outside the dura mater

g. Level of intensity at which pain becomes appreciable or perceptible

h. An intervention with additive effects on pain management designed to assist the primary pain management intervention

i. Physical need for increasing doses of pain medication to achieve therapeutic results

DEFINITIONS AND THEORIES OF PAIN

1. According to McCaffrey and Pasero, *pain* is _____

_____.

2. The International Association for the Study of Pain defines *pain* as _____

_____.

Answer as either true (T) or false (F).

3. _____ The gate control theory supports the use of physiologic and psychologic interventions in pain management.

4. _____ Rubbing a sprained ankle makes the pain worse.

5. _____ A child with arthritis typically experiences acute pain.

6. _____ Acute pain experienced by hospitalized children is often procedural pain.

7. _____ Neuropathic pain is usually easier to manage than acute pain.

RESEARCH ON PAIN IN CHILDREN

Answer as either true (T) or false (F).

1. _____ There are no long-term consequences of pain experiences in the newborn period.

2. _____ Guidelines for managing pain in sickle cell disease were developed by the World Health Organization.

MYTHS ABOUT PAIN AND PAIN MANAGEMENT IN CHILDREN

Answer as either true (T) or false (F).

1. _____ Myelinization is not necessary for pain perception.

2. _____ Children are at greater risk for respiratory depression from narcotics than adults.

3. _____ Premature infants lack the neurologic structures required for pain perception.

4. _____ Emotional factors contribute to the pain experience.

5. _____ How present pain experiences are managed will influence future pain experiences.

ASSESSMENT OF PAIN IN CHILDREN

Fill in the blanks.

1. To assess pain in infants, the nurse looks for _____ and _____ responses.

2. As infants get older, their responses to pain change from generalized to _____ responses.

3. It is important for the nurse to distinguish between cries of pain and cries associated with _____ in infants.

4. Toddlers may react to pain with generalized _____.

5. Preschoolers may think that pain is a _____.

6. Give two reasons why a school-age child might overreact to pain.

   a. _____

   b. _____

7. How does adolescent egocentrism affect how adolescents communicate about pain?

8. Why is it imperative to use pain assessment tools with children?

9. Pain self-report tools are usually appropriate for children older than _____ years.

10. Which pain assessment tool uses a photographic scale as well as a numeric scale?

1. What are the benefits of regulated breathing techniques?

2. Explain how children who are using distraction are not necessarily pain free.

3. Guided imagery involves _____, _____, and _____.

4. What is biofeedback?

5. What are the benefits of progressive muscle relaxation in older children?

6. What is hypnosis?

7. A transcutaneous electrical nerve stimulator (TENS) unit interferes with the _____.

8. For children receiving patient-controlled analgesia (PCA) therapy, what drug should be readily available?

9. If naloxone (Narcan) is administered too rapidly, _____ may result.

Answer as either true (T) or false (F).

10. _____ Eutectic mixture of local anesthetic(s) (EMLA) cream is effective within 10 minutes of application.

11. _____ Nonsteroidal anti-inflammatory drugs (NSAIDs) reduce pain and inflammation.

12. _____ Acetaminophen does not inhibit prostaglandin.

13. _____ Opioid analgesics can cause sedation and respiratory depression.

14. _____ Meperidine (Demerol) is more effective than morphine in children.

15. _____ Midazolam (Versed) is used for conscious sedation.

16. _____ Epidural opioid analgesia has fewer side effects than intravenous (IV) opioid analgesia.

17. _____ Narcan may need to be repeated after 30 to 60 minutes because of its short half-life.

SUGGESTED LEARNING ACTIVITIES

1. Interview a pediatric nurse about his or her experiences with managing pain in children. Discover how the nurse assesses pain in children who have chronic pain. Ask the nurse to explain how he or she designs a plan for managing chronic pain in children.

2. Interview the parent of an infant or a toddler. Learn how the parent knows that the child is in pain.

STUDENT LEARNING APPLICATIONS

Enhance your learning by discussing your answers with other students.

An 8-year-old boy who weighs 30 kg is experiencing acute pain. The physician orders 3 mg of morphine sulfate intravenously every 4 hours for pain. The child receives 3 mg at 9 A.M. At 9:30 A.M., and he rates his pain as 0 on a 0-to-5 rating scale. At noon, he complains of "bad pain" and rates his pain as 5 on the same scale.

1. What do think about the child's order for pain medication? What changes may be required?

2. What other questions would you ask the child about his pain?

3. What questions would you ask the child about what else might be helpful in managing his pain?

4. How would you present your findings to the child's physician?

REVIEW QUESTIONS

Choose the correct answer.

1. The best indicator of pain in a 15-month-old toddler is:
   a. behavioral changes.
   b. changes in vital signs.
   c. the child's parents' assessment of the child's pain.
   d. the child's verbal response.

2. The side effects of opioid analgesics include:
   a. constipation.
   b. nausea.
   c. sedation.
   d. all of the above.

3. A 12-year-old had abdominal surgery at 10 A.M. She last received a dose of morphine at 5 P.M. At 8 P.M., the nurse enters her room and finds her playing a video game. When asked about her pain, the child rates it as 1 on a 0-to-5 rating scale. In this situation, playing a video game is an example of:
   a. imagery.
   b. distraction.
   c. play therapy.
   d. obsession.

4. A child's perception of pain is influenced by the:
   a. parental response to the child's pain.
   b. child's ethnic background.
   c. child's developmental stage.
   d. all of the above.

5. Postoperative pain is an example of:
   a. acute pain.
   b. conscious pain.
   c. chronic pain.
   d. objective pain.

6. Which drug is classified as an NSAID?
   a. Acetaminophen
   b. Codeine
   c. Ibuprofen
   d. Midazolam

7. Which statement about children and pain and its management is true?
   a. Children can easily become addicted to opioid analgesics.
   b. Children who are playing are not in pain.
   c. Past pain experiences affect how a child experiences pain.
   d. Children are more likely than adults to experience respiratory depression from narcotics.

8. Respiratory depression is a side effect of:
   a. acetaminophen.
   b. fentanyl.
   c. ketorolac.
   d. naloxone.

9. The drug Narcan:
   a. causes respiratory depression at high doses.
   b. is used as an antidote to an ibuprofen overdose.
   c. is a topical anesthetic.
   d. is used to reverse the sedative effects of morphine.

10. IV fentanyl is prescribed for a child who is about to have a chest tube placed. Fentanyl is an appropriate analgesic choice for this procedure because:
    a. it is more potent than meperidine.
    b. it releases less histamine than other analgesics.
    c. it is shorter acting than morphine.
    d. all of these reasons apply.

40 The Child with a Fluid and Electrolyte Alteration

Review the concepts of fluid and electrolyte balance in a biochemistry textbook.

MATCHING KEY TERMS

Match the term with its description.

1. _____ Acidosis

2. _____ Alkalosis

3. _____ Anuria

4. _____ Extracellular fluid (ECF)

5. _____ Hypernatremic (hypertonic) dehydration

6. _____ Hyponatremic (hypotonic) dehydration

7. _____ Intracellular fluid (ICF)

8. _____ Interstitial fluid

9. _____ Intravascular fluid

10. _____ Isonatremic (isotonic) dehydration

11. _____ Oliguria

a. Serum pH <7.35

b. Serum sodium >150 mEq/L

c. Serum pH >7.45

d. Fluid found within cells

e. Absence of urine formation

f. Condition that occurs when sodium concentration decreases below that of normal body fluids

g. Fluid found outside the cell

h. Fluid surrounding the cells, including lymph fluid

i. Fluid within the blood vessels

j. Diminished amounts of urine output

k. Condition that occurs when the sodium concentration is identical to that of the body fluids

REVIEW OF FLUID AND ELECTROLYTE IMBALANCES IN CHILDREN

Answer as either true (T) or false (F).

1. _____ Sensible water loss is water that is lost through the respiratory tract and the skin.

2. _____ Infants' higher metabolic rates make them more prone to fluid loss than older children.

3. _____ Infants' immature renal function increases their ability to concentrate urine.

4. _____ In a newborn, approximately 60% of body water is located in the extracellular compartment.

5. _____ Burns, fever, gastroenteritis, and respiratory infections can all result in a fluid volume deficit.

Fill in the blanks.

6. Children are more likely to lose _____ fluid when they have a fever.

7. Body fluids are composed of _____ and _____.

8. The primary electrolyte in the ECF is _____; the primary electrolytes in the ICF are _____ and _____.

9. The normal serum pH ranges from _____ to _____.

10. What three mechanisms operate to keep the serum pH within the normal range?

 a. _____

 b. _____

 c. _____

11. Two buffers that help maintain normal serum pH are _____ and _____.

12. If the serum pH drops below normal, the rate and depth of respirations will _____.

13. The kidneys help maintain normal serum pH by regulating _____ and _____ in the blood.

Match each disorder with its clinical manifestations.

14. _____ Hyponatremia

15. _____ Hypernatremia

16. _____ Hypokalemia

17. _____ Hyperkalemia

18. _____ Hypocalcemia

19. _____ Hypercalcemia

 a. Muscle weakness, leg cramps, and ileus

 b. Abdominal cramping; tachycardia; and cold, clammy skin

 c. Tetany, positive Chvostek's sign, and hypotension

 d. Itching, weakness, and bradycardia

 e. Flaccid paralysis and cardiac and respiratory arrest

 f. Thirst, peripheral edema, and seizures

Match each condition with its causes.

20. _____ Metabolic acidosis

21. _____ Metabolic alkalosis

22. _____ Respiratory acidosis

23. _____ Respiratory alkalosis

 a. Ketosis, tissue hypoxia, and bicarbonate loss

 b. Hyperventilation, sepsis, and compensation for metabolic acidosis

 c. Airway obstruction and respiratory failure

 d. Volume depletion and increased alkali intake

DEHYDRATION

Answer as either true (T) or false (F).

1. _____ Isotonic dehydration occurs when water and electrolytes are lost in the same proportion as they occur in the body.

2. _____ In dehydration, fluid loss occurs first in the ICF.

3. _____ An infant who has lost 7% of his body weight has moderate dehydration.

4. _____ Initial therapy in severe dehydration is aimed at preventing shock.

5. _____ When a child is severely dehydrated, electrolytes such as potassium are replaced by administering them via a slow IV push.

6. _____ Either Ringer's lactate solution or 0.9% sodium chloride is an appropriate fluid choice for parenteral rehydration.

7. _____ Diluted Gatorade is an acceptable oral rehydrating solution for a toddler.

227

DIARRHEA

1. Define *diarrhea*.

2. Diarrhea caused by infection is usually called _____.

3. List four other causes of diarrhea.

   a. _____

   b. _____

   c. _____

   d. _____

4. Why are sports drinks and colas inappropriate fluid choices for a child with diarrhea?

5. Explain why an infant with diarrhea should continue to receive breast milk or full-strength formula.

6. What common foods are generally well tolerated during diarrhea?

7. How can skin breakdown be prevented in infants with diarrhea?

VOMITING

Answer as either true (T) or false (F).

1. _____ Vomiting can result from allergic reactions.

2. _____ Emesis with a fecal odor may indicate a lower intestinal obstruction.

3. _____ Projectile vomiting is usually a result of overfeeding.

4. _____ Oral rehydrating solutions cannot be used when a child has vomited.

SUGGESTED LEARNING ACTIVITIES

1. Design an information sheet describing dehydration for new parents. Be sure to include the following information about dehydration: what causes it, what to look for, what to do if it occurs, when to call the physician, and other important information. Make your information sheet attractive, accurate, and concise.

2. Compare the ingredients in Pedialyte with those in Gatorade. How are they alike? How are they different?

Enhance your learning by discussing your answers with other students.

A 2-month-old boy is admitted to the hospital with severe dehydration.

1. As the child's nurse, what would you expect to find when assessing the following?

   Skin turgor

   Urine output

   Anterior fontanel

   Mucous membranes

   Pulse

   Blood pressure

   Sensorium

   Skin color

2. Because the child is not drinking, the physician orders IV fluids. The child presently weighs 9 lb, 4 oz. What are his 24-hour fluid maintenance requirements?

3. The child has not voided for at least 4 hours. The physician has included potassium chloride in the IV order. What problem does this pose? How would you handle it?

4. How will you recognize when the child is improving?

REVIEW QUESTIONS

Choose the correct answer.

1. An otherwise healthy infant is admitted to the hospital with dehydration and diarrhea. She is hyperirritable and agitated, and she has flushed skin and dry mucous membranes. The nurse suspects:
   a. hypercalcemia.
   b. hypokalemia.
   c. hyperkalemia.
   d. hypernatremia.

2. An infant who has been vomiting frequently is at risk for:
   a. metabolic acidosis.
   b. metabolic alkalosis.
   c. respiratory acidosis.
   d. respiratory alkalosis.

3. Which statement about the compensatory mechanisms that maintain a normal serum pH is true?
   a. If the serum pH increases above normal, the respiratory rate and depth increase.
   b. If the serum pH increases above normal, the kidneys conserve hydrogen ions.
   c. Bicarbonate is a chemical that buffers the ICF.
   d. Respiratory compensatory mechanisms work more slowly than renal mechanisms.

4. Indicators of dehydration in a 4-year-old child include:
   a. a heart rate of 120 beats/min (bpm) and sunken fontanel.
   b. a specific gravity of 1.010 and oliguria.
   c. weight gain and the absence of tears.
   d. thirst and specific gravity of 1.038.

5. Infants with dehydration must be monitored for signs of impending shock. A late sign of shock in the infant is:
   a. decreased blood pressure.
   b. elevated heart rate.
   c. change in skin color.
   d. change in sensorium.

6. A preschooler with moderate diarrhea who is just admitted to the hospital and who is not nothing-by-mouth (NPO) status wants something to drink. The nurse's best choice is to offer:
   a. an oral rehydrating solution.
   b. bottled water.
   c. diluted apple juice.
   d. low-fat milk.

229

7. An infant with diarrhea has tolerated clear liquids but begins having diarrhea again when she returns to her regular formula. Her diet should be changed to:
   a. boiled skim milk.
   b. soy formula.
   c. IV fluids.
   d. Pedialyte.

8. A child weighing 14 kg is receiving maintenance IV fluids. How many milliliters per hour should the child receive?
   a. 14
   b. 24
   c. 50
   d. 100

9. An infant weighed 6.4 kg at the pediatrician's office 2 days ago. He has had diarrhea since then. He now weighs 5.9 kg. His mucous membranes are dry, his fontanel is sunken, and his capillary refill is approximately five seconds. The infant has:
   a. hypotonic dehydration.
   b. moderate dehydration.
   c. hypernatremic dehydration.
   d. severe dehydration.

10. An infant has viral gastroenteritis. To prevent its spread to other family members, the nurse teaches the family:
    a. proper handwashing techniques.
    b. how to administer antidiarrheal medications.
    c. how to administer antibiotics.
    d. how to calculate daily fluid requirements.

41 The Child with an Infectious Disease

MATCHING KEY TERMS

Match the term with the correct definition.

1. _____ Antitoxin

2. _____ Exanthem

3. _____ Host

4. _____ Immunoglobulin

5. _____ Immunity

6. _____ Infection

7. _____ Inflammation

8. _____ Pathogen

9. _____ Prodrome

10. _____ Toxin

11. _____ Vector

12. _____ Virulence

a. Poison produced by a pathogenic microorganism

b. Invasion of the body by another organism

c. Organism from which a parasite obtains its nourishment

d. Strength of the effect produced by a pathogenic organism

e. Eruption or rash on the skin

f. Resistance of the body to the effects of harmful organisms

g. Microorganism that causes a disease

h. Carrier that transfers an infective agent from one host to another

i. Vaccine made from the pooled blood of a large number of people to ensure a broad spectrum of antibodies

j. Initial stage of a disease

k. A tissue response to injury or the destruction of cells

l. A particular type of antibody produced by the body in response to the presence of a toxin

13. What is epidemiology?

REVIEW OF DISEASE TRANSMISSION

Match each mode of infection transmission with its corresponding example.

1. Airborne route

2. Fecal-oral transmission

3. Direct contact transmission

4. Vector-borne route

5. Direct inoculation

a. Infection contracted through the use of contaminated needles

b. Transmission of disease through sexual activity

c. Illness that results from a deer tick bite

d. Infection caused by pathogens shed through sneezing or coughing

e. Illness that results from poor handwashing practices

INFECTION AND HOST DEFENSES

1. The first lines of defense in an intact immune system are the _____ and

   _____ .

IMMUNITY

Match each vaccine with its description.

1. _____ Live or attenuated

2. _____ Killed or inactivated

3. _____ Toxoid

4. _____ Human immunoglobulin

5. _____ Antitoxin

a. Bacterial toxins that have been inactivated by either chemicals or heat

b. Vaccine derived from the sera of immunized animals

c. Vaccine that contains a pathogen that has had its virulence diminished

d. Vaccine made from the pooled blood of many donors

e. Contains pathogens inactivated by either chemicals or heat

VIRAL INFECTIONS

Match each virus with its description.

1. _____ Cytomegalovirus (CMV)

2. _____ Epstein–Barr virus

3. _____ Fifth disease

4. _____ Mumps

5. _____ Poliomyelitis

6. _____ Rabies

7. _____ Roseola infantum

8. _____ Rubella

9. _____ Rubeola

10. _____ Varicella-zoster

11. _____ Variola

a. Infection may proceed to flaccid paralysis.

b. Rash appears after fever subsides.

c. Acute signs of fever, pharyngitis, lymphadenopathy, and hepatospleno-megaly continue for 2 to 4 weeks, followed by a gradual recovery.

d. Virus remains latent in a sensory nerve ending and the dorsal root ganglion and may be reactivated at a later time.

e. The vaccine can be administered after exposure to the virus.

f. This is a common cause of congenital infections in infants.

g. Koplik spots in the buccal mucosa appear 2 days before the red, macu-lopapular rash.

h. Its classic sign is parotid glandular swelling.

i. This is a mild systemic disease with a fiery red edematous facial rash followed by a maculopapular rash on the trunk and extremities.

j. Infection during the first trimester of pregnancy has serious conse-quences for the fetus.

k. Although eradicated worldwide, it has the potential for being used as a bioterrorism weapon.

12. Why is the inactivated polio vaccine (IPV) the only polio vaccine available in the United States?

BACTERIAL, RICKETTSIAL, BORRELIA, HELMINTH, AND FUNGAL INFECTIONS

Answer as either true (T) or false (F).

1. _____ Pertussis is a highly contagious disease associated with a high infant mortality rate.

2. _____ Scarlet fever is caused by group A beta-hemolytic streptococci.

3. _____ In both Lyme disease and Rocky Mountain spotted fever, the vector is a tick.

4. _____ When a child is diagnosed with a helminthic infection, treatment is usually administered to the entire family.

5. _____ Frequent handwashing can prevent the spread of parasitic infections.

6. _____ Manifestations of fungal infections quickly appear after the child contracts the organism.

7. _____ A bullseye rash may be a manifestation of diphtheria.

8. _____ Children should receive a pertussis booster (Tdap) at 11 to 12 years of age.

SEXUALLY TRANSMITTED DISEASES (STDs)

Match each disease with its treatment(s). Diseases may have more than one treatment.

1. _____ Gonorrhea

2. _____ Syphilis

3. _____ Chlamydia

4. _____ Trichomoniasis

5. _____ Human papilloma virus (HPV)

6. _____ Bacterial vaginosis

7. _____ Herpes simplex virus, type 2 (HSV 2)

a. Metronidazole

b. Erythromycin

c. Clindamycin

d. Ceftriaxone

e. Acyclovir

f. Penicillin G

g. Surgical removal of the lesions

h. Doxycycline

Answer as either true (T) or false (F).

8. _____ Many teens are not aware that participating in oral sex places them at risk for STDs.

9. _____ The HPV vaccine is administered in a three-dose series.

10. _____ Bacterial vaginosis in a child who is not sexually active indicates that the child has been sexually abused.

11. _____ There is no cure for HSV 2.

SUGGESTED LEARNING ACTIVITIES

1. Obtain information from the local health department on STDs. Plan a presentation to adolescents on preventing STDs with the information you gather.

STUDENT LEARNING APPLICATIONS

Seven-year-old Jodie has been admitted to the hospital for oxygen therapy and IV antibiotics for the treatment of pneumonia. Ten days ago, her best friend presented with chickenpox. Jodie has never had chickenpox and has not yet received the varicella vaccine. Two days after admission, Jodie develops a macular rash on her trunk and scalp, and her fever returns.

1. Will Jodie require isolation?

2. Will she be administered acyclovir? Why or why not?

3. Will she be administered the varicella-zoster immunoglobulin? Why or why not?

When entering Jodie's room to take vital signs, the nurse finds her crying. She refuses to eat her lunch, saying she wants to go to the playroom.

4. How should the nurse handle this situation?

Jodie is uncomfortable from the itching caused by the skin lesions. You find her scratching her arms and trunk.

5. What interventions would you implement to relieve the itching and prevent Jodie from scratching?

REVIEW QUESTIONS

Choose the correct answer.

1. Congenital rubella may result in:
   a. encephalitis.
   b. cardiac anomalies.
   c. hydronephrosis.
   d. neural tube defects.

2. Splenic rupture is a complication of:
   a. CMV infection.
   b. Epstein–Barr virus.
   c. erythema infectiosum.
   d. varicella-zoster.

3. Which intervention is appropriate when caring for a child with pertussis?
   a. Monitoring intake and output
   b. Administering a cough suppressant
   c. Providing the child with periods of uninterrupted rest
   d. Administering erythromycin

4. A "white strawberry tongue" is a clinical manifestation of which infectious disease?
   a. Poliomyelitis
   b. Roseola
   c. Rubeola
   d. Scarlet fever

5. Using an insect repellent when in the woods can help prevent:
   a. CMV infection.
   b. helminth infections.
   c. Rocky Mountain spotted fever.
   d. scarlet fever.

6. An adolescent comes to the clinic because she has dysuria, urinary frequency, and a mucopurulent discharge. These signs are manifestations of which STD?
   a. HSV 2
   b. Syphilis
   c. Chlamydia
   d. HPV

7. Which statement regarding STDs is false?
   a. Sexual abuse is suspected when a toddler has a gonorrheal infection.
   b. Syphilis can be transmitted to the fetus through the placenta.
   c. Males with trichomoniasis usually have urethral discharge and dysuria.
   d. Chronic respiratory problems are complications of a neonatal chlamydial infection.

8. Which statement describes the rash associated with Lyme disease?
   a. Erythematous maculopapular rash surrounded by a whitish ring
   b. Fine, red papular rash that appears within 24 hours of the tick bite
   c. Petechial rash that begins on extremities and spreads to the rest of the body
   d. Erythematous macula or papule with a clearing in the center

42 The Child with an Immunologic Alteration

HELPFUL HINT

Review the immune system in an anatomy and physiology textbook.

MATCHING KEY TERMS

Match the term with the correct definition.

1. _____ Active immunity

2. _____ Allergy

3. _____ Antibody

4. _____ Antigen

5. _____ Autoimmune disease

6. _____ Complement

7. _____ Immune system

8. _____ Immunodeficiency

9. _____ Leukocytes

10. _____ Lymphocytes

11. _____ Nonspecific immune functions

12. _____ Passive immunity

13. _____ Specific immune functions

a. Blood cells that mainly function to protect the body against foreign substances

b. Production of autoantibodies against cells of the body by the immune system

c. Protection that occurs when serum containing an antibody is administered to someone without the antibody

d. Protection that follows an exposure to an antigen

e. A defect in the immune system that places a person at a high risk for an infection

f. Hypersensitivity reaction

g. Primary white blood cells of the immune system

h. Body's internal defense against foreign substances

i. Substance identified by the immune system as foreign

j. Protein produced by the immune system that binds to specific antigens and eliminates them from the body

k. Accessory system to a humoral response composed of proteins that facilitate enzyme action and antigen death

l. Humoral- and cell-mediated responses that are activated in a highly discriminatory manner

m. Protective barriers that are activated in the presence of an antigen but are not specific to that antigen

REVIEW OF THE IMMUNE SYSTEM

Match the cells with their functions.

1. _____ Neutrophils

2. _____ Eosinophils

3. _____ Basophils

4. _____ Monocytes

5. _____ B lymphocytes

6. _____ T lymphocytes

7. _____ Helper (CD4+) T cells

8. _____ Suppressor T cells

9. _____ Cytotoxic (CD8+) T cells

a. Directly kill target cells

b. Are responsible for cellular immunity

c. Are the first leukocytes to respond to tissue damage

d. Ingest and introduce antigens into the circulation

e. Inhibit the actions of helper T and B cells

f. Neutralize histamine

g. Are responsible for humoral immunity

h. Secrete lymphokines that stimulate B cells to manufacture antibodies

i. Secrete histamine, heparin, and serotonin in inflammatory and hypersensitivity reactions

Answer as either true (T) or false (F).

10. _____ The production of antibodies signals the beginning of the nonspecific immune response.

11. _____ The immune complexes include the bone marrow, thymus, spleen, and lymph nodes and tissues.

12. _____ Antibodies are also called immunoglobulins.

13. _____ Transfer of maternal antibodies to the fetus via the placenta is an example of active immunity.

HUMAN IMMUNODEFICIENCY VIRUS (HIV) INFECTION

1. Name three ways HIV infection can be transmitted from a mother to child.

   a. _____

   b. _____

   c. _____

2. The rate of HIV transmission from a mother to child decreases when both receive _____.

3. Describe the prophylaxis for *Pneumocystis jirovecii* (formerly *Pneumocystis carinii*) pneumonia (PCP) for an infant exposed to HIV.

4. List the four goals of HIV treatment.

   a. _____

   b. _____

   c. _____

   d. _____

CORTICOSTEROID THERAPY

1. How do corticosteroids cause immunosuppression?

2. Why is it dangerous to abruptly discontinue the administration of corticosteroid medication?

3. Corticosteroid excess is diagnosed by administering a bolus of _____.

4. If long-term use of corticosteroids is required, they are usually prescribed to be taken _____.

5. In a child receiving corticosteroids, what can be done to minimize the risk for gastrointestinal (GI) bleeding?

   What can be done to deal with an increased appetite?

IMMUNE COMPLEX AND AUTOIMMUNE DISORDERS

1. Give two examples of immune complex disorders.

   a. _____

   b. _____

2. What are autoantibodies?

Answer as either true (T) or false (F).

3. _____ Systemic lupus erythematosus (SLE) has periods of remission and exacerbation.

4. _____ SLE affects more males than females.

5. _____ In SLE, antinuclear antibodies are present.

6. _____ In SLE, systemic corticosteroids are used to control the inflammatory process.

7. _____ The clinical manifestations of SLE depend on which body systems are affected.

8. _____ Antimalarial drugs are used to treat renal disorders in SLE.

ALLERGIC REACTIONS AND ANAPHYLAXIS

1. What is an allergy?

Match each allergic reaction with its example.

2. _____ Immediate hypersensitivity

3. _____ Cytotoxic hypersensitivity

4. _____ Arthus hypersensitivity

5. _____ Delayed cell-mediated hypersensitivity

a. Transfusion reaction

b. Asthma

c. Poison ivy

d. Post-streptococcal glomerulonephritis

237

6. List the most serious features of anaphylaxis.

7. What is an *EpiPen?*

8. What is a *biphasic reaction?*

9. What is the primary cause of anaphylaxis in children?

SUGGESTED LEARNING ACTIVITIES

1. Many communities have support groups for people with SLE. Contact one in your community and arrange to attend a meeting. Report on the meeting to your class.

STUDENT LEARNING APPLICATIONS

Caring for a child with an HIV infection or AIDS can be very challenging from both physical and psychosocial perspectives. It is important for health care professionals to be aware of their own feelings regarding the disease. Think about the following questions and then discuss them with a family member, friend, or another student.

1. Which aspects of caring for a child with HIV or AIDS would you personally find the most difficult?
   - Providing physical care

   - Worrying about contracting HIV from the child

   - Dealing with the child's family

   - Knowing that the child has a life-threatening illness

   - Meeting the child's psychosocial needs

2. If the child prenatally contracted HIV, how would you feel about the child's mother? Could you remain non-judgmental and supportive?

3. Which of the following HIV-positive adolescents would be most difficult for you to care for? The least difficult? Why?
   - A 14-year-old who uses illegal intravenous drugs

   - A 16-year-old who is a teenage prostitute

   - A 17-year-old who is homosexual

REVIEW QUESTIONS

Choose the correct answer.

1. When the immune system fails to differentiate the body's cells from foreign cells, which event occurs?
   a. Active immunity
   b. Autoimmune response
   c. Cell-mediated response
   d. Humoral response

2. IgA:
   a. crosses the placenta.
   b. provides antibacterial protection.
   c. passes to the neonate through breast milk.
   d. influences B-cell differentiation.

3. The test used to assess the immune status of an HIV-positive child is:
   a. CD4+count.
   b. enzyme-linked immunosorbent assay (ELISA).
   c. HIV culture.
   d. p24 antigen.

4. In teaching a family about corticosteroids, which statement should the nurse *not* include?
   a. "Take the medication with food or milk."
   b. "Do not abruptly discontinue the medication."
   c. "The drug may mask usual signs of infection."
   d. "Changes in physical appearance are permanent but minor."

5. Signs of SLE include:
   a. erythema marginatum, carditis, and chorea.
   b. discoid rash, photosensitivity, and positive antinuclear antibody (ANA) test.
   c. fever, erythematous rash, and strawberry tongue.
   d. laryngospasm, edema, and hypotension.

6. The antibody involved in allergic reactions is:
   a. IgA.
   b. IgD.
   c. IgE.
   d. IgG.

7. Most children with HIV are infected:
   a. through blood and blood products.
   b. perinatally.
   c. through sexual abuse.
   d. through the failure to use standard precautions.

8. Prophylaxis for PCP includes:
   a. trimethoprim-sulfamethoxazole.
   b. corticosteroids.
   c. immunoglobulins.
   d. all of the above.

9. The school nurse is discussing an upcoming field trip to the zoo with two sixth graders who are allergic to bees. Which statement indicates that the students need further clarification about their condition?
   a. "I'll make sure that I wear khakis instead of jeans that day."
   b. "When bees come near me, I run away as fast as I can."
   c. "If I have to use my EpiPen, I can inject it right into my thigh without pulling down my sweat pants."
   d. "I'll keep the windows on the bus closed."

43 The Child with a Gastrointestinal Alteration

HELPFUL HINT

Review the anatomy and physiology of the gastrointestinal (GI) tract in an anatomy and physiology textbook.

MATCHING KEY TERMS

Match the term with the correct definition.

1. _____ Achalasia
2. _____ Atresia
3. _____ Azotemia
4. _____ Dysphagia
5. _____ Encopresis
6. _____ Fistula
7. _____ Fundoplication
8. _____ Hematemesis
9. _____ Melena
10. _____ Occult bleeding
11. _____ Peristalsis
12. _____ Projectile vomiting
13. _____ Pylorus
14. _____ Tenesmus

a. Presence of urea in the blood

b. Distal opening of the stomach

c. Black, tarry stools, indicating bleeding

d. Abnormal passage between two organs

e. Progressive wave-like motions that propel fluid and food through the GI tract

f. Failure of the smooth muscle fibers of the GI tract to relax

g. Incontinence of feces

h. Surgical wrapping of the stomach fundus around the distal esophagus to prevent gastric reflux

i. Forceful vomiting

j. Abnormal closure or the absence of a body passage or orifice

k. Vomiting of blood, either red or "coffee grounds"

l. Inability to swallow or difficulty in swallowing

m. Bleeding that is detectable only by microscopic or chemical means

n. Ineffective, painful, or continuous urge to defecate

REVIEW OF THE GASTROINTESTINAL SYSTEM

1. What are the primary functions of the upper GI system?

2. What are the primary functions of the lower GI system?

3. What are the functions of the liver?

4. Prenatally, how are nutrients brought to and waste products removed from the fetus?

DISORDERS OF PRENATAL DEVELOPMENT

Answer as either true (T) or false (F).

1. _____ The diagnosis of cleft lip and palate can be determined through inspection.

2. _____ Infants with a cleft lip are at risk for problems that involve parent–infant attachment.

3. _____ Cleft palate repair precedes a cleft lip repair.

4. _____ To keep a cleft palate repair incision site clean, the nurse gives water after all feedings.

5. _____ Children with cleft palates require frequent hearing tests.

Fill in the blanks.

6. _____ is a significant prenatal clue in the diagnosis of a tracheoesophageal fistula (TEF).

7. An infant with TEF is at constant risk for _____.

8. What are the "3 Cs" that suggest TEF?

    a. _____

    b. _____

    c. _____

9. How does an infant with TEF receive nutrition before surgery?

10. Describe how to care for an esophagostomy.

Match each disorder with its description.

11. _____ Hiatal hernia

12. _____ Congenital diaphragmatic hernia

13. _____ Imperforate anus

14. _____ Gastroschisis

15. _____ Omphalocele

16. _____ Umbilical hernia

a. Condition in which the viscera are outside of the abdominal cavity and not covered with a sac

b. Incomplete development of the anus

c. Protrusion of a portion of the stomach through the esophageal hiatus of the diaphragm

d. Herniation of the gut into the umbilical cord

e. Herniation of abdominal contents into the thoracic cavity through the diaphragm

f. Condition in which the gut pushes outward at the umbilicus during straining or crying

MOTILITY DISORDERS

1. Describe the home dietary management of gastroesophageal reflux (GER) in a 5-month-old infant.

2. List the drugs used to treat GER that have the following actions:

   a. Decrease acid secretions

   b. Accelerate gastric emptying

   c. Offer barrier protection

   d. Suppress gastric acid secretion

3. Describe how chronic constipation can lead to encopresis.

4. _____ is considered to be a common cause of irritable bowel syndrome (IBS).

5. List the clinical manifestations of IBS.

INFLAMMATORY AND INFECTIOUS DISEASES

Answer as either true (T) or false (F).

1. _____ Stress ulcers are considered primary ulcers.

2. _____ Dietary management of ulcers includes a bland diet with added milk.

3. _____ *Helicobacter pylori* is a bacteria associated with duodenal ulcers.

4. _____ *Giardia* is the most common pathogen that causes gastroenteritis in daycare settings.

5. _____ Antimicrobials are used to treat infections caused by rotavirus.

6. _____ In gastroenteritis, dehydration and electrolyte imbalances must be promptly corrected.

7. _____ Headache, irritability, nuchal rigidity, and seizures are manifestations of *Salmonella*.

8. _____ The cardinal symptom of appendicitis is pain that eventually localizes at the McBurney point.

9. _____ Sudden cessation of pain in a child with appendicitis is indicative of spontaneous remission.

10. Describe the differences between Crohn disease and ulcerative colitis.

11. Which four categories of drugs are used to treat IBS?

   a.

   b.

   c.

   d.

OBSTRUCTIVE DISORDERS

1. Describe the vomiting that occurs with pyloric stenosis.

2. The classic signs of intussusception include _____.

3. How is hydrostatic reduction of an intussusception attempted?

4. _____ is caused by a malrotation of the bowel.

5. What is the cardinal sign of Hirschsprung disease in the newborn?

6. A life-threatening complication of Hirschsprung disease is _____.

MALABSORPTION DISORDERS

Answer as either true (T) or false (F).

1. _____ Isomil is an appropriate formula for an infant with lactose intolerance.

2. _____ Celiac disease results from the inability to digest celiac.

3. _____ Corn and rice products must be avoided in celiac disease.

4. _____ Corticosteroids are used to decrease mucosal inflammation in celiac disease.

HEPATIC DISORDERS

For each type of hepatitis, list its mode(s) of transmission.

1. Hepatitis A (HAV)

2. Hepatitis B (HBV)

3. Hepatitis C (HCV)

4. Hepatitis D (HDV)

5. Hepatitis E (HEV)

6. Hepatitis G (HGV)

7. List the clinical manifestations for each of the following:

    a. Anicteric phase of acute hepatitis

    b. Icteric phase of acute hepatitis

    c. Fulminating hepatitis

8. Vaccinations are currently available for which forms of hepatitis?

Answer as either true (T) or false (F).

9. _____ The hepatitis B vaccine protects against both HBV and HDV.

10. _____ The available hepatitis vaccines are recommended for all infants and children who are not immunocompromised.

11. _____ HCV is the major indication for liver transplantation in children.

12. _____ The Kasai procedure corrects biliary atresia.

13. _____ In biliary atresia, fat-soluble vitamins are not absorbed.

14. _____ Pruritus can be alleviated with colloidal oatmeal baths.

15. _____ Manifestations of portal hypertension include ascites, GI bleeding, and splenomegaly.

Fill in the blanks.

16. The three major complications of cirrhosis are _____, _____,

    and _____.

17. _____ is the definitive therapy for cirrhosis.

SUGGESTED LEARNING ACTIVITIES

1. Role play with another student. In this scenario, one of you is the nurse and the other is the parent of a newborn with a cleft lip and palate. The "parent" refuses to hold or even look at the infant. How would the "nurse" promote parent–infant attachment in this situation? You may want to include another student as an observer/"coach."

2. Observe one of the diagnostic procedures discussed in this chapter, such as fiberoptic endoscopy, abdominal flat plate X-ray, or colonoscopy. Based on your observations and readings, design a teaching plan for the observed procedure for an 8-year-old child.

STUDENT LEARNING APPLICATIONS

Enhance your learning by discussing your answers with other students.
    Melissa, aged 16 years, has just been diagnosed with Crohn disease.

1. From what you know about adolescent development, what would you guess Melissa's chief concerns are about this diagnosis?

2. As her nurse, how would you determine whether your guesses are accurate?

3. How might this disease affect Melissa's physical and psychosocial development?

4. Melissa tells you, "Well, I guess this means that I won't be going to college." How would you respond to this statement?

Choose the correct answer.

1. At his 1-year-old checkup, you note that Jason has thin arms and legs and abdominal distention. His mother reports that he has been irritable, has lost his appetite, and has foul-smelling stools. He has fallen behind on the growth chart. Jason probably has:
   a. Crohn disease.
   b. Hirschsprung disease.
   c. IBS.
   d. celiac disease.

2. Which intervention is *not* appropriate following surgery for Hirschsprung disease?
   a. Assessing the surgical site for swelling, redness, and drainage
   b. Monitoring the rectal temperature every four hours for evidence of a fever
   c. Reuniting the parents with the child as soon as possible
   d. Keeping the child nothing by mouth (NPO) until bowel sounds return

3. A 5-year-old, admitted to rule out appendicitis, tells the nurse, "It doesn't hurt anymore." The nurse suspects that the child:
   a. is afraid of surgery.
   b. has a ruptured appendix.
   c. wants to please the nurse.
   d. cannot accurately communicate about the pain.

4. A 6-year-old is admitted to the hospital with severe abdominal pain, bloody diarrhea, high fever, headache, and nuchal rigidity. The child probably has:
   a. an intussusception.
   b. cirrhosis.
   c. a perforated appendix.
   d. a *Shigella* infection.

5. For the child with encopresis, mineral oil is often prescribed to:
   a. facilitate the absorption of fat-soluble vitamins.
   b. eliminate pain associated with bowel movements.
   c. evacuate fecal impactions.
   d. initiate normal gastrocolic reflex.

6. An adolescent has just been diagnosed with an ulcer. Which statement indicates that she requires clarification about her therapeutic regimen?
   a. "I won't take my ulcer medication and milk of magnesia close together."
   b. "I'll switch to orange soda from cola."
   c. "I'll take two Motrin when the pain comes back."
   d. "I'll stay away from cigarette smoke."

7. When performing a newborn assessment, the nurse observes that the infant is cyanotic and has nasal flaring and retractions. In addition, no breath sounds can be auscultated on the left side, and an apical pulse is palpated on the right side of the sternum. The nurse immediately notifies the physician because which condition is suspected?
   a. A tracheoesophageal fistula
   b. A cleft palate
   c. Pyloric stenosis
   d. A diaphragmatic hernia

8. Careful handwashing before and after patient contact can prevent the spread of:
   a. hepatitis A.
   b. volvulus.
   c. ulcerative colitis.
   d. all of the above.

9. A child with lactose intolerance may be able to drink milk if it is taken with:
   a. Colace.
   b. Lactaid.
   c. lactulose.
   d. Lomotil.

10. In teaching parents about the use of elbow restraints following the surgical repair of a cleft lip, which statement should the nurse *not* include?
    a. "Restraints may be removed for sleep."
    b. "Remove the restraints for 10 or 15 minutes every 2 hours."
    c. "Apply the restraints loosely but tight enough to prevent elbow bending."
    d. "Continue to use the restraints for 8 days."

11. A newborn with a TEF is waiting for a transfer to a neonatal intensive care unit. The nurse's priority intervention is:
    a. arranging for transportation.
    b. preventing aspiration.
    c. providing psychosocial support for the parents.
    d. providing small, frequent feedings.

12. Which test is not typically ordered when GER is suspected?
    a. Fiberoptic endoscopy
    b. Barium enema
    c. pH studies
    d. Scintigraphy

13. Which dietary modification is appropriate for GER?
    a. An infant is given small, frequent, thickened feedings.
    b. A toddler eats solid foods before drinking liquids.
    c. A school-age child avoids colas and chocolate.
    d. All of the above are appropriate.

14. Which vaccine is currently being developed but is not yet available?
    a. Vaccine for hepatitis A
    b. Vaccine for rotavirus
    c. Vaccine for *H. pylori*
    d. All of these vaccines are currently available.

44 The Child with a Genitourinary Alteration

HELPFUL HINT

Review the anatomy and physiology of the renal system in an anatomy and physiology textbook.

MATCHING KEY TERMS

Match the term with the correct definition.

1. _____ Arteriovenous fistula
2. _____ Arteriovenous graft
3. _____ Dysuria
4. _____ Edema
5. _____ Frequency
6. _____ Hypercalciuria
7. _____ Hyperlipidemia
8. _____ Hypoalbuminemia
9. _____ Proteinuria
10. _____ Urgency

a. Sudden urge to urinate
b. Excessive calcium in the urine
c. Presence of protein in the urine
d. Tube inserted between an artery and a vein for hemodialysis
e. Presence of abnormally large amounts of fluid in intercellular spaces of the body
f. Connection between an artery and a vein
g. Low levels of albumin in the blood
h. High levels of serum cholesterol and triglycerides
i. Pain when urinating
j. Urination at short time intervals

REVIEW OF THE GENITOURINARY SYSTEM

1. The newborn's bladder is located in the _____ cavity.

2. Children's shorter urethras predispose them to _____.

3. The _____ is the kidney's functional unit.

4. A child's bladder capacity is approximately equal to _____ mL/kg of body weight.

5. Normal urine pH ranges from _____ to _____.

ENURESIS

Answer as either true (T) or false (F).

1. _____ Nocturnal enuresis in a 4-year-old requires medical evaluation.

2. _____ Diurnal enuresis may be helped by biofeedback.

3. _____ Primary enuresis results from excessive calcium loss in the urine.

4. _____ Imipramine, an antidepressant, may be prescribed for nocturnal enuresis.

5. _____ Secondary enuresis may be the result of stress.

URINARY TRACT INFECTIONS (UTIs)

Match each disorder with its description.

1. _____ Cystitis

2. _____ Pyelonephritis

3. _____ Hydronephrosis

4. _____ Vesicoureteral reflux

a. Structural defect that allows urine to backflow into the ureters

b. Inflammation of the bladder

c. Kidney infection

d. Dilation of the renal pelvis

Fill in the blanks.

5. The diagnostic study for an UTI is _____.

6. Bladder catheterization and _____ are two invasive ways of collecting a urine specimen that will accurately detect bacteria in the urine.

7. A voiding cystourethrogram is ordered to detect _____.

8. Pyelonephritis is treated with _____ antibiotics.

9. Hypertension in childhood might result from renal scarring caused by _____.

10. List five ways of preventing UTIs in young children.

    a. _____

    b. _____

    c. _____

    d. _____

    e. _____

CRYPTORCHIDISM

Answer as either true (T) or false (F).

1. _____ Preterm infants have a higher incidence of cryptorchidism.

2. _____ Most infants with cryptorchidism require surgery.

3. _____ Orchidopexy is the surgical correction for cryptorchidism.

4. _____ Children with cryptorchidism are at an increased risk for testicular cancer.

HYPOSPADIAS AND EPISPADIAS

Fill in the blanks.

1. Infants with hypospadias should not be _____ before surgical correction.

2. Dorsal placement of the urethral opening in males is called _____; ventral placement is called _____.

3. _____ is a downward curvature of the penile shaft.

4. After surgery, urinary diversions, such as indwelling catheters or_____, are used to allow the meatus to heal.

MISCELLANEOUS DISORDERS AND ANOMALIES OF THE GENITOURINARY TRACT

Match each disorder with its description.

1. _____ Hydrocele

2. _____ Phimosis

3. _____ Testicular torsion

4. _____ Bladder exstrophy

5. _____ True hermaphroditism

a. Inability to retract the prepuce after approximately the age of 3 years

b. Presence of both ovarian and testicular tissues with abnormal genitalia

c. Painless swelling of the scrotum

d. Urinary bladder located outside of the body at birth

e. Surgical emergency presenting with the sudden onset of severe pain in the scrotum

ACUTE POST-STREPTOCOCCAL GLOMERULONEPHRITIS

1. List the clinical manifestations of acute post-streptococcal glomerulonephritis.

2. Describe the role that antigen–antibody complexes play in acute post-streptococcal glomerulonephritis.

3. In severe renal insufficiency, blood urea nitrogen (BUN) and creatinine levels _____.

4. _____ indicates that acute post-streptococcal glomerulonephritis is starting to resolve.

NEPHROTIC SYNDROME

1. List the clinical manifestations of nephrotic syndrome.

2. Which drug is initially used to achieve remission in nephrotic syndrome?

3. When is a child with nephrotic syndrome considered to be in remission?

ACUTE RENAL FAILURE

Match each disorder with the type of acute renal failure it causes. (Answers may be used more than once.)

1. _____ Glomerulonephritis   a. Prerenal

2. _____ Pyelonephritis   b. Intrarenal

3. _____ Dehydration   c. Postrenal

4. _____ Hemolytic uremic syndrome

5. _____ Hemorrhagic shock

6. _____ Neurogenic bladder

7. _____ Kidney stones

Answer as either true (T) or false (F).

8. _____ Hemolytic uremic syndrome is the most common cause of acute renal failure in children.

9. _____ Kayexalate is administered to manage hypokalemia.

10. _____ Hyponatremia results from a fluid overload in acute renal failure.

11. _____ In acute renal failure, children develop metabolic alkalosis.

CHRONIC RENAL FAILURE AND END-STAGE RENAL DISEASE (ESRD)

1. Dialysis removes _____ and _____ from the blood and regulates _____ and _____.

2. Vascular access for hemodialysis is achieved through a double-lumen central line or a(n) _____.

3. The chief hazard of peritoneal dialysis is _____.

4. Manifestations of ESRD include _____.

5. Children with ESRD require either dialysis or _____.

6. _____ is the most common complication of kidney transplantation.

7. Children with kidney transplants are at a higher risk for infection because of _____.

SUGGESTED LEARNING ACTIVITIES

1. Visit a dialysis center and interview one of the nurses. Report to your class on the most challenging aspects of the nurse's work.

2. Contact a medical supply company. Find out the cost of the equipment and supplies needed for peritoneal dialysis. Calculate the approximate cost per month. Find out whether the costs are covered entirely by medical insurance. Report to your class.

STUDENT LEARNING APPLICATIONS

Enhance your learning by discussing your answers with other students.

A 5-year-old is brought to the pediatrician by his parents, who have noticed that their son has "puffiness" around his eyes and ankles and that his "belly is getting bigger." They also report that "he's just not himself" and that he has no appetite. You find that his vital signs are within the normal limits for his age and sex. You note pitting edema of his lower extremities and abdomen. Urine tests are negative for occult blood and are +4 for protein.

1. Based on these findings, what would you expect the child's diagnosis to be?

After a brief hospitalization, the child is discharged home. He will be treated with prednisone, penicillin, and a no-added-salt diet.

2. What will you teach the family about the actions and side effects of prednisone and how to administer it?

3. The child's mother does not understand the need for penicillin "because the doctor said he does not have an infection." How will you explain this?

4. What will you teach the family about the reason for the no-added-salt diet?

After 2 weeks, the child goes into remission. At this point, the physician recommends a pneumococcal vaccination. The child's father responds to this recommendation by saying, "Why? All of my son's shots are up to date."

5. How will you address this?

REVIEW QUESTIONS

Choose the correct answer.

1. A 7-year-old with cystitis will require:
   a. a renal ultrasound.
   b. oral antibiotics.
   c. a suprapubic aspiration.
   d. all of the above.

2. A 9-year-old is admitted to the hospital with acute glomerulonephritis. In taking the child's history, the nurse is not surprised to find that the child has had:
   a. back pain for a few days.
   b. dysuria since the previous night.
   c. a history of hypertension.
   d. a sore throat last week.

3. A child with nephrotic syndrome who is steroid dependent:
   a. will have an antibiotic added to the steroid.
   b. initially responds well to prednisone but relapses while on a tapering schedule.
   c. requires a kidney biopsy to determine the exact cause of the disease.
   d. will eventually require dialysis.

4. A child with grade I vesicoureteral reflux is treated with:
   a. antibiotics.
   b. diuretics.
   c. muscle relaxants.
   d. surgery.

5. Recurrent UTIs are clinical manifestations of:
   a. enuresis.
   b. hypospadias.
   c. glomerulonephritis.
   d. vesicoureteral reflux.

6. Acute renal failure is suspected when a child presents with:
   a. dysuria and fever.
   b. oliguria and elevated BUN.
   c. edema and proteinuria.
   d. fatigue and hypertension.

7. A pale, listless 5-year-old is brought to the emergency department. The child has many bruises, decreased urine output, and bloody diarrhea. The nurse plans emergency care based on a suspicion of:
   a. child abuse.
   b. glomerulonephritis.
   c. hemolytic uremic syndrome.
   d. hemorrhagic shock.

8. The most common cause of chronic renal failure in children is:
   a. congenital renal abnormalities.
   b. insulin-dependent diabetes.
   c. hemolytic uremic syndrome.
   d. nephrotoxic antibiotic use.

9. Corticosteroids are used in the treatment of:
   a. glomerulonephritis.
   b. nephrotic syndrome.
   c. phimosis.
   d. vesicoureteral reflux.

10. In a child with ESRD, recombinant erythropoietin is used to treat:
    a. the rejection of a transplanted kidney.
    b. renal osteodystrophy.
    c. hypertension.
    d. anemia.

Review the anatomy and physiology of the respiratory system in an anatomy and physiology textbook.

MATCHING KEY TERMS

Match the term with the correct definition.

1. _____ Atelectasis		a. Abnormal movement of the chest wall during inspiration
2. _____ Crackles		b. Sound, similar to a grunting noise, that can be heard with or without a stethoscope
3. _____ Dysphagia		c. Shrill, harsh sound heard during inspiration, expiration, or both
4. _____ Dyspnea		d. Increased respiratory rate
5. _____ Grunting		e. Widening of the nares that indicates air hunger
6. _____ Hypercapnia		f. Increased levels of carbon dioxide in the blood
7. _____ Hypocapnia		g. Difficulty breathing except in an upright position
8. _____ Hypoxemia		h. Collapsed or airless part of the lung
9. _____ Hypoxia		i. High-pitched musical whistles heard with or without a stethoscope
10. _____ Nasal flaring		j. Breath sounds caused by passage of air through thick secretions
11. _____ Nasal polyps		k. Difficulty breathing
12. _____ Orthopnea		l. Decreased levels of carbon dioxide in the blood
13. _____ Retractions		m. Rales
14. _____ Rhonchi		n. Decreased oxygenation of cells and tissues
15. _____ Stridor		o. Decreased levels of oxygen in the blood
16. _____ Tachypnea		p. Difficulty swallowing
17. _____ Wheezing		q. Semitransparent herniations of respiratory epithelium

REVIEW OF THE RESPIRATORY SYSTEM AND DIAGNOSTIC TESTS

Answer as either true (T) or false (F).

1. _____ Lack of surfactant places a preterm infant at risk for respiratory distress syndrome.

2. _____ Diffusion of gases occurs in the upper airway.

3. _____ The tonsils help filter circulating lymph fluid.

4. _____ Arterial blood gases are mainly used to assess acid–base balance.

5. _____ A sweat test is used to diagnose allergies.

6. _____ Pulse oximetry is used to measure oxygen saturation.

ALLERGIC RHINITIS

Fill in the blanks.

1. The onset of allergic rhinitis rarely occurs before the age of _____.

2. Classic manifestations of allergic rhinitis include: _____.

3. Describe how parents can prepare saline solutions.

SINUSITIS

Fill in the blanks.

1. Acute sinusitis often follows a(n) _____.

2. Chronic sinusitis is associated with allergic rhinitis and _____.

3. Pain associated with sinusitis may be relieved by administering _____ and

   applying _____.

OTITIS MEDIA

Answer as either true (T) or false (F).

1. _____ Risk factors for otitis media include using a pacifier after 6 months of age, attending a daycare center, and bottle feeding.

2. _____ Ear drainage indicates otitis media with effusion.

3. _____ Tympanostomy tubes usually spontaneously fall out.

PHARYNGITIS AND TONSILLITIS

Answer as either true (T) or false (F).

1. _____ Children with allergies to penicillin are usually administered erythromycin for viral pharyngitis.

2. _____ Abdominal pain and vomiting are manifestations of bacterial pharyngitis.

3. _____ Tonsillectomy reduces the incidence of recurrent pharyngitis.

LARYNGOMALACIA

1. The hallmark of laryngomalacia is _____.

CROUP

Match each type of croup with its description.

1. _____ Acute spasmodic croup   a. Occurs more often in anxious, excitable children

2. _____ Laryngotracheobronchitis   b. Bacterial form of croup

3. _____ Epiglottitis   c. Most common form of croup

4. _____ Tracheitis   d. Usually follows an upper respiratory infection

Answer as either true (T) or false (F).

5. _____ Children with laryngotracheobronchitis are typically afebrile.

6. _____ The Hib (*Haemophilus influenzae* type B) vaccine has reduced the incidence of tracheitis.

7. _____ Children who receive racemic epinephrine in the emergency department should be observed for at least 3 hours after treatment.

8. _____ Sedatives are frequently used to keep a child with croup calm.

EPIGLOTTITIS

Fill in the blanks.

1. Manifestations of epiglottitis include: _____

_____.

2. When epiglottitis is suspected, never use a _____ to inspect the child's throat.

BRONCHITIS

Fill in the blanks.

1. Bronchitis is usually caused by a _____.

2. Treatment includes _____, _____, and _____.

BRONCHIOLITIS

1. Respiratory syncytial virus (RSV) is the causative agent in bronchiolitis in more than _____% of cases.

2. Why is RSV so easily communicable?

3. Why do health care professionals maintain contact precautions when caring for infants with RSV?

4. What product is intramuscularly administered monthly during RSV season as an RSV prophylaxis in preterm infants?

PNEUMONIA

1. What can be done to promote pulmonary drainage in a child with pneumonia?

2. The oxygen saturation of a child with pneumonia, who has no underlying chronic pulmonary disease, should be maintained at >_____ SaO2 %.

FOREIGN BODY ASPIRATION

1. List six foods that are commonly aspirated by young children.

   a. _____

   b. _____

   c. _____

   d. _____

   e. _____

   f. _____

2. Manifestations of an obstructed airway in a child who has aspirated are _____ and _____.

PULMONARY NONINFECTIOUS IRRITATION

1. Acute respiratory distress syndrome can be precipitated by _____, _____, _____, _____, and _____.

2. _____ is associated with bronchial hyperresponsiveness in children.

3. _____ poisoning is a complication of smoke inhalation.

APNEA

Match each term with its description.

1. _____ Apnea

2. _____ Periodic breathing

3. _____ Apparent life-threatening event

a. Three or more respiratory pauses lasting longer than 3 seconds with less than 20 seconds of respiration between pauses

b. Cessation of breathing for at least 20 seconds or for a shorter period if accompanied by bradycardia and cyanosis

c. Sudden episode of apnea with changes in color and muscle tone accompanied by coughing or gagging

4. What should a nurse witnessing an apneic episode note?

5. When home apnea monitoring is prescribed, parents need instruction about _____ and _____.

SUDDEN INFANT DEATH SYNDROME (SIDS)

Answer as either true (T) or false (F).

1. _____ SIDS usually occurs during sleep.

2. _____ SIDS usually occurs after the age of 6 months.

3. _____ Healthy infants should be placed in the supine position to sleep.

4. _____ Most parents of an infant who has died from SIDS will experience guilt, anger, and emotional distress.

ASTHMA

1. In recent years, the incidence and mortality rates for asthma have both _____.

2. Wheezing is typically heard on _____.

3. Tachypnea _____ carbon dioxide levels in the blood.

4. Beta$_2$-adrenergic agonists are used to _____.

5. Increasingly severe asthma that does not respond to vigorous treatment is called _____.

6. _____ is an ideal sport for children with asthma.

7. Corticosteroids are used during an acute asthma attack to _____.

8. Children with asthma monitor their condition at home using _____.

9. Mast cell inhibitors are administered 30 minutes before _____.

10. Two breathing exercises to slow the respiratory rate are _____ and _____.

BRONCHOPULMONARY DYSPLASIA (BPD)/CHRONIC LUNG DISEASE OF INFANCY (CLD)

Answer as either true (T) or false (F).

1. _____ BPD results from lung injury related to receiving supplemental oxygen and mechanical ventilation.

2. _____ Pursing of the lips and nasal flaring are early signs of impending respiratory distress.

3. _____ In BPD, diuretics are used to treat hypertension related to BPD.

4. _____ Infants with BPD tend to have irreversible developmental delays.

CYSTIC FIBROSIS (CF)

Answer as either true (T) or false (F).

1. _____ CF is an autosomal-dominant inherited disorder.

2. _____ CF affects the functioning of the exocrine glands.

3. _____ Children with CF present with malnutrition because of a poor diet.

4. _____ Meconium ileus may be the first indicator of CF.

5. _____ Aerosolized antibiotics may be used in place of intravenous antibiotics.

6. _____ Aerobic exercise may be as effective as chest physiotherapy in relieving pulmonary obstruction in CF.

7. _____ Enzyme dosage is adjusted according to weight gain.

8. _____ A child with CF requires extra salt and fluids when the weather is hot.

TUBERCULOSIS (TB)

Match each term with its description.

1. _____ TB exposure   a. Recent contact with a person who has contagious TB

2. _____ TB infection   b. Positive skin test with signs and symptoms of TB

3. _____ TB disease   c. Positive skin test with no signs and symptoms

Answer as either true (T) or false (F).

4. _____ Children with TB are rarely contagious.

5. _____ The Mantoux test is the preferred method of screening for TB.

6. _____ Children with a TB infection are treated with bacille Calmette-Guérin for 9 months.

7. _____ In infants, a negative tuberculin skin test rules out a TB infection.

SUGGESTED LEARNING ACTIVITIES

1. Interview a public health nurse about the incidence of TB in your community. Has your community observed an increase in new cases of TB? If yes, to what does the nurse attribute this increase? Share your findings with the class.

2. Investigate an asthma self-help group for children in your community. How does it meet the child's informational and psychosocial needs? Report to your class.

STUDENT LEARNING APPLICATIONS

Enhance your learning by discussing your answers with other students.

Parents bring their 2-month-old daughter, Tina, to the pediatrician. They are very anxious because she has been crying "all the time and won't eat or sleep." They also tell you that she feels "very hot." Tina is diagnosed with acute otitis media and amoxicillin is prescribed for 10 days.

1. What would you teach the parents about the causes, risk factors, and course of acute otitis media?

2. What would you teach them about the treatment and follow-up?

Tina's parents remain extremely anxious. Their anxiety seems out of proportion to the situation. You are tempted to say, "It's just an ear infection. Lighten up."

3. Why would you *not* say that?

4. Why do you think the parents are so upset?

5. How can you determine whether you are correct?

In talking with Tina's parents, you discover that both of them had siblings who died before their first birthdays.

6. How does this information change your perception of their anxiety?

7. How can you effectively intervene with this family?

REVIEW QUESTIONS

Choose the correct answer.

1. A toddler is admitted to the hospital with croup. He is tachypneic with substernal retracting and nasal flaring. He has a harsh, bark-like cough. His pulse oximetry reading on room air is 98%. The most accurate nursing diagnosis for him is:
   a. ineffective breathing pattern.
   b. ineffective airway clearance.
   c. impaired gas exchange.
   d. all of the above.

2. In preparing a 6-year-old child for a tonsillectomy, the nurse should not:
   a. direct the teaching at the child's parents.
   b. reassure the child that she will be able to talk following the surgery.
   c. explain that her throat will be sore after surgery.
   d. explain that she will have to drink a lot after surgery.

3. A preschooler arrives in the emergency department. She is very anxious and irritable and refuses to lie down to be examined. She is sitting up, leaning forward on her hands, and drooling saliva. She is warm to the touch and her color is pale. The nurse should:
   a. take the child's vital signs.
   b. immediately notify the physician.
   c. ask the parents to wait outside the examining room.
   d. start an intravenous line.

4. Parents bring their 8-month-old son to the emergency department because "He's breathing so fast that he can't even eat, and he's so hot." Physical examination reveals nasal flaring, intercostal retracting, and moderate expiratory wheezing. The nurse suspects that the infant has:
   a. acute spasmodic croup.
   b. bronchiolitis.
   c. epiglottitis.
   d. aspirated a foreign body.

5. The nurse is preparing a child for a bronchoscopy. The child most likely has:
   a. apnea.
   b. bronchiolitis.
   c. aspirated a foreign body.
   d. pneumonia.

6. Which drug is a respiratory stimulant?
   a. Isoniazid
   b. Albuterol
   c. Caffeine
   d. Ribavirin

7. Active bleeding in a child following a tonsillectomy is indicated by:
   a. refusal to drink fluids.
   b. frequent swallowing.
   c. "coffee grounds" emesis.
   d. all of the above.

8. A child experiences bronchoconstriction 5 hours after an acute asthma attack. This is an example of which kind of inflammatory response?
   a. Immediate
   b. Intermediate
   c. Delayed

9. A nurse teaching a family about the use of pancreatic enzymes for the treatment of CF should include:
   a. "Administer the preparation thrice a day and before bedtime."
   b. "Dissolve the enzymes in warm whole milk."
   c. "Increase the dosage if the child has loose, fatty stools."
   d. "Chewing the enzymes will increase their efficacy."

10. A test used in the diagnosis of CF is:
    a. radioallergosorbent test (RAST).
    b. sweat chloride.
    c. culture for *Pseudomonas*.
    d. Mantoux.

11. Which therapy is least likely to be used for a child with CF who is hospitalized with a respiratory infection?
    a. Chest physiotherapy every 3 hours
    b. Intravenous antibiotics
    c. Cough-suppressant medications
    d. Postural drainage

12. An infant is hospitalized following an apparent life-threatening event. The apnea monitor suddenly alarms. The nurse should first:
    a. assess the infant.
    b. question witnesses about the triggering event.
    c. initiate cardiopulmonary resuscitation (CPR).
    d. reset the monitor.

46 The Child with a Cardiovascular Alteration

HELPFUL HINT

Review the anatomy and physiology of the heart and fetal circulation in an anatomy and physiology textbook.

MATCHING KEY TERMS

Match the term with the correct definition.

1. _____ Angioplasty

2. _____ Cardiomegaly

3. _____ Compensation

4. _____ Decompensation

5. _____ Dysrhythmia

6. _____ Palpitation

7. _____ Pulmonary edema

8. _____ Pulmonary hypertension

9. _____ Pulmonary venous congestion

10. _____ Shunt

11. _____ Systemic venous congestion

12. _____ Valvuloplasty

a. Increased systemic venous pressure, leading to excessive fluid in the systemic veins

b. Abnormal blood flow from one part of the circulatory system to another

c. Maintenance of adequate blood flow accomplished by cardiac and circulatory adjustments

d. Procedure to open a valve

e. Increased pulmonary pressure, leading to excessive fluid in the pulmonary veins

f. Procedure that dilates vessels

g. Disturbance of rhythm

h. Enlarged heart

i. Collection of excess fluid in the alveoli

j. Sensation of a rapid or irregular heartbeat

k. Inability of the heart to maintain adequate circulation

l. Increased pressure in the pulmonary arteries and arterioles

MORE DEFINITIONS

Recall the definitions of the terms in italics in the following statements. Then, apply your knowledge and determine whether each statement is true (T) or false (F).

1. _____ *Afterload* is the amount of force against which the ventricles contract.

2. _____ *Central venous pressure* (CVP) is measured in the left ventricle.

3. _____ A drug's *chronotropic* effect has an effect on the heart's rate.

4. _____ A drug's *inotropic* effect has an effect on *myocardial contractility*.

5. _____ *Preload* is measured by determining CVP.

6. _____ *Pulmonary vascular resistance* affects the left ventricle.

7. _____ *Regurgitation* is the result of turbulent blood flow.

8. _____ *Systemic vascular resistance* is the amount of pressure exerted by the systemic vascular bed.

REVIEW OF THE CARDIOVASCULAR SYSTEM

Fill in the blanks.

1. In fetal circulation, gas exchange occurs at the _____.

2. In fetal circulation, oxygenated blood from the placenta flows from the right atrium into the left atrium through the

   _____.

3. After birth, the fetal shunt between the pulmonary artery and the aorta, called the _____,
   closes.

4. After birth, pulmonary vascular resistance _____ and the systemic arterial pressure _____.

CARDIOVASCULAR ASSESSMENT

Answer as either true (T) or false (F).

1. _____ Clubbing of nail beds indicates chronic hypoxia.

2. _____ A gallop is a missing heart sound.

3. _____ The point of maximal impulse (PMI) at the seventh intercostal space indicates cardiomegaly.

4. _____ Cool extremities in a warm room may indicate decreased cardiac output.

5. _____ Dyspnea is an indicator of congestive heart failure (CHF).

6. _____ S_2 is auscultated at the heart's apex and correlates with the palpable pulse.

7. _____ Squatting may be an attempt to improve cardiac circulation.

8. _____ Cardiac catheterization can be an interventional as well as a diagnostic procedure.

PHYSIOLOGIC CONSEQUENCES OF CONGENITAL HEART DISEASE

1. In infants, early manifestations of CHF include: _____.

Match each drug or class of drugs with its description.

2. _____ Furosemide

3. _____ Spironolactone

4. _____ Thiazide diuretic

5. _____ Digoxin

6. _____ Vasodilator

a. Acts on distal renal tubules

b. Potassium-sparing diuretic

c. Relaxes smooth muscles; decreases afterload

d. Increases cardiac output; has positive inotropic and negative chronotropic effects

e. Potent loop diuretic

7. In an infant, fluid retention is monitored by _____.

8. Before administering digoxin, the nurse should count _____, check _____,
   and observe _____.

9. Polycythemia compensates for _____.

10. Treatment of hypercyanotic episodes includes: _____

    _____.

LEFT-TO-RIGHT SHUNTING LESIONS AND OBSTRUCTIVE LESIONS

Fill in the blanks.

1. _____ can be medically managed with indomethacin in some cases.

2. Classic signs of _____ are decreased pulses and blood pressure in the lower extremities.

3. _____ is an abnormal opening between the ventricles, whereas _____ is an abnormal opening between the atria.

4. Endocardial cushion defect is also known as _____.

5. Narrowing at the entrance of the pulmonary artery is called _____.

6. Thickening of the aortic valve is known as _____.

CYANOTIC LESIONS WITH ALTERED PULMONARY BLOOD FLOW

Match each defect with its description.

1. _____ Total anomalous pulmonary venous return

2. _____ Transposition of the great arteries

3. _____ Hypoplastic left heart syndrome

4. _____ Pulmonary atresia

5. _____ Tetralogy of Fallot

6. _____ Tricuspid atresia

7. _____ Truncus arteriosus

a. Defect composed of four distinct lesions

b. Condition in which pulmonary artery and aorta are one vessel

c. Failure of the pulmonary valve to develop

d. Absence of the tricuspid valve

e. Inadequate development of the left side of the heart

f. Reversal of the aorta and pulmonary artery

g. Absence of direct communication between the pulmonary veins and the left atrium

ACQUIRED HEART DISEASE

Answer as either true (T) or false (F).

1. _____ Gram-positive microorganisms are usually responsible for infective endocarditis.

2. _____ Immune complexes play a role in rheumatic fever.

3. _____ Kawasaki disease is an immune-mediated condition, resulting in vasculitis.

4. _____ Antibiotic prophylaxis with penicillin for at least 5 years is part of the management of rheumatic fever without cardiac complications.

5. _____ Vegetation observed on an echocardiogram suggests Kawasaki disease.

6. _____ Congenital heart malformations require infective endocarditis prophylaxis.

7. _____ Normal blood pressure for a child is defined as a systolic and/or diastolic blood pressure less than the 90th percentile for age and gender.

8. _____ Children with essential hypertension often have a family history of the disease.

9. _____ Renal disease is a complication of secondary hypertension.

10. _____ Nonpharmacologic therapies for hypertension are usually not effective.

CARDIOMYOPATHIES

1. Which type of cardiomyopathy is a major cause of sudden cardiac death in adolescents?

2. Which type of cardiomyopathy results from an infection or exposure to a toxin?

3. Drugs used to decrease ventricular hypercontractility and outflow tract obstruction are _____

   and _____ blockers.

DYSRHYTHMIAS

Fill in the blanks.

1. Vagal maneuvers may be used to terminate an episode of _____.

2. Bradydysrhythmias are associated with _____.

3. In _____, there is no cardiac output.

4. Briefly placing an ice bag over an infant's face may stimulate a _____ response.

5. In asystole, _____ is administered to stimulate cardiac activity.

HIGH CHOLESTEROL IN CHILDREN AND ADOLESCENTS

1. List the risk factors for coronary artery disease in children and adolescents.

2. In children, borderline levels for low-density lipoprotein (LDL) cholesterol are _____ mg/dL,

   and a high level for LDL is greater than _____ mg/dL.

SUGGESTED LEARNING ACTIVITIES

1. Role play with two other students. Have one student act as the nurse and another act as a parent who has just been told that his or her child has a cardiac defect and will require surgery. The third student should observe the interaction. After 10 minutes, discuss the role play. The "nurse" can describe how it felt to deal with the "parent." The "parent" can describe which of the "nurse's" interventions were effective and which could use improvement. The observer can describe the interchange from an objective viewpoint.

2. Interview the parent of a child who has had cardiac surgery in the past. Try to discover what the health care team did that was helpful for the family during the child's hospitalization. What could have been done better?

3. Observe a cardiac catheterization. Design a teaching plan used to describe to a 12-year-old child what to expect.

STUDENT LEARNING APPLICATIONS

Enhance your learning by discussing your answers with other students.

Michael is a healthy 10-year-old African-American boy undergoing a routine physical. His height and weight are at the 75th percentile. His blood pressure is at the 95th percentile for his age and gender, but a review of his chart reveals that his blood pressure has been slightly below the 90th percentile on previous visits.

1. Based on these findings, what questions would you, as his nurse, ask Michael and his parents?

2. How would you further assess his blood pressure?

The physician makes the diagnosis of essential hypertension and decides to initiate nonpharmacologic therapy.

3. How would you assess the family's need for information about the following treatments?

 - Weight control

 - Physical conditioning

 - Dietary modifications

 - Relaxation techniques

4. What key features of these treatments would you stress when you present the information?

5. How would you evaluate the effectiveness of your presentation?

REVIEW QUESTIONS

Choose the correct answer.

1. In a physical assessment of an infant with a ventricular septal defect (VSD), the nurse notices dyspnea, hepatosplenomegaly, and periorbital edema and understands that these are clinical manifestations of:
   a. heart failure.
   b. endocarditis.
   c. fluid overload.
   d. decreased central venous pressure.

2. Percentiles for average blood pressure are based on a child's:
   a. weight and gender.
   b. age and gender.
   c. gender and race.
   d. age and weight.

3. Which nursing intervention is *not* appropriate when caring for an infant with cardiovascular alterations?
   a. Discouraging breastfeeding
   b. Limiting bottle feedings to no longer than 30 minutes
   c. Maintaining a neutral thermal environment
   d. Providing periods of uninterrupted rest

4. Children with hypertension who are receiving loop diuretics are at risk for imbalances of:
   a. calcium.
   b. chloride.
   c. potassium.
   d. sodium.

5. A toddler is hospitalized with CHF and is receiving digoxin and furosemide. She has vomited twice in the past 4 hours. The nurse's best action is to:
   a. increase the child's fluid intake.
   b. omit the next dose of furosemide.
   c. check the child's blood pressure before the next dose of digoxin.
   d. get an order to draw a digoxin level.

6. An infant with a left-to-right shunt is admitted to the hospital in CHF. Yesterday, she weighed 3.6 kg. A finding that indicates a worsening of her condition today is:
   a. weight of 3.67 kg.
   b. urine output of 40 mL in the past 8 hours.
   c. rales in the lower lobes.
   d. all of the above.

7. While the nurse is performing a newborn assessment, he finds that the infant's blood pressure in her arms is much higher than in her legs. The nurse suspects that the infant has:
   a. aortic stenosis.
   b. atrioventricular canal.
   c. coarctation of the aorta.
   d. truncus arteriosus.

8. Parents of a toddler with tetralogy of Fallot explain that they do not want him to overexert himself, so they always keep him in his playpen or crib to limit his mobility. Based on this information, the most appropriate nursing diagnosis is:
   a. activity intolerance.
   b. risk for impaired parenting.
   c. caregiver role strain.
   d. risk for delayed growth and development.

9. While the nurse is taking routine vital signs, she notices that the infant is having a hypercyanotic episode. What should the nurse do first?
   a. Continue getting vital signs for a baseline comparison.
   b. Place the infant in a knee–chest position.
   c. Get a pulse oximetry reading.
   d. Administer morphine sulfate.

10. Parents of children with congenital heart problems often experience a loss of control when the child is hospitalized. The nurse who understands this will:
    a. encourage parents to participate in their child's care.
    b. explain procedures before performing them.
    c. answer questions honestly.
    d. do all of the above.

11. The father of a child with a congenital heart defect asks the nurse why his daughter has to take penicillin before she gets her teeth cleaned by the dentist. The nurse explains that this is necessary to prevent:
    a. infective endocarditis.
    b. CHF.
    c. rheumatic fever.
    d. infected gums.

12. An indicator of infective endocarditis is:
    a. positive blood cultures.
    b. vegetation seen via Holter monitoring.
    c. decreased erythrocyte sedimentation rate.
    d. all of the above.

47 The Child with a Hematologic Alteration

HELPFUL HINT

Review the anatomy and physiology of the hematologic system in an anatomy and physiology textbook.

MATCHING KEY TERMS

Match the term with the correct definition.

1. _____ Autoimmune disorder
2. _____ Chelation
3. _____ Erythropoiesis
4. _____ Extramedullary
5. _____ Granulocytes
6. _____ Hematopoiesis
7. _____ Hemolysis
8. _____ Hemosiderosis
9. _____ Pancytopenia
10. _____ Reticulocytes
11. _____ Reticuloendothelial system

a. Outside the bone marrow
b. Collection of cells capable of phagocytosis
c. Reduction in all types of blood cells
d. Breakdown of red blood cells (RBCs)
e. Increase in tissue iron stores
f. Production of RBCs
g. Immature RBCs
h. Production of blood cells
i. Disorder in which the body launches an immunologic response against itself
j. Neutrophils, eosinophils, or basophils
k. Binding of a metallic ion with a structure that results in the inactivation of the ion

REVIEW OF THE HEMATOLOGIC SYSTEM

1. Explain the function of the following:

   a. RBCs

   b. White blood cells (WBCs)

   c. Platelets

2. Define each term.

   a. Anemia

   b. Polycythemia

   c. Lymphopenia

   d. Megakaryocytes

IRON DEFICIENCY ANEMIA (IDA)

1. How does the introduction of cow's milk into the diet before 1 year of age affect the development of IDA?

2. Why are infants with IDA lethargic?

3. Give two reasons why adolescents are prone to IDA.

4. What foods can interfere with iron absorption?

SICKLE CELL DISEASE (SCD)

1. Under what three conditions do RBCs change to a sickle shape?

   a.

   b.

   c.

2. Sickled RBCs cause microvascular occlusion. What does this lead to?

Match each complication of SCD with its clinical manifestation.

3. _____ Vaso-occlusive crisis   a. Altered level of consciousness

4. _____ Acute chest syndrome   b. Painful, persistent erection of the penis

5. _____ Dactylitis   c. Pallor, lethargy, and fainting

6. _____ Stroke   d. Swelling of the hands and feet

7. _____ Acute splenic sequestration   e. Signs of hypovolemic shock

8. _____ Aplastic crises   f. Fever, cough, and chest pain

9. _____ Priapism   g. Pain depending on the organ or tissues affected

BETA-THALASSEMIA

Fill in the blanks.

1. β-Thalassemia is inherited in a(n) _____ pattern.

2. The major complication of the treatment of β-thalassemia is _____.

3. In β-thalassemia, chelation removes _____ from the body.

4. The drug used to manage hemosiderosis is _____.

HEMOPHILIA

1. Describe the parents of a girl with hemophilia.

2. In hemophilia A, the missing blood clotting component is _____; in hemophilia B, the missing component is _____.

3. What are the manifestations of bleeding into the joints?

4. Hemophilia is a genetic disorder carried on the _____ chromosome.

VON WILLEBRAND DISEASE (VWD)

Answer as either true (T) or false (F).

1. _____ VWD is an acquired bleeding disorder.

2. _____ Prolonged and excessive bleeding and menorrhagia are signs of VWD.

3. _____ The von Willebrand protein carries coagulation factor IX.

4. _____ VWD is sometimes treated with desmopressin acetate (DDAVP).

IMMUNE THROMBOCYTOPENIC PURPURA (ITP)

Answer as either true (T) or false (F).

1. _____ In ITP, autoantibodies are responsible for the destruction of platelets.

2. _____ Children will undergo bone marrow aspirations as part of the diagnostic workup for ITP.

3. _____ Thrombocytopenia, petechiae, and bruising are manifestations of ITP.

4. _____ Splenectomy is the treatment of choice for acute ITP.

5. _____ Chronic ITP is more prevalent among adolescents.

DISSEMINATED INTRAVASCULAR COAGULATION (DIC)

Answer as either true (T) or false (F).

1. _____ Excessive bleeding and clotting occur at the same time in DIC.

2. _____ In DIC, bleeding occurs because of the depletion of platelets and clotting factors.

3. _____ Excessive bruising and oozing from venipuncture sites are late signs of DIC.

APLASTIC ANEMIA

1. In aplastic anemia, the bone marrow stops producing _____, _____, and _____.

2. What are the clinical manifestations of aplastic anemia?

3. Medications used to treat aplastic anemia include steroids, cyclosporin, antithymocyte/antilymphocyte globulin, and

_____.

ABO INCOMPATIBILITY AND HEMOLYTIC DISEASES OF THE NEWBORN

Fill in the blanks.

1. ABO incompatibility results when the mother has blood type O and the fetus has either blood type

_____ or _____.

2. Rh incompatibility results when the mother's blood is Rh _____ and the fetal blood is

Rh _____.

3. Rh incompatibility can be prevented by administering Rho (D) immunoglobulin (RhoGAM) to Rh-negative mothers

after _____.

HYPERBILIRUBINEMIA

Answer as either true (T) or false (F).

1. _____ Neonatal hyperbilirubinemia is referred to as physiologic jaundice.

2. _____ Kernicterus refers to damage to the liver cells.

3. _____ Hyperbilirubinemia is more common in term infants.

4. _____ Phototherapy allows unconjugated bilirubin to be removed by the liver and spleen.

5. _____ After an exchange transfusion, phototherapy is no longer necessary.

270

SUGGESTED LEARNING ACTIVITIES

With one or several other students in a discussion group, review the genetic implications of inherited hematologic disorders by discussing the following questions.

1. Sickle cell disease is an autosomal-recessive disorder.

   a. When both parents have the trait, what are the chances that:

      - a child will have neither the trait nor the disease?

      - a child will have the disease?

      - a child will have the trait?

   b. When one parent has the disease and the other has the trait, what are the chances that:

      - a child will have neither the trait nor the disease?

      - a child will have the disease?

      - a child will have the trait?

   c. When neither parent has the disease but one has the trait, what are the chances that:

      - a child will have neither the trait nor the disease?

      - a child will have the disease?

      - a child will have the trait?

2. Hemophilia is an inherited X-linked recessive disorder.

   a. When the mother is a carrier and the father does not have hemophilia, what are the chances that:

      - a daughter will have the disease?

      - a daughter will be a carrier?

      - a son will have the disease?

      - a son will be a carrier?

   b. When the mother is a carrier and the father has hemophilia, what are the chances that:

      - a daughter will have the disease?

      - a daughter will be a carrier?

      - a son will have the disease?

      - a son will be a carrier?

271

STUDENT LEARNING APPLICATIONS

Enhance your learning by discussing your answers with other students.

A 12-year-old girl was admitted to the hospital in a vaso-occlusive sickle cell crisis. Her pain is localized in her right arm and shoulder, and she rates it as 3.5 on a 0-to-5 scale. Her vital signs are slightly elevated, with an oral temperature of 38.2°C. She weighs 40 kg.

1. She is receiving morphine sulfate for pain. As her nurse, what nonpharmacologic measures for pain management might you also suggest to the child?

The physician orders intravenous (IV) fluids to run at 2× maintenance.

2. What are the child's basic fluid maintenance requirements for a 24-hour period? What should her hourly IV rate be to provide 2× maintenance fluids?

3. You want to assess the child's knowledge about the prevention of sickle cell crises. How would you do this?

4. While caring for the child, you notice that she has a productive cough. She also starts to complain about pain in her chest. How would you address this new problem?

REVIEW QUESTIONS

Choose the correct answer.

1. An example of an autoimmune disorder is:
   a. hemolytic disease of the newborn.
   b. DIC.
   c. ITP.
   d. VWD.

2. If a preschooler with mild hemophilia is experiencing joint pain, the nurse should:
   a. administer children's aspirin.
   b. apply cold compresses.
   c. do passive range-of-motion exercises.
   d. give the child a warm bath in the tub.

3. Which statement about chelation therapy is true?
   a. It is used to rid the body of excess sulfate.
   b. It is used to treat one of the complications of factor VIII therapy.
   c. It is used to manage hemosiderosis.
   d. It often results in increased bleeding.

4. An example of a disorder inherited in an autosomal-inherited pattern is:
   a. hemophilia A.
   b. β-thalassemia.
   c. VWD.
   d. ABO-Rh incompatibility.

5. Which statement by an adolescent with iron deficiency anemia indicates that she needs more teaching about her iron supplement?
   a. "I'll take my pill with orange juice."
   b. "I'll keep the pills out of reach of my younger brother and sister."
   c. "I'll double the dose during my periods."
   d. "It's normal for my bowel movements to be black while I'm taking iron."

6. A 4-year-old is admitted to the hospital with SCD. Her vital signs are a temperature of 37.2°C, heart rate of 124 beats/min (bpm), a respiratory rate of 38 breaths/min, and blood pressure of 70/40 mm Hg. She is pale and listless and has splenomegaly. She is experiencing:
   a. aplastic crisis.
   b. acute chest syndrome.
   c. a cerebrovascular accident (CVA).
   d. acute sequestration crisis.

7. An infant receiving phototherapy for hyperbilirubinemia is at increased risk for:
   a. hyperthermia.
   b. hypothermia.
   c. dehydration.
   d. all of the above.

8. A 6-year-old hospital patient complains of a headache. This could be a sign of a serious complication if the child has:
   a. aplastic anemia.
   b. hemophilia.
   c. SCD.
   d. any of the above.

9. A toddler with hemophilia is at risk for:
   a. altered growth related to poor appetite.
   b. developmental delay related to activity restrictions.
   c. infection related to decreased WBCs.
   d. all of the above.

10. In taking the history of a child with ITP, the nurse is not surprised to discover that:
   a. the child's father has classic hemophilia.
   b. the child had the flu 2 weeks ago.
   c. the child fell off a bike last week.
   d. the child suddenly had a red, raised rash appear today.

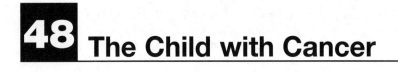

48 The Child with Cancer

HELPFUL HINT

A pharmacology textbook will provide a more extensive discussion of chemotherapy.

MATCHING KEY TERMS

Match the term with the correct definition.

1. _____ Benign cells
2. _____ Blast cells
3. _____ Clean margins
4. _____ Extramedullary
5. _____ Immunosuppression
6. _____ Intrathecal
7. _____ Malignant cells
8. _____ Neutropenia
9. _____ Protocol
10. _____ Thrombocytopenia

a. Immature lymphocytes
b. Plan of research-based care outlining drug therapy and follow-up interventions
c. Within the spinal column
d. Decrease in number of white blood cells (WBCs) that results in a reduced ability to fight infection
e. Reduction in platelet count
f. Slow-growing cells forming a tumor with distinct borders
g. Outside the bone marrow
h. Evidence of normal, disease-free tissue in the outermost layer of cells of a surgical sample
i. Abnormal cells that have invasive and unregulated growth
j. Weakening of the body's normal immune response

REVIEW OF CANCER

1. Any tumor that arises from a new, abnormal growth is called a _____.

2. The two ways that cancer cells spread are _____ and _____.

3. Why is staging done for tumors?

Answer as either true (T) or false (F).

4. _____ The cause of most childhood cancers is unknown.

5. _____ Screening tests for cancer in childhood are the same as adult cancer screening tests.

6. _____ Cancer in children is a common occurrence.

7. _____ Symptoms of cancer in children resemble those of common childhood illnesses.

8. _____ How is a child positioned for a bone marrow aspiration?

THE CHILD WITH CANCER

1. Identify the three primary treatment modalities for children with cancer.

   a. _____

   b. _____

   c. _____

2. Chemotherapy is the use of _____ to kill cancer cells.

3. Identify the three body systems whose cells are most often affected by chemotherapy.

   a. _____

   b. _____

   c. _____

4. Define *nadir*.

5. _____ places the child with cancer at risk for the development of opportunistic infections.

   Identify each of the following signs and symptoms as a side effect of chemotherapy (C), radiotherapy (R), or both (B).

6. Skin reactions

7. Nausea and vomiting

8. Alopecia

9. Bone marrow suppression

10. Stomatitis

11. Fatigue

12. Which class of antiemetic drugs has been found to be more effective than other antiemetics in treating chemotherapy-induced nausea and vomiting?

13. What is the purpose of a biopsy?

14. How would a central venous catheter facilitate chemotherapy administration?

15. The side effects of radiotherapy are specific to the _____ and _____.

16. The side effects of radiotherapy usually appear _____ days after treatment is initiated.

17. _____ is the most common side effect of radiotherapy.

18. What is the difference between hematopoietic stem cell transplantation (HSCT) and bone marrow transplantation (BMT)?

19. Hematopoietic stem cells are able to differentiate into _____.

Match each term with its description.

20. _____ Autologous transplant

21. _____ Allogenic transplant

22. _____ Umbilical cord blood

23. _____ Graft-versus-host disease (GVHD)

24. _____ Engraftment

25. _____ Conditioning

26. _____ Colony-stimulating factors (CSFs)

27. _____ Peripheral blood stem cells (PBSCs)

a. Occurs when transplanted bone marrow recognizes the recipient's tissue as foreign

b. Occurs when the transplanted cells produce WBCs, red blood cells (RBCs), and platelets

c. Goal is to eradicate any disease from the body with high-dose chemotherapy and radiotherapy

d. Source of stem cells for transplantation

e. Source of stem cells for autologous transplants

f. Transplanted cells come from a related or unrelated donor

g. Naturally occurring biologic agents that stimulate the recovery of WBCs, RBCs, and platelets

h. Transplanted cells come from the patient

LEUKEMIA

1. Leukemia is caused by the proliferation of _____.

2. List five clinical manifestations of leukemia.

   a. _____

   b. _____

   c. _____

   d. _____

   e. _____

3. The diagnostic test that confirms a diagnosis of leukemia is _____.

4. The preferred treatment for leukemia is _____.

5. When is a child with acute lymphocytic leukemia considered to be in remission?

6. Why are allopurinol and intravenous (IV) fluids with sodium bicarbonate administered before chemotherapy?

7. List two sanctuary sites.

   a. _____

   b. _____

8. Why are rectal temperatures contraindicated for a child with neutropenia?

9. A child is at severe risk for infection when his or her absolute neutrophil level is: _____.

10. What should the nurse teach the child with leukemia and his or her family about oral hygiene?

11. What action is indicated if an immunosuppressed child is exposed to someone with chickenpox?

12. What precautions should be taken for a child who is thrombocytopenic?

BRAIN TUMORS

1. Manifestations of brain tumors vary with _____ and _____.

2. What are the two hallmark symptoms of brain tumors in children?

   a. _____

   b. _____

3. Currently, the imaging modality used to evaluate brain tumors is _____.

4. Which treatment modalities are used to treat brain tumors in children younger than 3 years?

OTHER CHILDHOOD CANCERS

Answer as either true (T) or false (F).

1. _____ The abdominal mass on a child with Wilms' tumor should be palpated every shift for changes.

2. _____ Treatment for tumor lysis syndrome includes allopurinol and hydration with IV fluids containing potassium.

3. _____ The primary treatment modality for non-Hodgkin lymphoma is surgery.

4. _____ Neuroblastoma is a solid tumor that is found in infants and children.

5. _____ In most cases, neuroblastoma manifests as a primary abdominal mass.

6. _____ Ewing sarcoma is the most common primary bone malignancy in children.

7. _____ Tumors in Ewing sarcoma are sensitive to radiotherapy.

8. _____ Treatment of osteogenic sarcoma involves surgery and chemotherapy.

9. _____ Leukocoria and strabismus are common findings in most cases of retinoblastoma.

Provide the description/pathophysiologic information for each condition or tumor listed in the following table.

	Description/Pathophysiology
Wilms' tumor	
Hodgkin disease	
Non-Hodgkin lymphoma	
Brain tumor	
Neuroblastoma	
Osteosarcoma	
Ewing sarcoma	
Rhabdomyosarcoma	
Retinoblastoma	

CREATE YOUR OWN STUDY GUIDE

Describe the clinical manifestations and treatment for each condition or tumor listed in the following table.

	Clinical Manifestations	Treatment
Wilms' tumor		
Hodgkin disease		
Non-Hodgkin lymphoma		
Brain tumor		
Neuroblastoma		
Osteosarcoma		
Ewing sarcoma		
Rhabdomyosarcoma		
Retinoblastoma		

SUGGESTED LEARNING ACTIVITIES

1. What are the guidelines for administering chemotherapy at your clinical site?

2. If there is an oncology clinic at your clinical site, discuss with the nurses about their responsibilities in the oncology clinic. Do the nurses need more advanced preparation in pediatric oncology?

STUDENT LEARNING APPLICATIONS

Enhance your learning by discussing your answers with other students.

The parents of a 12-year-old are concerned because he has had a low-grade fever for a week. His appetite and energy levels have decreased. They have also noticed bruises on his legs even though he has not been physically active. A complete blood count shows blast cells on the differential. The child is referred to a pediatric oncologist because leukemia is suspected. He is then admitted to the hospital. This is his first day in the hospital, and you are caring for him.

1. What diagnostic studies would you expect to be ordered for the child?

2. Respond to the following questions asked by his father: "What is a bone marrow biopsy? Why does my son need this test?"

When a bone marrow biopsy confirms acute lymphocytic leukemia (ALL), chemotherapy is initiated.

3. What are the nurse's responsibilities when caring for a child receiving chemotherapy?

4. What nursing assessments will you make while the child is receiving chemotherapy?

When his parents leave the room to go to the cafeteria for lunch, the child asks you several questions. How would you respond when the child asks the following questions?

5. "Do I have to have a transplant?"

6. "Another boy in my class got leukemia last year and he died. Am I going to die too?"

7. "How long do I have to get chemo?"

8. "Will I lose my hair?"

REVIEW QUESTIONS

Choose the correct answer.

1. BMT is considered standard therapy for which childhood cancer?
   a. Acute myelocytic leukemia
   b. Wilms' tumor
   c. Osteosarcoma
   d. Hodgkin disease

2. The most common side effect of radiotherapy is:
   a. vomiting.
   b. bone marrow suppression.
   c. fatigue.
   d. erythema at the radiation site.

3. Which position is contraindicated for a child following surgery to remove a brain tumor?
   a. Supine
   b. Prone
   c. Trendelenburg
   d. Low Fowler

4. When a child's own bone marrow is used in a bone marrow transplant, it is called a(n):
   a. allogenic transplant.
   b. autologous transplant.
   c. homogenic transplant.
   d. none of these terms is correct.

5. A child with neutropenia following a round of chemotherapy is receiving a CSF. The purpose of the CSF is to stimulate the production of:
   a. blast cells.
   b. platelets.
   c. RBCs.
   d. WBCs.

6. A child has a history of a fever of unknown origin, excessive bruising, and fatigue. This combination of symptoms is suggestive of which childhood cancer?
   a. Leukemia
   b. Neuroblastoma
   c. Lymphoma
   d. Osteosarcoma

7. A diagnosis of leukemia is confirmed by which study?
   a. Lumbar puncture
   b. Bone scan
   c. Bone marrow biopsy
   d. Complete blood count

8. Which instruction would the nurse give to a 15-year-old with a platelet count of 18,000?
   a. Eat a low-bacteria diet.
   b. Use a soft-bristled toothbrush.
   c. Get extra rest.
   d. Make sure you take an iron supplement.

9. What is the best fluid choice for the child who is nauseated from chemotherapy?
   a. Child's favorite flavored milkshake
   b. Room temperature water
   c. Sips of cold soda
   d. Hot tea with honey

10. What should the nurse tell an adolescent receiving chemotherapy about alopecia?
    a. "Don't worry. Most chemotherapy does not cause hair loss."
    b. "Your hair will grow back but it might be a different color or texture."
    c. "Your hair will come back when you are finished with all of your chemotherapy."
    d. "Aren't you lucky. The bald look is in right now."

11. What should not be included in a plan of care for a child with Wilms' tumor?
    a. Palpate the abdominal mass for any changes.
    b. Teach the child and family about a nephrectomy.
    c. Talk with the family about postoperative chemotherapy.
    d. Assess the urine for microscopic or gross hematuria.

12. The prevention of tumor lysis syndrome includes:
    a. hydrating and alkalinizing the urine.
    b. administering bicarbonate to make the urine acidic.
    c. assessing the urine for hematuria.
    d. administering a leucovorin rescue.

13. What is the risk for an infection if a child's absolute neutrophil count is less than 400 cells/mm^3?
    a. Severe
    b. Moderate
    c. Minimal
    d. Not significant

14. What is considered a hallmark symptom of brain tumors in children?
    a. Ataxia
    b. Morning vomiting
    c. Visual changes
    d. Seizure

49 The Child with an Alteration in Tissue Integrity

HELPFUL HINT

Review skin assessment in Chapter 33 "Physical Assessment of Children." Review Chapter 39 "Pain Management for Children."

MATCHING KEY TERMS

Match the term with the correct definition.

1. _____ Débridement
2. _____ Desquamation
3. _____ Ecchymosis
4. _____ Eschar
5. _____ Erythema
6. _____ Excoriation
7. _____ Intertrigo
8. _____ Keratosis
9. _____ Lichenification
10. _____ Pruritus
11. _____ Urticaria

a. Thickening and hardening of the skin

b. Scratch or abrasion of the skin

c. Itching

d. Sloughing of the skin in scales or sheets

e. Redness of the skin

f. Overgrowth and thickening of the cornified epithelium

g. Hives

h. Dark plaque associated with tissue necrosis

i. Discoloration of the skin or mucous membranes caused by leakage of blood into the subcutaneous tissue

j. Maceration of two closely apposed skin surfaces

k. Removal of foreign material and devitalized or contaminated tissue from a traumatic or infected lesion to expose healthy tissue

REVIEW OF THE INTEGUMENTARY SYSTEM

1. List the five major functions of the skin.

   a. _____

   b. _____

   c. _____

   d. _____

   e. _____

Answer as either true (T) or false (F).

2. _____ The skin is the body's largest organ.

3. _____ The epidermis is completely replaced every 4 months.

4. _____ Mongolian spots are more commonly observed in infants of color.

5. _____ Vascular birthmarks are extremely uncommon.

IMPETIGO

1. Impetigo is the most common _____ skin infection of childhood.

2. The organisms responsible for most of the cases of impetigo are _____ and

   _____.

3. Describe the appearance of primary lesions of impetigo.

   a. Bullous

   b. Crusted

4. What is the treatment for impetigo?

5. What is a complication of impetigo caused by β-hemolytic streptococci?

6. What should parents be taught about preventing the spread of impetigo?

7. Failure to respond to treatment may indicate that the infection is caused by which organism?

CELLULITIS

1. What is cellulitis?

2. Which areas of the body are most commonly affected by cellulitis?

3. Name three clinical manifestations of cellulitis.

    a. _____

    b. _____

    c. _____

4. How is cellulitis treated?

5. Identify four nursing interventions for a child with cellulitis on his lower leg.

    a. _____

    b. _____

    c. _____

    d. _____

CANDIDIASIS

1. What is the organism responsible for causing thrush?

2. Describe the clinical manifestations of thrush.

3. During an assessment, what questions should the nurse ask the mother of an infant with oral candidiasis?

4. The medication used to treat oral candidiasis is _____.

5. How should the prescribed medication be administered to an infant with oral candidiasis?

TINEA INFECTIONS

1. Identify the body parts affected in the following tinea infections.

   a. Tinea capitis

   b. Tinea corporis

   c. Tinea pedis

2. What medications are used in the treatment of the following tinea infections, and how are they administered?

   a. Tinea capitis

   b. Tinea corporis

   c. Tinea cruris

   d. Tinea pedis

Answer as either true (T) or false (F).

3. _____ Children receiving a prolonged course of griseofulvin therapy should undergo liver function studies.

4. _____ Tinea infections are not contagious to others.

5. _____ Tinea infections heal more quickly if the affected area is kept warm and moist.

HERPES SIMPLEX VIRUS (HSV) INFECTION

1. What is herpetic whitlow?

2. What medication can lessen the severity of HSV 1?

3. How would the nurse advise the parents of a child with HSV 1 lesions on the lips who does not want to eat or drink?

LICE INFESTATIONS

Answer as either true (T) or false (F).

1. _____ Lice can be transmitted only by direct contact with an infested person.

2. _____ Clean hair is a deterrent to head lice.

3. Describe what the nurse is looking for when assessing a child for head lice.

4. What is the recommended treatment for killing active lice?

5. Give three interventions that should be taken if head lice are found.

a. _____

b. _____

c. _____

MITE INFESTATION (SCABIES)

1. How is scabies transmitted?

2. Name the clinical manifestations of scabies.

3. How should a scabicide lotion be applied to the skin?

ATOPIC DERMATITIS

1. What causes the intense pruritus associated with atopic dermatitis?

2. Describe the appearance of the skin in childhood-onset eczema.

3. List three interventions that can relieve itching for a child with atopic dermatitis.

a. _____

b. _____

c. _____

SEBORRHEIC DERMATITIS

1. Seborrheic dermatitis is also known as _____.

2. Name two clinical manifestations of seborrheic dermatitis.

a. _____

b. _____

3. Name two interventions used to treat seborrheic dermatitis of the scalp.

a. _____

b. _____

CONTACT DERMATITIS

1. What is contact dermatitis?

2. Name three interventions that can relieve itching from contact dermatitis.

   a. _____

   b. _____

   c. _____

3. What initial interventions should be taken if a child is exposed to poison ivy?

Answer as either true (T) or false (F).

4. _____ Diaper dermatitis is easier to prevent than to treat.

5. _____ The diaper area should be cleaned with water and mild soap after each voiding or bowel movement.

6. _____ Rubber pants should not be used because they hold in moisture and cause the skin to break down.

ACNE VULGARIS

1. What parts of the skin are involved in acne vulgaris?

2. Develop an explanation of acne for a young adolescent.

3. What should the nurse teach an adolescent about the following medications to prevent adverse effects?

   a. Tretinoin (Retin-A)

   b. Tetracycline

   c. Isotretinoin (Accutane)

4. What guidelines for daily skin care should be followed by the adolescent with acne?

MISCELLANEOUS SKIN DISORDERS

1. What precautions should be taken when a child is allergic to bee stings?

2. What intervention should be taken when a child gets a bee sting?

3. Why should insect repellents containing diethyltoluamide (DEET) not be used on small children?

4. Describe the management of frostbite.

5. What should children and parents know about preventing frostbite?

6. Describe the best method of removing a tick.

Match each skin disorder with its definition.

7. _____ Stevens-Johnson syndrome

8. _____ Molluscum contagiosum

9. _____ Psoriasis

10. _____ Warts

a. Viral infection of the skin and mucous membranes

b. Chronic inflammatory condition caused by the rapid proliferation of keratinocytes

c. Skin infection caused by a human papilloma virus

d. Autoimmune disease that may be triggered by infections or medications

BURN INJURIES

Match each description of burn injury with the corresponding level of burn depth. (Answers may be used more than once.)

1. _____ Blisters within minutes of burn injury

2. _____ Peels after 24 to 48 hours

3. _____ Has a mottled, waxy, white, dry surface

4. _____ White, cherry red, or black appearance

a. Superficial

b. Partial thickness

c. Full thickness

Match each description of burn injury with the corresponding levels of severity. (Answers may be used more than once.)

5. _____ Partial-thickness burns of greater than 20% of total body surface area (TBSA)

6. _____ Full-thickness burn of less than 2% TBSA, not involving special areas

7. _____ Partial-thickness burns of 10% to 20% TBSA

8. _____ Burns of eyes, ears, face, hands, feet, perineum, or joints

a. Minor

b. Moderate

c. Major

9. What should the nurse teach parents about preventing a sunburn in children?

10. List the three commonly used topical antimicrobial agents for burns.

a. _____

b. _____

c. _____

11. Define *burn shock*.

12. Name the four possible complications of an electrical injury.

a. _____

b. _____

c. _____

d. _____

SUGGESTED LEARNING ACTIVITIES

1. Develop a one-page instruction sheet for the parents of children with any of the disorders presented in this chapter.

2. If possible, arrange an observational experience at a pediatric burn center.

3. What are your fears and concerns about caring for a child who has had a major burn injury?

Enhance your learning by discussing the following two scenarios with other students.

Scenario A

A first grader was sent to the school nurse because her teacher noticed that she had been scratching her head for the past few days.

1. How should the school nurse check the child for head lice?

The examination of the child's head revealed nits throughout her hair. When the nurse called the child's mother to discuss the matter, her mother comments, "I wash her hair almost every day. She is a neat child. How could she get lice?"

2. How should the nurse respond to this comment?

3. What are the implications of this problem for the other children in the classroom? For other members of the child's family?

4. How should the nurse explain the treatment for head lice to the mother?

5. What measures should be taken in the child's classroom?

6. What can children be taught about preventing head lice?

Scenario B

A 2-year-old was burned when she pulled on a tablecloth and hot coffee spilled on her chest. On arrival at the emergency department, the child is alert. Her vital signs are temperature 98.4°F, heart rate is 102 beats/min (bpm), respiratory rate is 24 breaths/min, and blood pressure is 86/54 mm Hg. A 5- $\times$ 10-cm area on her upper chest area is red, and there are four fluid-filled blisters.

1. How would you classify the depth and severity of the child's injury?

2. What would you expect to be included in the child's treatment?

The child will be discharged to home where her parents will take care of the burned area until it heals.

3. What will you teach them about caring for a burn wound?

4. What concerns do you have about preventing burns in the child's home?

5. How should you respond to the mother when she asks you, "Will she have a scar?"

REVIEW QUESTIONS

Choose the correct answer.

1. A child cut his hand a few days ago. Now the area is swollen and painful, and a red streak extends from it up to the forearm. These are signs of:
   a. impetigo.
   b. cellulitis.
   c. contact dermatitis.
   d. eczema.

2. Which medication is appropriate for the treatment of tinea capitis?
   a. Griseofulvin orally for 6 to 8 weeks
   b. Lotrimin cream to affected areas thrice a day until lesions are healed
   c. Tinactin spray twice a day to the affected lesions
   d. Penicillin four times a day for 10 days

3. The stinger of a honeybee should be removed by:
   a. squeezing it out of the skin.
   b. using tweezers to lift it out.
   c. scraping it out horizontally.
   d. applying heat to draw out the stinger.

4. What should an adolescent female with severe acne know about Accutane before treatment is initiated?
   a. She will need to use sunscreen to reduce photosensitivity.
   b. Accutane can cause menstrual irregularities.
   c. Accutane is teratogenic if taken during pregnancy.
   d. Exposure to sunlight should be avoided while taking Accutane.

5. What should the nurse teach parents about skin care for the child with atopic dermatitis?
   a. After bathing, apply moisturizing cream when the skin has been thoroughly dried.
   b. Avoid clothing made of cotton and polyester because these materials are irritating.
   c. Dress the child warmly at bedtime to prevent itching due to coldness.
   d. Moisturizing creams can be applied whenever the skin looks dry.

6. Which action is appropriate for the prevention of diaper dermatitis?
   a. Apply medicated powder to the perineum after each diaper change.
   b. Wash the diaper area with a mild soap and water after each voiding or bowel movement.
   c. Keep the diaper area open to air during rest periods.
   d. Change diapers at least every 4 hours.

7. Assessment of the skin of a child with allergic dermatitis is likely to reveal:
   a. keratosis.
   b. ecchymoses.
   c. lichenification.
   d. pruritus.

8. Assessment of a child with nits would reveal:
   a. very small black bugs jumping throughout the hair.
   b. white specks firmly attached to the hair shaft.
   c. small flakes, resembling dandruff, that are easily removed from the hair.
   d. clusters of nits at the crown of the head and front hairline.

9. The depth of a burn that appears red to pale ivory, with a moist surface and fluid-filled blisters, is most likely:
   a. superficial.
   b. superficial partial thickness.
   c. deep partial thickness.
   d. full thickness.

10. What is the first priority when initiating treatment on a child with a major burn injury?
    a. Fluid resuscitation
    b. Prevention of sepsis
    c. Airway assessment
    d. Correcting metabolic imbalances

11. What is the most common cause of burn injuries in children younger than 3 years?
    a. Flame
    b. Electrical
    c. Chemical
    d. Scald

12. Burn shock results from:
    a. hypovolemia.
    b. sepsis.
    c. toxins.
    d. metabolic acidosis.

50 The Child with a Musculoskeletal Alteration

HELPFUL HINT

Review the anatomy and physiology of the musculoskeletal system in an anatomy and physiology textbook.

MATCHING KEY TERMS

Match the term with the correct definition.

1. _____ Avascular necrosis
2. _____ Dislocation
3. _____ Dysplasia
4. _____ Ossification
5. _____ Osteoblasts
6. _____ Osteoclasts
7. _____ Osteotomy
8. _____ Paresthesia
9. _____ Polydactyly
10. _____ Pseudarthrosis
11. _____ Reduction
12. _____ Subluxation
13. _____ Syndactyly
14. _____ Valgum
15. _____ Varum

a. Failure of the bones to fuse
b. Abnormal bending away from the midline
c. Displacement of a bone from its normal articulation with a joint
d. Extra fingers or toes
e. Tissue damage resulting from inadequate blood supply to the area
f. Surgical cutting of the bone
g. Partial dislocation of a joint
h. Abnormal development of tissue
i. Abnormal bending toward the midline
j. Fusing or webbing of two or more fingers or toes
k. Repositioning of bone fragments into a neutral alignment
l. Mesodermal cells whose activity produces bone
m. Sensation of numbness and tingling
n. Bone cells that absorb and remove old bone tissue
o. Process of forming bone from osseous tissue or cartilage

16. Write the opposite of each of the following terms.

a. Abduction: _____

b. Eversion: _____

c. Internal rotation: _____

d. External fixation: _____

Recall the definition of the italicized term in each of the following. Then identify whether the statement is true (T) or false (F).

17. _____ Artificial limbs are called *orthoses*.

18. _____ *Arthroscopy* is a medical treatment for joint injuries.

19. _____ *Callus* becomes hardened through osteoclastic activity.

20. _____ *Superior mesenteric artery syndrome* resembles intestinal obstruction.

21. _____ In an *autologous blood transfusion,* a person receives blood from a close relative.

294

3. Improper positioning of an infant's hip in a Pavlik harness can interrupt the blood supply to the head of the femur, resulting in _____.

4. List five actual or potential problems encountered when caring for a child in a spica cast.

   a. _____

   b. _____

   c. _____

   d. _____

   e. _____

LEGG–CALVÉ–PERTHES DISEASE

Answer as either true (T) or false (F).

1. _____ Legg–Calvé–Perthes disease can result in arthritis and skeletal deformities.

2. _____ In Legg–Calvé–Perthes disease, there is avascular necrosis of the femoral head.

3. _____ Surgical correction increases the overall treatment time.

4. _____ In Legg–Calvé–Perthes disease, both hips are usually affected.

SLIPPED CAPITAL FEMORAL EPIPHYSIS (SCFE)

1. Most adolescents with SCFE are _____ average for height and weight.

2. The adolescent with SCFE often presents with _____ pain.

3. In SCFE, the _____ plate thins in response to hormonal changes during adolescence.

4. Surgical correction involves inserting a screw across the _____.

FRACTURES

1. A compound fracture is _____.

2. Describe compartment syndrome.

3. A child with a compound fracture is at risk for _____.

4. Proper healing of a fracture requires correct reduction and _____.

5. Open reduction requires the surgical insertion of a(n) _____ device.

6. Fractures in infants usually result from birth trauma or _____ trauma.

7. The most common sites for fractures in children are the_____, _____, _____, and _____.

8. Epiphyseal injuries are fractures that occur between the shaft of a long bone and the _____.

9. Fat emboli occur most commonly after _____ injuries or fractures of _____ bones.

Chapter **50** **The Child with a Musculoskeletal Alteration**

SOFT TISSUE INJURIES

Match each term with its description.

1. _____ Sprain

2. _____ Strain

3. _____ Contusion

4. _____ Dislocation

a. Articulating surfaces of the joint are no longer in contact

b. Damage to soft tissue, muscle, or subcutaneous tissue

c. Excessive muscle stretch, resulting in tears and pulls

d. Stretched or torn ligaments

OSGOOD–SCHLATTER DISEASE

1. To what is Osgood–Schlatter disease thought to be related?

2. List three clinical manifestations of Osgood–Schlatter disease.

   a. _____

   b. _____

   c. _____

OSTEOGENESIS IMPERFECTA

1. Describe osteogenesis imperfecta.

2. Identify three clinical manifestations of osteogenesis imperfecta.

   a. _____

   b. _____

   c. _____

OSTEOMYELITIS

Answer as either true (T) or false (F).

1. _____ Osteomyelitis may follow otitis media.

2. _____ Cellulitis can result in osteomyelitis.

3. _____ Osteomyelitis occurs most often in infants.

4. _____ Children with osteomyelitis require complete bed rest.

5. _____ Areas of sequestrum are highly susceptible to antibiotics.

JUVENILE ARTHRITIS (JA)

1. Briefly describe juvenile arthritis.

2. What is uveitis?

3. When are cytotoxic drugs used in the management of JA?

4. JA is the leading cause of _____ in children.

MUSCULAR DYSTROPHIES

1. Muscular dystrophies are _____
   _____.

2. What is the most common type of muscular dystrophy?

3. What is the most common cause of death resulting from muscular dystrophy?

SCOLIOSIS, KYPHOSIS, AND LORDOSIS

Answer as either true (T) or false (F).

1. _____ Paralytic scoliosis is the predominant form of scoliosis.

2. _____ Uneven shoulder height is an indicator of scoliosis.

3. _____ Bracing is used to correct existing curves in scoliosis.

4. _____ Spinal fusion is used to treat severe scoliosis.

5. _____ Superior mesenteric artery syndrome is a complication of bracing for scoliosis.

6. _____ After washing and drying the skin, Keri lotion should be applied before putting on a tee shirt and brace for scoliosis.

7. _____ Lordosis is a lateral curvature of the spine.

8. _____ Kyphosis is a convex curvature of the spine, usually in the thoracic area.

SUGGESTED LEARNING ACTIVITIES

1. Spend some time with a school nurse doing scoliosis screening. Report on the procedure, the reactions of the students, and the screening results to your class.

2. Arrange to observe in a newborn nursery. Observe the nurses' techniques for assessing skeletal abnormalities.

STUDENT LEARNING APPLICATIONS

Enhance your learning by discussing your answers with other students.

Twelve-year-old Kai is admitted to the hospital with a fractured femur. He is in Russell traction, and he says to you, "I hate this thing! Why are you doing this to me?"

1. How would you explain to Kai about traction and why he needs it?

2. How would you address the "doing this to me" aspect of Kai's question?

3. How would you facilitate trust?

4. How would you enlist Kai's cooperation in maintaining proper alignment and in doing range-of-motion exercises and neurovascular assessments?

REVIEW QUESTIONS

Choose the correct answer.

1. Screening for idiopathic scoliosis is performed:
   a. prenatally.
   b. during the newborn period.
   c. during the school-age years.
   d. during middle adolescence.

2. A disorder that is obvious in the newborn period is:
   a. clubfoot.
   b. polydactyly.
   c. syndactyly.
   d. all of the above.

3. When developmental dysplasia of the hip is diagnosed:
   a. treatment is immediately initiated.
   b. treatment is postponed until the child is able to bear weight.
   c. surgery is scheduled as soon as the child weighs 10 lb.
   d. bilateral casting is done at 1 month of age.

4. Uncorrected scoliosis can result in:
   a. superior mesenteric artery syndrome.
   b. reduced respiratory function.
   c. fusion of the vertebrae.
   d. none of the above.

5. A child with lordosis may present with:
   a. a concave deformity and obesity.
   b. scoliosis and kyphosis.
   c. a convex deformity and pain in the lower back.
   d. unequal shoulder height and leg-length discrepancy.

6. A newborn has been casted for a clubfoot. Parents should be taught about:
   a. assessing for genu varum.
   b. preventing pathologic fractures.
   c. frequent follow-up visits.
   d. preventing deformities of the hands.

7. A child has a closed fracture of the right radius, with slight ecchymosis below the elbow. She always rates her pain as either 9 or 10 on a 10-point scale. Her right hand is cooler than her left, and she cannot extend the fingers of her hand because they "burn." She is probably experiencing:
   a. compartment syndrome.
   b. epiphyseal injuries.
   c. early signs of an infection.
   d. all the above.

8. In taking the history of a child with JA, the nurse would probably discover that the child is taking:
   a. acetaminophen.
   b. aspirin.
   c. morphine.
   d. prednisone.

9. A male adolescent is diagnosed with Osgood–Schlatter disease. In taking a history, the nurse is not surprised to find that he:
   a. is below the 20th percentile for height and weight.
   b. is a medal-winning swimmer.
   c. is on the football team.
   d. has a family history of arthritis.

10. A painful limp, pain in the knee and hip joints, and quadriceps muscle atrophy are clinical manifestations of:
    a. Legg–Calvé–Perthes disease.
    b. Osgood–Schlatter disease.
    c. osteogenesis imperfecta.
    d. Duchenne muscular dystrophy.

11. An appropriate intervention for a child's sprained ankle is:
    a. ibuprofen.
    b. ice packs applied for 20 minutes.
    c. elastic bandage wrap.
    d. all of the above.

12. What is the best way to assess sensory function in a 6-year-old child with a lower leg cast?
    a. Ask "Do you feel this?" when pressing down on the little toe.
    b. Check the capillary refill in the middle toe.
    c. Tell the child to wiggle his toes.
    d. Ask "Which toe am I pinching?" when pinching the great toe.

13. A child is hospitalized with musculoskeletal trauma following a severe scooter crash. The nurse expects to find:
    a. elevated alkaline phosphatase (ALP) level.
    b. positive rheumatoid factor (RF).
    c. decreased erythrocyte sedimentation rate (ESR).
    d. all of the above.

14. A musculoskeletal condition that typically results in death in late adolescence is:
    a. osteogenesis imperfecta.
    b. Legg–Calvé–Perthes disease.
    c. JA.
    d. Duchenne muscular dystrophy.

51 The Child with an Endocrine or Metabolic Alteration

Refer to an anatomy and physiology textbook for a more extensive discussion of the endocrine system.

MATCHING KEY TERMS

Match the term with the correct definition.

1. _____ Hormone

2. _____ Gland

3. _____ Pituitary

4. _____ Euthyroid

5. _____ Glucagon

6. _____ Hyperglycemia

7. _____ Hypoglycemia

8. _____ Hypothalamus

a. An endocrine gland attached to the base of the brain that secretes many hormones

b. Chemical substance produced by one gland or tissue and transported by the blood to other tissues, where it causes a specific effect

c. Blood glucose levels less than 70 mg/dL

d. Portion of the brain that secretes releasing factors

e. Organ or structure that secretes a substance to be used in some other part of the body

f. Normal thyroid function

g. In a non-diabetic person, fasting blood glucose level greater than or equal to 110 mg/dL

h. Counteracts the action of insulin

REVIEW OF THE ENDOCRINE SYSTEM

Match each hormone with the pituitary lobe that produces it. (Answers may be used more than once.)

1. _____ Oxytocin

2. _____ Adrenocorticotropic hormone (ACTH)

3. _____ Thyroid-stimulating hormone (TSH)

4. _____ Luteinizing hormone (LH)

5. _____ Antidiuretic hormone (ADH)

6. _____ Growth hormone (GH)

7. _____ Prolactin

a. Anterior pituitary lobe

b. Posterior pituitary lobe

DIAGNOSTIC TESTS AND PROCEDURES

1. How are alterations in endocrine functioning usually diagnosed?

2. Accurate measurements of _____ and _____ are essential when assessing a child for endocrine function.

Neonatal Hypoglycemia

1. Hypoglycemia in the neonate is defined as a plasma glucose concentration of less than _____.

2. The neonates who are most likely to experience hypoglycemia are _____ infants and infants who are _____.

3. List five signs that indicate a neonate is hypoglycemic.

   a. _____

   b. _____

   c. _____

   d. _____

   e. _____

4. What is the intervention for a neonate who is hypoglycemic but asymptomatic?

5. What assessments are indicated if a neonate is at an increased risk for hypoglycemia?

6. What complication can occur when a neonate is receiving intravenous (IV) glucose?

HYPOCALCEMIA

1. *Neonatal hypocalcemia* is defined as the total serum calcium concentration lower than _____.

2. Why does neonatal hypocalcemia occur most often in infants of diabetic mothers?

3. What is the best time to administer an oral calcium supplement?

PHENYLKETONURIA AND INBORN ERRORS OF METABOLISM

1. What is the genetic transmission pattern of phenylketonuria?

2. Phenylketonuria results in damage to which body system?

3. When should the neonate be screened for phenylketonuria?

4. What is the treatment of phenylketonuria?

Answer as either true (T) or false (F).

5. _____ The child with galactosemia must be on a lifelong low-protein, limited amino acid diet.

6. _____ Maple syrup urine disease causes ketoacidosis 2 to 3 days after birth.

7. _____ Tay–Sachs disease can be treated through dietary modifications.

CONGENITAL ADRENAL HYPERPLASIA

1. In congenital adrenal hyperplasia, the adrenal gland is not able to manufacture _____ but
   instead produces excess _____.

2. What finding in the newborn infant should raise suspicion of congenital adrenal hyperplasia?

3. The treatment of congenital adrenal hyperplasia involves lifelong _____.

CONGENITAL AND ACQUIRED HYPOTHYROIDISM

Answer as either true (T) or false (F).

1. _____ Newborn screening for hypothyroidism should be performed between 10 and 14 days of age.

2. _____ If untreated, congenital hypothyroidism can result in intellectual disability.

3. _____ Treatment of congenital hypothyroidism requires lifelong thyroid hormone replacement.

4. _____ The most common cause of acquired hypothyroidism in children is an autoimmune process.

5. _____ A decreased TSH level is the most sensitive indicator of primary hypothyroidism.

Match each disorder with its characteristic signs and symptoms. (Disorders may be used more than once.)

6. _____ Decreased activity   a. Hypothyroidism

7. _____ Nervousness   b. Hyperthyroidism

8. _____ Increased appetite

9. _____ Weight gain

10. _____ Edema of face, hands, and eyes

11. _____ Cold intolerance

12. What should parents be taught about administering levothyroxine to their infant?

8. Hunger

9. Weight loss

10. A fasting serum glucose level exceeding _____ and a random level exceeding _____ are indicative of type 1 diabetes mellitus.

Answer as either true (T) or false (F).

11. _____ The child in the "honeymoon" phase requires increased insulin therapy to prevent hyperglycemia.

12. _____ The goal of insulin therapy is to assist the beta cells with insulin production.

13. _____ Oral hypoglycemic agents are not effective in the management of type 1 diabetes mellitus.

14. _____ Food intake should be balanced with insulin dosage.

15. _____ The family should adhere to a consistent schedule for mealtimes and the amount of food intake.

16. _____ Exercise increases blood sugar levels.

17. _____ Exercise should be scheduled to coincide with insulin peak times.

18. _____ A 15- to 30-g carbohydrate snack can be eaten when the child is planning 1 hour of exercise.

19. Give three examples of a 15-g serving of carbohydrates for the treatment of hypoglycemia.

   a. _____

   b. _____

   c. _____

20. What situations could result in hypoglycemia?

21. What intervention for hypoglycemia should be taken if the child is unconscious?

22. Why is rehydration the initial step in resolving diabetic ketoacidosis (DKA)?

23. In the treatment of DKA, what type of insulin is used and how is it administered?

Chapter **51** **The Child with an Endocrine or Metabolic Alteration**

24. In DKA, what values would you expect the following laboratory test results to be?

Blood glucose _____

Urinary ketones _____

Arterial pH _____

25. The increase in the incidence of overweight and obese children is directly related to the number of cases of _____ in children.

26. What is metabolic syndrome?

27. Describe acanthosis nigricans.

28. For how many minutes a day should children with type 2 diabetes participate in moderate physical activity?

SUGGESTED LEARNING ACTIVITIES

1. Arrange an observational experience in an outpatient endocrine clinic. Because many children with endocrine alterations are treated in outpatient settings, this would provide firsthand knowledge of pediatric endocrine alterations.

2. Develop a teaching plan for the parents of a newborn diagnosed with congenital hypothyroidism.

3. Review the teaching materials for type 1 diabetes mellitus used at your clinical site. Compare them with the teaching materials at another site.

4. Talk with children who have type 1 diabetes mellitus and their families about management and living with this chronic disease.

Enhance your learning by discussing your answers with other students.

A 7-year-old child has been sent to the emergency department from a pediatrician's office for possible DKA. Her parents brought her to the pediatrician because she has had increased urination and abdominal pain. She has lost weight over the past few weeks. The emergency department nurse observes that the child is rapidly and deeply breathing and that her breath has a fruity odor. Her blood glucose is 580 mg/dL. Her parents are shocked when they are told that their daughter is experiencing DKA. Her father says, "We thought she might have a urinary tract infection."

1. Why might her parents have thought that their daughter had such an infection?

2. What is the basis for the child's symptoms?

3. What would you expect the child's insulin schedule to be?

The child and her parents receive intensive teaching about type 1 diabetes mellitus management. She is placed on a schedule of three insulin injections per day. A few days later, her mother calls the nurse because the child is pale, shaky, and diaphoretic.

4. What do you think is happening to the child?

5. What action would you take?

The child has been active in soccer and softball at her school, and she wants to continue to play.

6. What can the child do to prevent problems during a game or practice?

REVIEW QUESTIONS

Choose the correct answer.

1. Which statement about congenital hypothyroidism is correct?
   a. Intellectual disability caused by hypothyroidism is reversible with treatment.
   b. The most common cause of congenital hypothyroidism is thyroiditis.
   c. The child with congenital hypothyroidism requires lifelong thyroid hormone replacement.
   d. Screening for this disorder is usually performed between 3 and 6 months of age.

2. The child with precocious puberty is at risk for:
   a. altered reproductive ability.
   b. delayed development of secondary sex characteristics.
   c. short adult stature.
   d. endocrine tumors.

3. A clinical manifestation of GH deficiency is:
   a. weight less than fifth percentile for age.
   b. hyperglycemia.
   c. precocious puberty.
   d. height less than fifth percentile for age and gender.

4. A nursing intervention for a child with SIADH is to:
   a. offer fluids frequently to increase fluid intake.
   b. explain the reason for restricting fluids.
   c. assist the child in selecting low-sodium foods.
   d. assess the child for dehydration.

5. When performing a physical assessment on a child with hyperthyroidism, the nurse should be alert for:
   a. coarse hair.
   b. dry, thick skin.
   c. cold intolerance.
   d. tremors.

6. The child experiencing SIADH should be assessed for signs of the electrolyte imbalance called:
   a. hyponatremia.
   b. hypernatremia.
   c. hypocalcemia.
   d. hypokalemia.

7. The cause of type 1 diabetes mellitus is thought to be:
   a. viral.
   b. genetic.
   c. environmental.
   d. autoimmune.

8. A child received regular insulin subcutaneously at 8:00 A.M. At what time is this child most likely to become hypoglycemic?
   a. 8 to 9 A.M.
   b. 10 to 11 A.M.
   c. 12 noon to 2 P.M.
   d. 3 to 5 P.M.

9. Which situation could lead to hypoglycemia?
   a. Insufficient insulin
   b. Decreased exercise
   c. Missed meal
   d. Minor illness

10. An appropriate diabetes task for the preschool child is to include:
    a. performing finger puncture for blood.
    b. choosing injection sites according to a rotation schedule.
    c. pushing the plunger on the syringe.
    d. identifying a "code" word to describe hypoglycemia.

11. Sick day rules for the child with type 1 diabetes mellitus include:
    a. do not administer insulin if the child is nauseated or vomiting.
    b. test blood glucose levels at least twice a day.
    c. test urine for ketones with each void.
    d. offer fluids with calories if the child is not eating.

12. One adrenergic sign of hypoglycemia is:
    a. blurred vision.
    b. clammy skin.
    c. irritability.
    d. increased respiratory rate.

13. If not properly balanced with insulin and diet, exercise can lead to:
    a. hypoglycemia.
    b. hyperglycemia.
    c. ketoacidosis.
    d. hypokalemia.

14. The best action for a child who is experiencing hypoglycemia is to:
    a. drink 4 oz of fruit juice.
    b. eat a chocolate bar.
    c. drink a can of diet soda.
    d. get some exercise.

15. Type 2 diabetes in children is associated with:
    a. intrauterine growth restriction.
    b. obesity.
    c. family history of type 2 diabetes.
    d. all of the above.

52 The Child with a Neurologic Alteration

HELPFUL HINT

Review the physiology of the nervous system in an anatomy and physiology textbook. In addition, refer to a pharmacology textbook for a more detailed discussion of anticonvulsant medications.

MATCHING KEY TERMS

Match the term with the correct definition.

1. _____ Blood–brain barrier
2. _____ Cerebral herniation
3. _____ Cushing response
4. _____ Decerebrate posture
5. _____ Decorticate posture
6. _____ Monro–Kellie doctrine
7. _____ Myelinization

a. Abnormal flexion of the upper extremities and extension of the lower extremities

b. Formation of the proteolipid coating of the nerves

c. Separation between the brain tissue and blood

d. Shift of brain tissue sideways or downward, causing severe neurologic dysfunction

e. Abnormal extension of upper extremities with the internal rotation of upper arms and wrists

f. Compensatory mechanism of cranial contents that maintains a steady volume and pressure

g. Late sign of increased intracranial pressure (ICP)

REVIEW OF THE CENTRAL NERVOUS SYSTEM

1. Identify the week(s) during gestation when the following occur:

   a. Neural tube closes

   b. First period of rapid brain cell growth

   c. Second period of rapid brain cell growth

   d. Myelin sheath begins to form

2. Name the three main sections of the brain.

   a. _____

   b. _____

   c. _____

3. What is the function of the cerebrospinal fluid (CSF)?

Match each term with its description.

4. _____ Dura mater

5. _____ Tentorium

6. _____ Pia mater

7. _____ Axial skeleton

8. _____ Cerebrum

9. _____ Brainstem

a. Fills the upper portion of the skull

b. Outer layer of meninges

c. Contains the pons, medulla, midbrain, thalamus, and third ventricle

d. Tent-like structure separating the cerebellum from the occipital lobe

e. Innermost layer of the meninges

f. Protects the structures of the central nervous system

INCREASED INTRACRANIAL PRESSURE (ICP)

1. How does the brain compensate for increased ICP?

2. Identify two clinical manifestations of increased ICP for each of the following age groups:

   a. Infants

   b. Children

3. What three assessments are included in the Glasgow Coma Scale?

   a. _____

   b. _____

   c. _____

Match each level of consciousness with its description.

4. _____ Confused

5. _____ Disoriented

6. _____ Lethargic

7. _____ Obtunded

8. _____ Stupor

9. _____ Coma

a. Person requires considerable stimulation to arouse

b. Ability to clearly and rapidly think is lost

c. Person easily awakens but exhibits limited responsiveness

d. Person is unable to recognize a place or person

e. Vigorous stimulation produces no motor or verbal response.

f. Person sleeps unless aroused

Answer as either true (T) or false (F).

10. _____ Changes in a child's normal behavior are important indicators of increased ICP.

11. _____ The pupils constrict as ICP increases.

12. _____ The progression from decerebrate to decorticate posturing indicates the deterioration of the child's condition.

13. _____ The appearance of the Cushing reflex is an early sign of increased ICP.

SPINA BIFIDA

1. Spina bifida results from _____

_____.

2. Define the following terms.

   a. Meningocele

   b. Myelomeningocele

   c. Spina bifida occulta

Answer as either true (T) or false (F).

3. _____ Degree of impairment is related to the level of the defect on the spinal cord.

4. _____ Folic acid deficiency in the mother has been linked to neural tube defects in the child.

5. _____ A child with a myelomeningocele below S3 will have a serious motor impairment.

6. _____ Prenatal closure of myelomeningocele reduces the severity of Chiari II malformations.

7. _____ Before surgery, the neonate with a myelomeningocele is at risk for infection.

8. _____ Children with spina bifida are at a high risk for developing a latex allergy.

HYDROCEPHALUS

1. The treatment for hydrocephalus is

_____.

2. How should the infant or child with hydrocephalus be positioned postoperatively?

3. What are the signs of a shunt infection?

Match each clinical manifestation with the corresponding age group. (Answers may be used more than once.)

4. _____ Full, bulging anterior fontanel

a. Infant early sign

5. _____ Nausea and vomiting that may be projectile

b. Infant late sign

6. _____ "setting sun" eyes

c. Child early sign

7. _____ Shrill, high-pitched cry

d. Child late sign

8. _____ Widely separated cranial sutures

9. _____ Frontal headache in the morning relieved by vomiting or sitting upright

10. _____ Seizures

CEREBRAL PALSY

Answer as either true (T) or false (F).

1. _____ Almost all children with cerebral palsy will have some degree of intellectual disability and other handicaps.

2. _____ In cerebral palsy, the damage to the motor system can occur in the prenatal, perinatal, or postnatal periods.

3. _____ A delay in motor development is an indicator of cerebral palsy.

4. _____ A child with dyskinetic cerebral palsy exhibits slow, writhing movement of the extremities.

5. _____ What equipment is kept at the bedside of a child on seizure precautions?

HEAD INJURY

1. What is included in the initial assessment of a child with a head injury?

2. What guidelines should parents follow in determining when to notify the physician of a child's head injury?

Match each type of head injury with its description.

3. _____ Contusion

a. Transient and reversible neuronal dysfunction with an instantaneous loss of responsiveness

4. _____ Concussion

5. _____ Closed head injury

b. Accumulation of blood between the dura and skull

6. _____ Epidural hemorrhage

c. Petechial hemorrhages along the superficial aspects of the brain

7. _____ Subdural hemorrhage

d. Accumulation of blood between the dura and the cerebrum

8. _____ Missile injury

e. Nonpenetrating injury to the head

f. Penetrating injury of the skull or brain

9. Describe postconcussion syndrome.

SPINAL CORD INJURY

Answer as either true (T) or false (F).

1. _____ Spinal shock is accompanied by flaccid paralysis.

2. _____ A common cause of spinal cord injury in an infant is aggressive shaking by an adult or older child.

3. _____ Most spinal cord injuries in children occur in the cervical spine.

4. _____ Before any attempt is made to move a child with a neck or spinal cord injury, the spine must be immobilized.

5. _____ After a spinal cord injury, the spine is immobilized by tongs or traction.

6. _____ If steroid treatment is used, it must be started within 2 hours of the spinal cord injury.

SEIZURE DISORDERS

Match each classification of seizure with its description.

1. _____ Tonic-clonic

2. _____ Atonic

3. _____ Myoclonic

4. _____ Absence

a. Sustained, generalized contraction of the muscles followed by alternating the contraction and relaxation of major muscle groups

b. Brief, random contractions of a muscle group

c. Brief episodes of altered consciousness characterized by a blank facial expression

d. Abrupt loss of postural tone, impaired consciousness, and confusion

5. Differentiate between a seizure and epilepsy.

6. Precipitating factors in febrile seizures are the _____ and _____ of temperature elevation.

7. What information should the nurse get from a parent or caregiver when a child has a seizure?

8. List five nursing interventions to maintain a child's safety during a generalized tonic-clonic seizure.

a. _____

b. _____

c. _____

d. _____

e. _____

9. What should the nurse teach parents about the use of the antiepileptic medication phenytoin (Dilantin)?

10. Define *status epilepticus*.

11. The most common cause of neonatal seizures is _____.

MENINGITIS

1. What diagnostic test confirms that a child has meningitis?

2. Describe a positive Kernig sign.

3. Describe a positive Brudzinski sign.

4. How is acute bacterial meningitis treated?

Answer as either true (T) or false (F).

5. _____ Signs of meningitis in young children may be vague and nonspecific.

6. _____ The child with bacterial meningitis should be kept in isolation for 7 days.

7. _____ The treatment of viral meningitis is symptomatic and supportive.

8. _____ Adolescents entering college should receive the Hib (*Haemophilus influenzae* type B) vaccine.

GUILLAIN–BARRÉ SYNDROME (GBS)

1. What causes inflammation in GBS?

2. What emergency equipment belongs at the bedside of a child with GBS?

3. Describe the progression of neuromuscular impairment in GBS.

HEADACHES

1. How are migraine headaches different from tension-type headaches?

SUGGESTED LEARNING ACTIVITIES

1. Assess the neurologic status of several children using the Glasgow Coma Scale.

Enhance your learning by discussing your answers with other students.

A mother brings her 4-year-old son to the emergency department because he has had a seizure. She explains that the child became unconscious, his body became rigid, and his back began systematically arching and relaxing. The child has also had a headache, sore neck, and fever for the past day.

1. What information in this situation is suggestive of meningitis?

2. What diagnostic study would confirm this diagnosis? What would you expect an analysis to reveal?

3. What other diagnostic study might be ordered for the child, given his history?

4. What additional information about the child's seizure should you gather from his mother?

5. The child's mother then asks, "What caused the seizure?" How would you respond?

As you are speaking with the mother, the child begins to have a seizure like the one his mother described.

6. How would you classify the seizure?

7. What nursing actions would you take to ensure the child's safety while he is having the seizure?

8. What would you document about the seizure?

9. What is the treatment for bacterial meningitis?

The child is admitted to the hospital.

10. As his nurse, what assessments would you make?

REVIEW QUESTIONS

Choose the correct answer.

1. What is used to monitor brain growth?
   a. CSF analysis
   b. Head circumference measurement
   c. Electroencephalogram (EEG)
   d. Computed tomography (CT) scan

2. A clinical manifestation of increased ICP in an infant is:
   a. slurred speech.
   b. headache.
   c. double vision.
   d. bulging fontanel.

3. Raccoon eyes and clear fluid draining from the ears are suggestive of which type of head injury?
   a. Basilar skull fracture
   b. Concussion
   c. Subdural hemorrhage
   d. Contusion

4. If a child awakens easily but exhibits limited responsiveness, his level of consciousness is described as:
   a. confused.
   b. disoriented.
   c. lethargic.
   d. stuporous.

5. What is not included in the Glasgow Coma Scale?
   a. Eye opening
   b. Motor response
   c. Verbal response
   d. Neurovascular status

6. Which change in vital signs is not associated with the Cushing reflex?
   a. Increased systolic pressure
   b. Decreased heart rate
   c. Increased temperature
   d. Irregular respiratory pattern

7. A newborn has a sac in the lumbosacral area containing CSF, meninges, nerve roots, and the spinal cord. This condition is referred to as:
   a. myelomeningocele.
   b. meningocele.
   c. Arnold Chiari malformation.
   d. spina bifida occulta.

8. Before surgery, the priority for care of a newborn with a myelomeningocele is:
   a. preventing infection.
   b. preserving urinary function.
   c. promoting nutrition.
   d. maximizing motor function.

9. An early sign of hydrocephalus in an infant is:
   a. "setting sun" eyes.
   b. frontal bone enlargement.
   c. shrill, high-pitched cry.
   d. widely separated cranial sutures.

10. Which type of cerebral palsy is characterized by increased deep tendon reflexes, hypertonia, and flexion of extremities?
    a. Spastic
    b. Ataxic
    c. Athetoid
    d. Rigid

11. An expected finding in an analysis of CSF in the child with bacterial meningitis is:
    a. low protein level.
    b. cloudy appearance.
    c. high glucose level.
    d. increased red blood cells.

12. An appropriate nursing action during a tonic-clonic seizure is:
    a. restraining flailing extremities.
    b. placing padding between the teeth.
    c. observing the type of movements and duration of the seizure.
    d. placing the child in a supine or prone position.

13. A parent describes his child as having a blank stare with eyelid twitching. This child is most likely experiencing which type of seizure?
    a. Complex partial
    b. Atonic
    c. Myoclonic
    d. Absence

14. What is the first priority when a child has sustained a spinal cord injury?
    a. Assess motor function.
    b. Assess sensory function.
    c. Immobilize the spine.
    d. Measure vital signs.

15. Which statement about febrile seizures is true?
    a. Most children who experience febrile seizures develop epilepsy.
    b. Febrile seizures most commonly occur after 5 years of age.
    c. Seizure activity occurs as the temperature rises.
    d. A prolonged temperature elevation usually precedes the febrile seizure.

HELPFUL HINT

Review a psychiatric nursing textbook for additional information about psychosocial disorders and psychotropic medications.

OVERVIEW OF CHILDHOOD PSYCHOPATHOLOGY

Answer as either true (T) or false (F).

1. _____ Cognitive development proceeds from abstract to concrete thinking.

2. _____ A significant factor that influences the effect of brain damage on the child is the maturational stage of the brain at the time the damage occurs.

3. _____ Most psychosocial disorders occur as the result of genetic or biologic and environmental factors.

ANXIETY AND MOOD DISORDERS

Match each disorder with its description.

1. _____ Adjustment disorder

2. _____ Dysthymic disorder

3. _____ Social anxiety

4. _____ Bipolar mood disorder

5. _____ School refusal

6. _____ Major depressive disorder

7. _____ Separation anxiety

8. _____ Posttraumatic stress disorder

9. _____ Obsessive–compulsive disorder

10. _____ Panic disorder

a. Episode of an irritable or depressed mood with disturbances in sleep, appetite, energy, and self-esteem lasting at least 2 weeks

b. Reactive depression

c. Most common anxiety disorder in children

d. Chronic mood disturbances fluctuating between depressive lows and highs lasting at least 1 year

e. May be precipitated by bullying

f. Irritable or depressed mood for at least 1 year

g. Rapid onset of symptoms that overwhelms a child's ability to cope

h. Cognitive and psychologic disorders following the exposure to a horrifying event

i. Disabling fear about being away from parents or home

j. Manifests as repetitive thoughts or ritualistic actions

Answer as either true (T) or false (F).

11. _____ Children with mood disorders have increased serotonin levels.

12. _____ Affective disorders have been shown to have a genetic basis.

13. _____ A child or an adolescent may have both anxiety and depression.

14. _____ Antidepressants predispose adolescents to suicide.

15. Which classification of medications is often prescribed for the treatment of anxiety and depression?

SUICIDE

1. Identify five manifestations that indicate a child is at risk for suicide.

   a. _____

   b. _____

   c. _____

   d. _____

   e. _____

2. List three questions a nurse could ask an adolescent when he says that his life is not worth living anymore.

   a. _____

   b. _____

   c. _____

3. Describe the best approach for the nurse to take when an adolescent has expressed thoughts of suicide.

Answer as either true (T) or false (F).

4. _____ Poor self-concept is a significant factor for suicide.

5. _____ Screening children for depression in the school system is a poor suicide prevention strategy.

6. _____ Most suicide statements by adolescents can be ignored.

7. _____ Gay and lesbian adolescents are more likely to attempt suicide than are their heterosexual peers.

EATING DISORDERS: ANOREXIA NERVOSA AND BULIMIA NERVOSA

1. Identify three distinguishing characteristics of anorexia nervosa.

   a. _____

   b. _____

   c. _____

2. Identify three distinguishing characteristics of bulimia nervosa.

   a. _____

   b. _____

   c. _____

Answer as either true (T) or false (F).

3. _____ Adolescents with eating disorders usually have a family history of affective disorders.

4. _____ Individuals with anorexia often exhibit ritualistic tendencies about food preparation and food consumption.

5. _____ Amenorrhea is commonly seen in females with bulimia.

6. _____ When assessing an adolescent with an eating disorder, it is best to use an unstructured format to elicit information.

ATTENTION-DEFICIT/HYPERACTIVITY DISORDER (ADHD)

1. Children with ADHD have problems in what three areas?

   a. _____

   b. _____

   c. _____

2. How is a diagnosis of ADHD established?

3. What is the primary nursing intervention for the child with ADHD?

Answer as either true (T) or false (F).

4. _____ Increased levels of norepinephrine in the brain have been associated with ADHD.

5. _____ ADHD affects boys more often than it affects girls.

6. _____ Children with ADHD tend to have fewer behavioral problems in chaotic environments.

SUBSTANCE ABUSE

1. List four behaviors that would alert the school nurse to a child's substance abuse.

   a. _____

   b. _____

   c. _____

   d. _____

Answer as either true (T) or false (F).

2. _____ The treatment of substance abuse includes individual, group, and family therapy.

3. _____ In a substance abuse treatment facility, the nurse's primary responsibility is to stabilize the child or adolescent's psychologic status.

4. _____ It is important for the child or adolescent and family to identify and develop social support systems.

CHILDHOOD PHYSICAL AND EMOTIONAL ABUSE AND NEGLECT

1. Identify three common characteristics of the abusive family.

   a. _____

   b. _____

   c. _____

2. Define *shaken baby syndrome.*

3. Define *Munchausen syndrome by proxy.*

4. How can the nurse establish trust with the child and family in suspected child abuse cases?

Answer as either true (T) or false (F).

5. _____ Family dysfunction underlies most forms of child abuse.

6. _____ In most cases of sexual abuse, a child is abused by someone who is not a family member.

7. _____ The most severe and frequent physical abuse occurs in children younger than 5 years of age.

8. _____ When child abuse is suspected, the nurse should write down verbatim any comments made by the child.

SUGGESTED LEARNING ACTIVITIES

1. Perform a mental status examination on a school-age child or an adolescent. Document your findings.

2. Complete the following table on the clinical manifestations of various forms of child abuse.

Type of Abuse	Physical Indicators	Behavioral Indicators
Physical abuse		
Physical neglect		
Emotional abuse		
Sexual abuse		

STUDENT LEARNING APPLICATIONS

Enhance your learning by discussing your answers with other students.

A child with ADHD is in the fifth grade. He began taking Ritalin thrice times a day in November. He is supposed to visit the school nurse's office at lunchtime for his second Ritalin dose of the day. He occasionally goes to the office for his midday dose but often does not. He explains to the school nurse that he just "forgets" to come for his medication.

1. Could there be other reasons why the child is not coming for his midday dose of Ritalin?

2. If you were the school nurse, what strategies might you use to help the child remember to come for his medication every day?

3. Before spring break, the child's teacher tells the school nurse that he is a "different child" on Ritalin. Why would this medication make such a difference in a child's behavior?

4. How else could you evaluate the effectiveness of Ritalin for a child with ADHD?

5. Why should the child take Ritalin after eating lunch instead of before lunch?

REVIEW QUESTIONS

Choose the correct answer.

1. A parent describes her child as irritable for the past month. The child has much less energy than usual, and her grades have declined. This child meets the criteria for:
   a. dysthymic disorder.
   b. cyclothymic disorder.
   c. school phobia.
   d. major depressive disorder.

2. One of the most significant risk factors for teen suicide is:
   a. poor self-concept.
   b. anxiety.
   c. heterosexual orientation.
   d. introverted personality.

3. An adolescent tells the school nurse that he has thought about killing himself. An appropriate response to the adolescent is:
   a. "I am going to call your parents about this ASAP."
   b. "I have the number of a suicide hotline."
   c. "How are you feeling right now?"
   d. "Why would you even think about killing yourself?"

4. Which is not a manifestation of anorexia nervosa?
   a. Recurring episodes of binge eating
   b. Secondary amenorrhea
   c. Extreme fear of obesity
   d. Thin extremities with muscle wasting

5. The nurse might expect a child with ADHD to be:
   a. a gifted student who is bored with school subjects.
   b. easily distracted by internal and external stimuli.
   c. able to complete one activity before moving to the next project.
   d. ritualistic about activities of daily living.

6. Which family characteristic puts an adolescent most at risk for substance abuse?
   a. Family practices an authoritarian parenting style
   b. Family participates in school and community projects
   c. Open communication among family members is encouraged.
   d. One parent has chronic physical and mental health problems.

323

7. An adolescent who uses drugs regularly and exhibits a physical dependence on the drug is considered to be in the phase of:
   a. experimentation.
   b. early drug use.
   c. true drug addiction.
   d. severe drug addiction.

8. A child has been coming to school early, staying late, and is seen stealing food from the cafeteria. These behaviors are suggestive of:
   a. physical abuse.
   b. physical neglect.
   c. emotional abuse.
   d. emotional neglect.
   e. sexual abuse.

54 The Child with a Developmental Disability

HELPFUL HINT

Review normal growth and development in Chapters 5 through 9 of your textbook.

MATCHING KEY TERMS

Match the term with the correct definition.

1. _____ Intelligence

2. _____ Pervasive developmental disorders

3. _____ Functional age

4. _____ Co-morbidity

a. Occurrence of two or more disorders in an individual

b. Disorders involving an impairment in several areas of development

c. Capacity of a child to learn, think, and solve the problem

d. Age equivalent at which a child is able to perform specific self-care or relational tasks

INTELLECTUAL AND DEVELOPMENTAL DISORDERS

1. Children with cognitive impairments have limitations in _____ and

   _____ abilities.

2. According to the *Diagnostic and Statistical Manual of Mental Disorders,* Fourth Edition, Text Revision (DSM-IV-TR), what criteria must be met for a diagnosis of intellectual impairment?

3. What term is now used to describe people with a significantly below-average intelligence quotient (IQ)?

4. Define the term *intellectual impairment.*

5. According to the Developmental Disabilities Assistance and Bill of Rights Act of 2000, a developmental disability is defined as having the following components:

6. What is an individualized education plan (IEP)?

INTELLECTUAL AND DEVELOPMENTAL DISORDERS

1. What places children with developmental disabilities at risk for child abuse?

2. What is the cardinal sign of developmental disorders?

3. Name the two most common genetic disorders in which intellectual impairment is a central feature.

   a.

   b.

Answer as either true (T) or false (F).

4. _____ Safety is a concern for intellectually impaired children.

5. _____ Disruptive behavior disorders or other psychiatric disorders often coexist with cognitive impairment.

6. _____ The diagnosis of intellectual disability is most often made during the neonatal period.

7. _____ Therapeutic management for children with cognitive impairments largely depends on community and educational resources.

DOWN SYNDROME

1. Down syndrome is also known as _____.

2. Down syndrome is generally diagnosed at birth as a result of the infant's _____.

3. List four areas to assess when caring for the child with Down syndrome.

   a.

   b.

   c.

   d.

Answer as either true (T) or false (F).

4. _____ Down syndrome is the most common genetic disorder causing moderate to severe intellectual disability.

5. _____ Most children with Down syndrome are born to women older than 35 years.

326

6. _____ In almost all instances, Down syndrome is the result of a translocation of chromosome 21 to chromosome 15.

7. _____ When caring for a child with Down syndrome in the hospital, it is important to keep the environment and schedule as close to the child's usual environment and routines as possible.

FRAGILE X SYNDROME

Answer as either true (T) or false (F).

1. _____ Fragile X syndrome is the most common inherited cause of an intellectual disability.

2. _____ Children with fragile X syndrome have no distinctive physical features.

3. _____ Fragile X syndrome is three times more common in girls than in boys.

FETAL ALCOHOL SYNDROME (FAS)

1. What are the clinical manifestations of FAS?

2. What is the cause of FAS?

AUTISM SPECTRUM DISORDERS (ASDs)

1. ASDs share the following characteristics:

2. Children with Asperger syndrome have the inability to _____ and

_____.

Answer as either true (T) or false (F).

3. _____ Family child-rearing practices and parental personalities are the basis of the development of autism.

4. _____ The incidence of autism is equal in males and females.

5. _____ Deoxyribonucleic acid (DNA) testing is the definitive method for diagnosing autism.

6. _____ Autism usually becomes apparent after the age of 3 years.

7. _____ Describe a child who is considered an autistic savant.

8. Rett syndrome and childhood disintegrative disorder are both ASDs. What other characteristic do they have in common?

FAILURE TO THRIVE

1. What causes organic failure to thrive?

2. What causes nonorganic failure to thrive?

3. What is the most commonly observed risk factor for nonorganic failure to thrive?

SUGGESTED LEARNING ACTIVITIES

1. Arrange an interview with a social worker or other member of the multidisciplinary team. Discuss early intervention programs for the child with an intellectual disability.

STUDENT LEARNING APPLICATIONS

Enhance your learning by discussing your answers with other students.

A 3-year-old is an outpatient at the pediatric clinic. Her routine well-child checkups indicate that she has consistently achieved developmental milestones, but she reaches them much later than children of the same chronologic age. She was a term infant, and her physical appearance is normal. Her weight and height are within the normal range for a child her age. She has been healthy throughout childhood, and her immunizations are up to date. Her mother concludes today's checkup by asking, "She's so much slower than her playmates, do you think she's retarded or autistic or something?"

1. How would you answer this inquiry?

2. What are the immediate needs of the mother?

3. What are the needs of the child?

4. Identify potential community resources that you could use for the child and her family at this stage of evaluation.

REVIEW QUESTIONS

Choose the correct answer.

1. A clinical manifestation of Down syndrome is:
   a. extremely soft and smooth skin.
   b. hypertonicity of large muscles.
   c. long, narrow face with large ears.
   d. single transverse palmar crease.

2. The best method of detecting intellectual disability at an early age is:
   a. neuropsychologic testing.
   b. using an IQ test for cognitive abilities.
   c. a developmental assessment at the well-child care.
   d. a radiographic evaluation of the brain.

3. The child with fragile X syndrome will likely exhibit:
   a. frustration with a change in routine.
   b. impairment in the rate of physical, social, and language skills.
   c. abnormal ways of relating to people.
   d. gaze avoidance, hand flapping, and abnormal speech patterns.

4. Which question, during a hospital admission assessment, best indicates that the nurse understands the needs of a child with Down syndrome?
   a. "Can you go over her daily routine with me?"
   b. "Does she require a special diet?"
   c. "Does she sleep through the night?"
   d. "Is she toilet trained?"

5. Injuries are less common among children with intellectual disabilities during:
   a. infancy.
   b. toddlerhood.
   c. preschool age.
   d. adolescence.

6. A child with autism will display:
   a. hyperkinetic behavior, poor coordination, and intellectual disabilities.
   b. absent or delayed speech and abnormal ways of relating to people.
   c. periods of remission and relapse.
   d. pubescent or adolescent onset of the disorder.

328

7. The goal for a child with an intellectual disability is to:
   a. find an appropriate facility to meet the long-term needs of the child.
   b. maximize the child's skill potential and provide safe, nurturing care in a supportive family.
   c. use community resources to support the family through stressful periods.
   d. assist the child to live within the child's limitations.

8. In developing a care plan for an infant with FAS, the nurse should anticipate parents to report difficulties with the infant's:
   a. feeding.
   b. mobility.
   c. speech.
   d. elimination.

55 The Child with a Sensory Alteration

HELPFUL HINT

Review vision, hearing, and language development in Chapters 5 through 9 in your textbook. In addition, refer to Chapter 33 "Physical Assessment of Children" for an overview of screening techniques.

REVIEW OF THE EYE AND THE EAR

Match each part of the eye or ear with its description.

1. _____ Eustachian tube
2. _____ Malleus, incus, and stapes
3. _____ Cochlea
4. _____ Tympanic membrane
5. _____ Retina
6. _____ Iris
7. _____ Cornea
8. _____ Macula
9. _____ Sclera

a. Small snail-shaped chamber in the inner ear
b. Clear area located in the front of the eye
c. Structure that separates the outer ear from the middle ear
d. Inner area of the eye containing rods and cones
e. Structure that contains the greatest concentration of nerve endings in the eye
f. Structure that connects the middle ear with the nasopharynx
g. Bones of the middle ear
h. Colored muscular ring located behind the cornea
i. White outer covering of the eye

Fill in the blanks.

10. The critical period of eye development is _____.

11. The critical period for ear development is _____.

12. Binocularity is established by _____.

13. A child usually develops 20/20 visual acuity by _____.

DISORDERS OF THE EYE

Match each disorder with its description.

1. _____ Refractive error
2. _____ Strabismus
3. _____ Color blindness
4. _____ Glaucoma
5. _____ Cataract
6. _____ Conjunctivitis
7. _____ Orbital cellulitis
8. _____ Corneal abrasion
9. _____ Hyphema

a. Infection of the soft tissues that surround the orbit
b. Misalignment of eyes because of a lack of coordination of the extraocular muscles
c. Disorder that results from a scraping of the lens
d. Alteration in the path of light rays through the eye
e. Inflammation of the clear membranous lining of the eyelid and sclera
f. Disorder caused by an increased intraocular pressure
g. Hemorrhage that results from a blow to the eye
h. Inability to distinguish between colors within certain groups
i. Opacity of the lens

10. What behaviors suggest that a child has a refractive error?

11. Define legal blindness.

12. What complications can develop if strabismus is not treated early?

13. Why is eye patching used to treat amblyopia?

14. What are the clinical signs of glaucoma?

15. The preferred treatment for glaucoma in children is _____.

16. For what signs of increased intraocular pressure must a child be postoperatively monitored?

17. How should the nurse position the infant after cataract surgery?

18. Identify four signs and symptoms of conjunctivitis.

   a.

   b.

   c.

   d.

19. What causes conjunctivitis during the first 24 hours of life?

20. What infection control measures should the family use when a child has conjunctivitis?

21. How can a parent recognize a blocked lacrimal duct in an infant?

22. What is the rationale for bed rest and eye patching for the treatment of hyphema?

23. A safety measure to prevent corneal abrasions and other eye injuries is _____.

24. What signs should the nurse assess for when caring for a child with a hyphema?

25. How should a chemical splash to the eye be irrigated?

Answer as either true (T) or false (F).

26. _____ A blocked lacrimal duct is usually opened surgically before 1 year of age.

27. _____ Strabismus is a normal finding up to 3 months of age.

28. _____ The child should be able to decide how long to wear the eye patch each day.

29. _____ If detected early, color blindness can be corrected.

30. _____ Intervention for the infant born with cataracts should be delayed until the infant is at least six months old.

31. _____ Chlamydia causes the majority of eye infections in infants.

32. _____ Untreated orbital cellulitis can result in meningitis.

33. _____ A chemical burn of the eyes should be irrigated immediately with water or saline.

34. _____ Of all sports activities, baseball and basketball are associated with the highest percentage of eye injuries.

HEARING LOSS IN CHILDREN

Match each type of hearing loss with its description.

1. _____ Central

2. _____ Conductive

3. _____ Mixed

4. _____ Sensorineural

a. Combination of conductive and sensorineural loss

b. Result of damage to the conduction system between the auditory nervous system and cerebral cortex

c. Result of damage or malformation of the structures of the inner ear and/or auditory nerve

d. Sound prevented from progressing across the middle ear

5. Identify three possible causes of conductive hearing loss.

   a.

   b.

   c.

6. Name three possible causes of sensorineural hearing loss.

   a.

   b.

   c.

7. The two hearing screening tests used to identify infants with hearing deficits are _____ and _____.

8. Hearing testing in a preschool or school-age child is done by _____.

9. List four guidelines for working with a hearing-impaired child.

   a.

   b.

   c.

   d.

Answer as either true (T) or false (F).

10. _____ The treatment for hearing loss depends on the type of loss.

11. _____ Sensorineural hearing loss is usually reversible.

12. _____ The recommended treatment for sensorineural hearing loss is a hearing aid.

13. _____ Deaf infants babble later than hearing infants.

14. A child with recurrent otitis media with an effusion lasting longer than 3 months should be evaluated for conductive hearing loss.

LANGUAGE DISORDERS

Match each language milestone with the age at which it normally occurs.

1. _____ Speaks first words   a. 12 months

2. _____ Speaks first sentences   b. 18 months

3. _____ Has a vocabulary of at least 50 words   c. 2 years

4. Expressive language disorders affect which three areas of speech?

   a.

   b.

   c.

5. Identify three guidelines for parents on being effective role models in the area of speech.

   a.

   b.

   c.

Answer as either true (T) or false (F).

6. _____ Girls have more rapid language development than boys until 3 years of age.

7. _____ There is strong evidence linking early talking with greater intelligence.

8. _____ Children with a receptive language disorder are unable to understand the spoken word.

9. _____ Parents should begin reading to their child during infancy.

334

SUGGESTED LEARNING ACTIVITIES

1. Arrange an observational experience with a pediatric ophthalmologist, audiologist, or speech therapist. What techniques do these professionals use to assess infants and children for sensory disorders? What are the most common disorders they encounter in their practice?

STUDENT LEARNING APPLICATIONS

Enhance your learning by discussing your answers with other students.

Twelve-year-old Jamie is developmentally delayed and blind. He was admitted to the hospital during the night for vomiting and abdominal pain. At the moment, he is moaning in pain. His intravenous (IV) line is infiltrated, and he needs to have another IV line placed. Jamie's parents are not present.

1. What do you think Jamie's fears might be at this time? How would you address each of these fears?

2. Write an explanation to Jamie for the experience of placing an IV line. What factors are you considering as you do this? What makes writing this explanation for Jamie difficult?

3. You learn that Jamie is going to the operating room for an appendectomy. How might preparing him for surgery differ from preparing a sighted child?

REVIEW QUESTIONS

Choose the correct answer.

1. At what age does a child normally develop 20/20 vision?
   a. 4 years
   b. 5 years
   c. 7 years
   d. 8 years

2. When assessing a 5-year-old's vision, a normal finding is:
   a. hyperopia.
   b. myopia.
   c. astigmatism.
   d. strabismus.

3. What is not a clinical sign of glaucoma?
   a. Blepharospasm
   b. Increased tearing
   c. Headache
   d. Light sensitivity

4. When several children in the same class have conjunctivitis, which type of eyedrops should be used to treat it?
   a. Steroid
   b. Antibiotic
   c. Mydriatic
   d. Myopic

5. The correct technique for a lacrimal massage is to:
   a. massage from the inner eye down to the nasal bone.
   b. press gently in a circular motion.
   c. massage from the lacrimal duct upward.
   d. press inward on the lacrimal duct.

6. The immediate intervention for a chemical burn to the eyes is to:
   a. flush with water or saline.
   b. apply an antibiotic ointment.
   c. patch the affected eye.
   d. instill mydriatic drops to constrict the pupil.

7. During a hearing assessment, a child failed to hear higher than 65 decibels. This hearing loss is considered to be:
   a. mild.
   b. moderate.
   c. severe.
   d. profound.

335

8. A cause of conductive hearing loss is:
   a. ototoxic medications.
   b. exposure to loud noises.
   c. otitis media.
   d. brain tumors.

9. An appropriate intervention to use when working with a child who has a hearing impairment is to:
   a. maintain a soft background noise.
   b. talk extremely slowly.
   c. speak louder than usual.
   d. use visual aids to assist your communication.

10. A delay in language development is suggested by:
    a. babbling at 6 months.
    b. saying three words at 18 months.
    c. having a vocabulary of 50 words at 2.5 years.
    d. beginning to use two-word sentences at 3 years.

11. What is not an expressive language disorder?
    a. Difficulty with fluency
    b. Difficulty with articulation
    c. Problem with pitch and articulation
    d. Problem with comprehending the spoken word

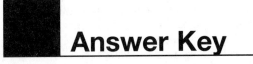

Answer Key

CHAPTER 1: FOUNDATIONS OF MATERNITY, WOMEN'S HEALTH, AND CHILD HEALTH NURSING

Matching Key Terms
1. b   3. c   5. d   7. f
2. e   4. a   6. g   8. h

Historical Perspectives
Maternity Nursing
1. a. Childbirth is usually a normal, healthy event in the life of a family.
   b. Childbirth affects the entire family, and family restructuring is required.
   c. Families are capable of making decisions about care, provided they are given adequate information and professional support.
2. a. In a traditional hospital setting, labor, birth, recovery, and postpartum care occur in separate rooms; delay of parent–infant contact.
   b. Labor and Delivery Room (LDR): labor, birth, and immediate recovery occur in a single room, with transfer to a postpartum room for continuing care; emphasis on keeping parents and infants together; liberal visiting.
   c. Labor and Delivery Room and Postpartum (LDRP) rooms: same as LDR rooms except that the mother and infant remain in the same room where the birth occurred.
   d. Birth centers: freestanding centers that provide antepartum, intrapartum, postpartum, and newborn care to low-risk mothers and babies; typically staffed with certified nurse-midwives.
   e. Home births: birth occurs in a familiar setting with support people the mother wants; fewer nurse-midwives now attend these births because of malpractice insurance problems.

Pediatric Nursing
1. F   3. T
2. T   4. T

Current Trends in Maternity and Pediatric Care
1. For maternity care, prospective payment plans have resulted in a shortened length of stay after delivery. This has created problems for some women and infants who require readmission following an early discharge. The legislation now mandates that the length of stay following a vaginal birth is 48 hours; following a cesarean birth, the length of stay is four days. Concerns about managed care in pediatrics include a delay in treatment authorization and pediatric referrals and limited coordination with community health, education, and social services.
2. F   4. F   6. T
3. T   5. T   7. F

Ethical Perspectives on Maternal and Child Nursing
1. Beneficence; nonmaleficence; autonomy; justice

Legal Issues
1. a. Duty
   b. Breach of duty
   c. Damage
   d. Proximate cause
2. a. Patient's competence to consent
   b. Full disclosure of information
   c. Patient's understanding of information
   d. Patient's voluntary consent

Review Questions
1. b   3. a
2. c   4. c

CHAPTER 2: THE NURSE'S ROLE IN MATERNITY, WOMEN'S HEALTH, AND PEDIATRIC NURSING

The Role of the Professional Nurse
1. T   2. T   3. F

Key Concepts
4. a. Care provider   d. Researcher
   b. Teacher   e. Advocate
   c. Collaborator   f. Manager
5. Developmental level, language, culture, previous experiences, physical environment, organization, and skill of the teacher
6. a. Certified nurse-midwives: registered nurses that complete a course of study and clinical experience and are certified by the American College of Nurse-Midwives; they are qualified to provide complete care during pregnancy, childbirth, and the postpartum period in uncomplicated pregnancies.
   b. Nurse practitioners: advanced practice nurses who provide care to specific groups of patients in various settings. They may collaboratively work with a physician or work independently, depending on the individual state's board of nursing mandates.
   c. Clinical nurse specialists: registered nurses with a graduate education to be experts in the care of childbearing families or pediatric patients. Their functions may include clinical leaders, role models, patient advocates, and change agents.

Implications of Changing Roles for Nurses
1. Therapeutic communication is purposeful, goal directed, and focused. It requires conscious effort and practice.
2. What is being said; nonverbal clues

337

3. a. Block: failure to acknowledge a child's feelings and providing false reassurance.

   Possible alternative response: "You will feel a prick when I give you the needle. You can cry or yell if you want. I do need you to keep your leg still. I will put a Band-Aid on it when I am done."

   b. Block: the failure to acknowledge comments or feelings.

   Possible alternative response: "This pregnancy has not gone as you expected. Tell me how being on bed rest has been difficult for you."

4. To help nurses make the best clinical judgments by identifying and overcoming habits that interfere with decision-making

5. a. Recognize assumptions.
   b. Examine personal biases.
   c. Analyze the need for closure.
   d. Collect and analyze data.
   e. Evaluate other factors (e.g., emotions, environment) that can impede critical thinking.

6. F   7. F   8. T

The Nursing Process in Maternity and Pediatric Care

1. Database assessment involves gathering data regarding all aspects of a patient's health to identify strengths and problems. Focused assessment involves gathering additional information relevant to an actual problem or one that the patient or family is at risk of acquiring.

2. Each outcome criterion is an example of how a nurse might word it; your answer may be different and still be accurate.
   a. Mrs. Lynch will ambulate in her room by 24 hours after surgery. She will ambulate the length of the hallway and back by 48 hours after surgery.
   b. By her next prenatal visit, Jane Starr will bring a diet journal for 1 day that demonstrates the correct number of servings from every food group.
   c. Andrew Franklin will be free of signs of infection, as evidenced by an afebrile state, no redness of integument, and negative cultures until his next examination in 2 weeks.

Review Questions

1. b   2. c   3. b   4. a

CHAPTER 3: THE CHILDBEARING AND CHILD-REARING FAMILY

Matching Key Terms

1. c   3. a   5. b   7. d
2. g   4. f   6. e

The Family and Nursing Care

1. a. Stress; child care
   b. Poverty; overwhelming child-rearing responsibilities
   c. Differences in parenting styles, values, and discipline

   d. Little time to prepare for the birth; little support afterward
   e. Generational conflicts
   f. Conflicts with community values
   g. Poverty; inability to seek higher education; high infant mortality rate
   h. Child neglect; risk-taking behaviors; possible criminal activity
   i. Financial hardship; marital stress; sibling resentment

2. a. I   d. I   g. E
   b. I   e. I   h. E
   c. E   f. E

Cultural Influences on Maternity and Pediatric Nursing

1. Southeast Asians
   a. Soft voice
   b. No prolonged eye contact
2. Hispanics: polite with preliminary small talk
3. Middle-Easterners
   a. Interpreters should be from an acceptable region; information is typically shared only with friends and family.
   b. A male's opinion or permission is often required.

Parenting

1. F   2. T   3. F   4. T
5. Distract the child with another object.
6. Explain why a behavior is not permitted.
7. Placing child in a nonstimulating environment for approximately 1 minute per year of age
8. Helps children see the direct result of their misbehavior
9. A technique that rewards positive behavior and ignores negative behavior
10. A controversial form of discipline usually involving spanking

Review Questions

1. b   3. d   5. a   7. c
2. a   4. c   6. a

CHAPTER 4: COMMUNICATING WITH CHILDREN AND FAMILIES

Matching Key Terms

1. c   3. e   5. a   7. h
2. f   4. d   6. b   8. g

Components of Effective Communication

1. T   4. F   7. F   10. T
2. F   5. T   8. T   11. T
3. T   6. T   9. T   12. F

Family Centered Communication

1. By creating partnerships with families and by recognizing that families have the right to fully participate in planning, implementing, and evaluating a child's care

2. Establish a rapport with the family; encourage questions; empower the parents to care for their children through education and support; effectively manage conflict with families; solicit feedback from families.
3. Understand the parents' perspective; determine a mutually agreed upon goal; look for win–win solutions; actively listen; openly express feelings; avoid blaming; summarize the discussion.

Transcultural Communication

1. Decision-making practices; child-rearing practices; extent of family support; communication practices; health and illness practices

Therapeutic Relationships: Developing and Maintaining Trust

1. Buying gifts; giving out home a phone number; accepting invitations to family gatherings; visiting the child on days off; lending or borrowing money; sharing personal information; making decisions for the family

Nursing Care: Communicating with Children and Families

1. T	3. F	5. F
2. T	4. F	6. T

Communicating with Children Who Have Special Needs

1. Assess the child's self-help skills; orient the child to landmarks in the room and typical environmental sounds; encourage parents to stay with child; keep objects in the immediate environment in the same place; explain all procedures.
2. Assess the child's self-help skills; identify how the family communicates; encourage the parents to stay with the child; develop a communication board; always face the child when speaking; do not exaggerate speech; be aware of your body language and nonverbal communication.

Review Questions

1. b	3. d	5. a	7. c
2. b	4. b	6. d	

CHAPTER 5: HEALTH PROMOTION FOR THE DEVELOPING CHILD

Matching Key Terms

1. d	4. h	7. i	10. e
2. g	5. c	8. a	
3. b	6. f	9. j	

Types of Play

1. c	2. b	3. a

Overview of Growth and Development

1. Meet the needs of their young patients
2. Growth
3. Maturation
4. Development
5. Learning

6. Delays
7. a. School aged
   b. Toddlerhood
   c. Adolescence
   d. Infancy
   e. Preschool
   f. Infancy
8. a. Weight
   b. Height
   c. Head circumference
9. 6 months, 1 year
10. Head circumference
11. 20; 32

Principles of Growth and Development

1. d	2. a	3. c	4. b

5. Under stress
6. Blocks of time during which children are ready to master specific developmental tasks

7. T	9. F	11. F	13. F
8. T	10. T	12. T	

Theories of Growth and Development

1. c	10. Mistrust
2. b	11. Autonomy
3. a	12. Initiative
4. d	13. Inferiority
5. Oral	14. Identity
6. Phallic	15. b
7. Genital	16. a
8. Anal	17. c
9. Latency	

Theories of Language Development

1. Cognitive
2. Understand the spoken word
3. Produce meaningful vocalizations

Assessment of Growth

1. Physical growth in infants and young children is an indicator of physical health.
2. Nutritional status
3. The earlier growth disorders are detected and treated, the better are the long-term prognoses.

Assessment of Development

1. a. Observing a child's behaviors and interactions
   b. Interviewing a child and his or her parents
   c. Physical examinations
   d. Standardized assessment tools
2. a. Ages and Stages questionnaire
   b. Parents' Evaluation of Developmental Status (PEDS)
   c. Infant Development Inventory
3. a. Gross motor
   b. Fine motor
   c. Language
   d. Personal–social

4. T	6. T	8. F
5. F	7. F	

339

The Nurse's Role in Promoting Optimal Growth and Development

1. Basic information about normal growth and development as a child approaches different ages

The Developmental Assessment

1. F   2. T   3. T
4. Work
5. Functional play
6. Represent an issue to be addressed
7. Rules
8. e   10. b   12. a
9. c   11. d

Health Promotion

1. T   3. F   5. T   7. F
2. F   4. T   6. T   8. F
9. Live
10. Epinephrine 1:1000
11. c   13. a   15. d
12. e   14. b
16. Infancy is a period of rapid growth, and infants need sufficient calories to support this growth.
17. 25 and 35
18. To ensure that the child will not be further stressed by unfamiliar foods in the hospital
19. a. 24-hour dietary recall
    b. Food frequency questionnaire
    c. Food diary
20. Unintentional injuries

Review Questions

1. a   4. d   7. b   10. c
2. c   5. c   8. d   11. d
3. d   6. b   9. d

CHAPTER 6: HEALTH PROMOTION FOR THE INFANT

Matching Key Terms

1. e   4. b   7. k   10. g
2. i   5. h   8. d   11. c
3. a   6. f   9. j

Growth and Development of the Infant

1. 8 to 9 months
2. 4 to 5 months
3. 6 to 7 months
4. 1 to 2 months
5. 6 to 7 months
6. 8 to 9 months
7. 6 to 7 months
8. 6 to 7 months
9. 1 to 2 months
10. 4 to 5 months
11. 8 to 9 months
12. 12 months
13. 4 to 5 months
14. 8 to 9 months

15. Immature immune systems; small, collapsible airways
16. Decreases; increases
17. Breast milk
18. 6 to 9 months
19. Fluid and electrolyte imbalances
20. d   23. b   26. T   29. F
21. c   24. F   27. T   30. F
22. a   25. F   28. T
31. When infants' needs are not consistently met, they perceive their environment as unsafe and develop a sense of mistrust.
32. Through mutually satisfying interactions in which parents meet their infants' dependency needs and provide nurturance and their infants respond positively to having their needs satisfied.
33. By this age, infants have developed strong feelings of attachment toward their caregivers and are now cognitively able to differentiate them from unfamiliar people.

Health Promotion for the Infant and Family

1. Three
2. Immunologic; digestibility
3. a. Mothers who use illegal or certain prescription drugs
   b. Mothers with untreated tuberculosis (TB)
   c. Mothers with human immunodeficiency virus (HIV)
4. Weaning is the transition from breastfeeding or bottle feeding to drinking from a cup.
5. When the infant has demonstrated readiness (see Box 6-3 in text), solid foods should be introduced in small amounts for several days before introducing a new solid.
6. F   8. F   10. T
7. F   9. T
11. a. Place infants on their backs to sleep.
    b. Use a firm mattress.
    c. Keep loose bedding and toys out of the crib.
    d. Do not expose infants to second-hand smoke.
    e. Avoid overheating.
12. Rear
13. 6 months
14. 120
15. Crawl
16. a. Hot dogs
    b. Hard candy
    c. Peanuts
    d. Grapes
    e. Raisins
    f. Chewing gum
17. a. Carrying the infant
    b. Taking the infant for a car ride
    c. Gently patting the infant on the back
    d. Placing the infant in an infant swing
18. To ascertain the appropriate dose and learn of possible allergic reactions

Review Questions

1. c   4. c   7. a   10. a
2. b   5. d   8. a
3. b   6. c   9. b

CHAPTER 7: HEALTH PROMOTION DURING EARLY CHILDHOOD

Matching Key Terms

1. i	5. k	9. h	13. g
2. d	6. b	10. a	14. c
3. f	7. m	11. j	
4. n	8. e	12. l	

Growth and Development During Early Childhood

1. 5	7. T	13. P	19. e
2. 2; 3	8. T	14. T	20. b
3. 3	9. T	15. P	21. c
4. T	10. P	16. T	
5. P	11. P	17. a	
6. P	12. P	18. d	

Health Promotion for the Toddler or Preschooler and Family

1. F	3. F	5. F
2. T	4. F	

6. Six months after the first tooth erupts
7. They provide the toddler with a sense of security.
8. Nightmares are frightening dreams that wake the child. Night terrors do not wake the child, although the child may scream out in his or her sleep and have the eyes open. The child does remember night terrors when awake.
9. Discipline; limit setting
10. a. Time-out
    b. Time-in
    c. Diversion
    d. Offering restricted choices
11. They should never leave young children alone in or near bathtubs or swimming pools or near buckets of water. They should keep toilet lids closed.
12. Booster seats raise the child high enough so that the car's lap belts and shoulder harnesses are correctly positioned over the child's smaller body.
13. They should be taught to "stop-drop-roll."
14. Guns should always be kept unloaded. They should be stored in locked cabinets with trigger guards in place.
15. After teaching the child about what is an inappropriate touching behavior, teach him or her to immediately tell an adult if someone inappropriately touches him or her. Reinforce that he or she should tell another adult even if the offending adult is a friend or a relative or tells the child not to tell anyone. Explain that he or she needs to keep telling as many adults as necessary until the inappropriate behavior stops.
16. By 24 to 30 months, children are less negative and more willing to please their caregivers. In addition, if the family is undergoing a change, such as moving or the birth of another child, it might be better to postpone toilet training until the child has adjusted to the change.
17. a. Limit exposure to situations that the child finds hard to handle.
    b. Anticipate the child's fatigue.
    c. Anticipate the child's hunger.
    d. Offer choices.
18. Before the birth of the sibling, include the child in preparations for the new baby. Read stories about new siblings. Talk about changes that may occur. Allow the child to express his or her feelings. Refer to the baby as "ours." After the birth, parents should spend a period of uninterrupted private time with the older sibling each day.
19. Speak slowly and pause frequently. Avoid pressuring the child to communicate immediately or rapidly. Notice what situations and environmental factors have a negative effect on the child's fluency. Do not complete the child's sentences. Do not draw attention to the child's speech.

Review Questions

1. c	5. d	9. c
2. b	6. b	10. a
3. d	7. c	11. b
4. a	8. c	12. d

CHAPTER 8: HEALTH PROMOTION FOR THE SCHOOL-AGE CHILD

Matching Key Terms

1. e	3. a	5. c
2. b	4. d	

Growth and Development for the School-age Child

1. F	3. F	5. F
2. T	4. F	

6. Active play increases coordination, refines motor skills, serves as a foundation for physical fitness as an adult, improves cardiovascular (CV) fitness, increases strength and flexibility, and aids in the prevention of obesity.
7. Children have higher metabolic rates and limited ability to sweat.
8. Actions
9. Weight; volume
10. Cognitively, they are able to arrange things in logical order and are able to recall similarities and differences.
11. Children learn that friendship is more than just being together. They begin to share problems and give each other emotional support. They develop a sense of loyalty.
12. Their eustachian tubes have grown.
13. By learning to do new things and by learning to do them well
14. As children learn to do things well, they become more confident and feel good about themselves.
15. Rules provide predictability and security. By conforming to external rules, children learn self-discipline and internalize values.
16. a. Child obeys to avoid punishment.
    b. Child obeys to avoid disapproval or to please others.
    c. Child obeys out of respect for authority.
17. a. Act
    b. Expectations
    c. Rewards; punishments

Health Promotion for the School-Age Child and Family

1. a. 5
   b. 2.5
   c. 1.5
   d. 5
   e. 3
2. 12; 9 to 10
3. By making children accountable for their actions and by allowing them to experience the consequences of their actions
4. Positively reinforce for effort; encourage self-discipline and good study habits; ensure adequate sleep; communicate with and support teachers; provide a quiet, well-lighted study area.
5. By knowing laws related to self-care children, by teaching specific strategies for staying safe at home alone, and by working to develop expanded after-school programs in their communities
6. They can set consistent times for meals and snacks; offer only nutritious food options; model good nutrition and exercise habits; plan physical activities for their child; limit TV and computer game time; avoid fast food restaurants; and not use food as a reward.

Review Questions

1. d	4. b	7. c	
2. a	5. b	8. d	
3. d	6. b	9. c	

CHAPTER 9: HEALTH PROMOTION FOR THE ADOLESCENT

Matching Key Terms

1. e	4. b	7. c	10. k
2. d	5. f	8. a	11. g
3. i	6. j	9. h	

Adolescent Growth and Development

1. Menstruation
2. Peak height velocity (PHV)
3. Breast buds (thelarche)
4. Gynecomastia
5. Tanner staging or sexual maturation rating (SMR)
6. Testicular enlargement
7. Estrogen; testosterone
8. Assure confidentiality; be patient; be flexible; remain nonjudgmental; assume nothing; use open-ended questions; encourage problem solving and analysis; be an advocate; do not side against the parents.
9. Period granted to teens as they are experimenting with roles and not yet ready to make permanent commitments
10. They provide safety and validation as teens emotionally move away from the family and experiment with new roles.
11. Early
12. Early
13. Late
14. Middle
15. Middle
16. Late
17. Early, middle
18. Middle

Health Promotion for the Adolescent and Family

1. T	3. T	5. T	7. T
2. F	4. F	6. T	

8. 1800; 2200
9. Eye injury; premature aging of the skin; increased risk of skin cancer of all types
10. Poor impulse control, poor school performance, poor mental health, family disorganization, conduct disorders, substance abuse, homosexuality, stress

11. T	13. T	15. F
12. T	14. T	16. T

Review Questions

1. d	3. c	5. b	7. c
2. d	4. c	6. d	8. b

CHAPTER 10: HEREDITARY AND ENVIRONMENTAL INFLUENCES ON DEVELOPMENT

Matching Key Terms

1. c	4. d	7. h	10. f
2. e	5. a	8. j	
3. i	6. b	9. g	

Hereditary Influences

1. Deoxyribonucleic acid (DNA) is the basic building block of genes. Specific segments of DNA form a gene, and many genes form a chromosome.
2. An international effort to map all genes contained in the 46 human chromosomes
3. a. Genetic information about an individual has implications for other family members. Should this information be shared with family, health insurance providers, employers?
   b. A person with a genetic problem may feel inferior or guilty about passing it on to his or her children.
   c. A person with a genetic abnormality who is currently asymptomatic may experience long-term anxiety waiting for the disease to occur.
   d. A person with a genetic abnormality may be denied insurance coverage or be forced to pay exorbitant premiums.
4. a. The child must receive a copy of autosomal-recessive gene from both parents; no sex difference
   b. The child may receive a copy of autosomal-dominant gene from either parent; no sex difference
   c. Because females are carriers, the child receives the abnormal gene from the mother. Males are affected because they do not have a compensating normal X chromosome. Affected fathers will pass on abnormal genes to their daughters, who become carriers, but not to their sons.

5. T	7. F	9. F
6. F	8. T	

Multifactorial Disorders

1. They are present and detectable at birth. They tend to be single, isolated defects.

2. The number of affected close relatives, severity of disorder in other family members, sex of affected person, geographic location, season of year

Environmental Influences

1. At least four weeks before conceiving
2. The woman's need for the therapeutic effects of the drug and how the drug will affect the fetus
3. Protected by a lead apron
4. Maternal hyperthermia is a teratogen.

Genetic Counseling

1. Family
2. Nondirective

Nursing Care of Families Concerned About Birth Defects

1. a. Identify women who may benefit from genetic counseling.
   b. Identify women who may benefit from genetic counseling; provide support if they receive abnormal results; support their decisions; teach.
   c. Evaluate family's perception of the problem; explain diagnostic tests and results; make referrals.
   d. Support family; make referrals.

Review Questions

1. b	3. b	5. b
2. d	4. c	

CHAPTER 11: REPRODUCTIVE ANATOMY AND PHYSIOLOGY

Matching Key Terms

1. a	5. d	9. a	13. f
2. b	6. d	10. h	14. b
3. e	7. c	11. e	15. g
4. c	8. a	12. i	

Key Concepts

1. An unknown area of the brain prevents the young child's hypothalamus from responding to estrogen and testosterone secretion by the ovaries or testes. Without the gonadotropin-releasing hormone from the hypothalamus, further estrogen or testosterone secretion ceases.
2. Puberty; 8 to 13 years; 9 to 17 years
3. Breast development; growth of the testes and penis
4. 2 to 2½ years
5. Boys begin puberty slightly later than girls. In addition, the effect of testosterone on closing the epiphyses of the long bones is not as strong as that of estrogen. Thus, boys start puberty later and continue growing in height longer than girls.
6. a. Longitudinal fibers
      Importance: expel the fetus at birth
      Location: fundus
   b. Interlacing fibers (Fig. 11-4)
      Importance: compresses the blood vessels to prevent hemorrhage after birth
      Location: the middle layer
   c. Circular fibers
      Importance: prevent the reflux of menstrual blood from the uterus into the tubes, control the entry of the embryo into the uterus for implantation, and retain the fetus until the proper time for birth
      Location: constriction around the fallopian tubes and internal cervical os
7. Fallopian tubes
8. Female ova are produced only during the prenatal life. Male spermatozoa are continuously produced after puberty.
9. a. Estrogen and progesterone decrease just before menstruation, increasing the secretion of follicle-stimulating hormone (FSH) and luteinizing hormone (LH) by the anterior pituitary; the follicles mature with increasing estrogen secretion until one follicle outgrows all others.
   b. Significant increases in LH secretion, a slight decrease in follicular estrogen, and an increase in follicular progesterone secretion; final maturation and the release of the most mature ovum
   c. The corpus luteum secretes progesterone to prepare the endometrium for a fertilized ovum; corpus luteum will persist and continue to secrete progesterone if it receives a signal (human chorionic gonadotropin) from a fertilized ovum. Otherwise, progesterone secretion increases, and menstruation occurs.
10. a. Cells of the basal layer of the endometrium multiply; endometrial glands form; spiral arteries and endometrial veins elongate.
    b. Endometrium continues to thicken; substances are secreted to nourish an embryo if one implants.
    c. Vasospasm occurs if the corpus luteum stops producing estrogen and progesterone, causing the endometrium to become necrotic; the necrotic layer separates from the basal layer to produce the menstrual flow.
11. Tight underwear keeps the testes near the body, possibly overheating them and preventing normal sperm formation.

Review Questions

1. b	4. b	7. c	10. a
2. d	5. d	8. d	11. b
3. b	6. a	9. d	12. c

CHAPTER 12: CONCEPTION AND PRENATAL DEVELOPMENT

Matching Key Terms

1. c	4. b	7. h	10. e
2. a	5. d	8. j	
3. g	6. i	9. f	

Key Concepts

1.

	Mitosis	**Meiosis**
Type of cell	Somatic cell	Gamete involved (reproductive cell)
Number and type of chromosomes in each resulting cell	46 Chromosomes (44 autosomes and 2 sex chromosomes [X and Y or 2 X])	23 Chromosomes (22 autosomes and an X plus either a Y [sperm] or an X [female])

2. See Table 12-1 in your textbook to complete this exercise.

3. The zona pellucida prevents other sperms from entering, and the ovum completes its second meiotic division.

4. Good blood supply; thick uterine lining; muscles to limit post-birth blood loss

5. See Table 12-3 in your textbook to complete this exercise.

6. a. 4 weeks
   b. 8 weeks
   c. 10 weeks
   d. 6 weeks
   e. 12 weeks
   f. 16 to 24 weeks
   g. 24 weeks

7. a. Creamy skin covering to lubricate and protect the fetal skin from amniotic fluid
   b. Fine, downy hair that helps vernix adhere to the skin
   c. Heat-producing fat found on the back of the neck, behind the sternum, and around kidneys
   d. Surface-active lipid substance that helps the alveoli remain slightly open between breaths to ease the work of breathing

8. Fertilization age is calculated in weeks from the actual time of conception. Gestational age is calculated from the first day of the woman's last menstrual period. Gestational age is approximately 2 weeks longer than the fertilization age.

9. a. High fetal hemoglobin and hematocrit give the fetus more oxygen-carrying capacity; fetal hemoglobin can carry 20% to 50% more oxygen than adult hemoglobin.
   b. Fetal carbon dioxide quickly diffuses into the mother's blood, causing her blood to become more acidic and the fetal blood to become more alkaline; this allows the fetal blood to more readily combine with oxygen.

10. a. Provides the newborn with temporary passive immunity to diseases to which the mother is immune
    b. Maternal blood-type antibodies may cross the placenta and destroy incompatible fetal erythrocytes.

11. a. Causes persistence of the corpus luteum to maintain estrogen and progesterone secretion during early pregnancy and causes the fetal testes to secrete testosterone to stimulate the development of normal male reproductive structures

   b. Promotes normal growth and nutrition of the fetus, stimulates maternal breast development, and makes more glucose available to the fetus by reducing maternal insulin sensitivity and glucose utilization
   c. Causes the enlargement of the uterine and breast, growth of the breasts' ductal system, and enlargement of the fetal external genitalia
   d. Changes the endometrium into decidua to nourish conceptus before the placenta is established, reduces uterine contractions, and stimulates breast growth and the development of the breast alveoli and ductal system

12. Cushions the fetus from impacts; provides a stable temperature; promotes normal fetal growth and development (promotes symmetrical development, prevents membrane adherence, and allows fetal movement)

13. a. Carries oxygenated blood and nutrients from the placenta to the fetus
    b. Carries deoxygenated blood and waste products from the fetus to the placenta
    c. Protects the cord vessels from stretching or pressure that would interrupt flow

14. a. As the infant breathes, resistance to blood flow to the lungs decreases and the foramen ovale closes; tissue proliferation causes it to fill the septum between the right and left atria.
    b. Increasing arterial oxygen levels cause constriction; becomes a ligament
    c. Cessation of umbilical cord blood flow with birth causes it to become nonfunctional; it becomes a ligament.

15.

	Monozygotic	**Dizygotic**
Number of ova and sperm involved	1 Ovum and 1 sperm	2 Ova and 2 sperm
Genetic component	Identical genes	Like any other siblings
Sex	Same sex	May be same or different sex
Hereditary tendency	No hereditary influence known	Hereditary (and ethnic) tendency often found
Number of amnions and chorions	Varies according to time when inner cell mass divides in two; but most often 2 amnions and 1 chorion	Always has 1 amnion and 2 chorions

Review Questions

1. c   2. a   3. c   4. b

CHAPTER 13: ADAPTATIONS TO PREGNANCY

Matching Key Terms

1. f	4. a	7. g	10. k
2. b	5. e	8. l	11. j
3. c	6. d	9. i	12. h

Key Concepts

1. a. 12 weeks
   b. 16 weeks
   c. 20 weeks
   d. 36 weeks

2. a. Bluish color that often extends to the vagina and labia; the cause is hyperemia.
   b. Cervical, uterine, and vaginal softening with an increased vascularity and softening of the connective tissue
   c. Plug caused by the increased secretion of mucus from cervical glands that block the ascent of bacteria from the vagina
   d. Mixture of cervical mucus and a small amount of blood; disruption of the mucous plug and small capillaries of the cervix

3. a. Bluish color (as in Chadwick's sign), thickening of the vaginal mucosa, prominence of rugae, heightened sexual interest
   b. Greater pliability of the vagina
   c. Increased acidic vaginal discharge that retards the growth of bacteria but favors the growth of *Candida albicans* (yeast)

4. Pregnancy cannot be maintained without progesterone.

5. Corpus luteum; placenta

6. The high levels of estrogen and progesterone inhibit the follicle-stimulating hormone (FSH) and luteinizing hormone (LH).

7. Darkening of the areolae, increased nipple and areolae size, areolae become more erect, Montgomery's tubercles become prominent

8. Changes in the heart sounds begin between 12 and 20 weeks and regress during the first week after childbirth. They may include the splitting of the first heart sound and a systolic murmur. Murmurs may persist beyond fourth week.

9. See "Cardiovascular System" in your text to complete this chart.

10. Lying in the supine position places the heavy uterus over the aorta and inferior vena cava, which temporarily occludes these vessels. Signs and symptoms include faintness, lightheadedness, dizziness, agitation, and sometimes brief unconsciousness. This position can reduce the placental blood flow. Prevention/treatment is to position the woman on her side or with a pillow under one hip.

11. Increased fibrinogen levels offer protection from excess blood loss but also predispose the woman to thrombus formation.

12. Vasocongestion from the effects of estrogen causes increased vascularity and edema, leading to nasal stuffiness, nosebleeds, and voice changes. It may also result in ear fullness or earaches.

13. The growing uterus eventually lifts the diaphragm and reduces lung expansion. Because the respiratory center becomes more sensitive to carbon dioxide, the minute volume increases and the partial pressure of carbon dioxide decreases.

14. Hypotonia prolongs emptying time and allows bile to become thicker.

15. The amount of calcium transferred to the fetus is small compared with maternal stores, and there is no loss of maternal bone density to supply fetal needs.

16. The fetus draws on maternal glucose and amino acids, reducing the mother's glucose levels and her ability to synthesize glucose. During the first trimester, the lower maternal blood glucose causes the pancreas to secrete less insulin. During the second trimester, hormones (human placental lactogen, prolactin, progesterone, and cortisol) reduce the maternal tissue sensitivity to insulin. Thus the mother's blood glucose levels increase to make more available for the fetus. The woman normally responds by increasing insulin production.

17. Edema of the legs and feet is not uncommon. Edema above the waist (face and fingers) may be an indication of pregnancy-induced hypertension and should be reported.

18. Presumptive: Some signs include amenorrhea, nausea, vomiting, fatigue, urinary frequency, and breast and skin changes. Probable: Some signs include abdominal enlargement, cervical softening, ballottement, Braxton–Hicks contractions, and a pregnancy test. Positive: Fetal heart sounds, fetal movements felt by examiner, and visualization of the fetus. The difference among the indications is that presumptive indicators are the least reliable because they are often caused by other conditions; probable indicators are stronger evidence but may still have other causes; positive indicators are those caused only by pregnancy.

19. Instructions not followed, too early, urine too dilute

20. 9 weeks

21. a. November 11, b. May 9

22. Later in the pregnancy, risk factors may appear that were not apparent at previous assessments.

23. protein, glucose, ketones

24. a. The uterine size is larger than expected for the length of gestation.
    b. Fetal movements are more numerous, which the woman who has had a previous pregnancy is more likely to notice.
    c. Greater weight gain occurs because of greater uterine growth, increased blood volume and amniotic fluid, and presence of two or more fetuses.

25. a. There is a 500-mL increase in blood volume over a singleton pregnancy.
    b. Cardiac workload is higher because of the increased blood volume.
    c. Greater diaphragm elevation increases dyspnea.
    d. Greater compression of the aorta and inferior vena cava causes earlier and more pronounced supine hypotension.
    e. Pressure on the bowels increases constipation.

345

26. See Patient-Centered Teaching: How to Overcome the Common Discomforts of Pregnancy in your textbook to complete this exercise.

27. See pp. 233-236 in your text to complete this exercise. Practice how you would actually say this teaching in real life.

28. a. Anxious to confirm pregnancy, ambivalence, focus on self
    b. Physical evidence of pregnancy, focus on fetus, narcissism, introversion, body image, sexual interest
    c. Feelings of vulnerability replaced by coming to terms with the situation, fantasies or nightmares, increased dependence, desire to see the baby, dread about labor or being anxious for the pregnancy to end

29. Increase in uterine size, weight gain, breast changes, fetal movements (quickening)

30. Sexual interest and activity may be heightened or reduced. The woman may be more responsive because pelvic vasocongestion heightens the sensitivity and lubricates the vaginal area. Fear of miscarriage, harming the fetus, or causing discomfort may suppress sexual desire in either partner. The woman may feel less attractive, or her partner may find her less attractive at this time.

31. a. Fetus seems vague and unreal rather than seeming like a baby to her
    b. Perceives the fetus as real and needing her protection, growing sense of the fetus as a separate person
    c. Wants to see her baby on the outside and as a separate being

32. It makes the fetus seem much more like a separate being rather than a part of the woman's body.

33. Grief may be caused by feelings of giving up life as a carefree woman and loss of spontaneity to go to places and do things.

34. a. Seeking safe passage for herself and the baby
    b. Securing acceptance of herself and the baby
    c. Learning to give of herself
    d. Developing an attachment and interconnection to the unknown child

35. a. Grappling with the reality of pregnancy and a new child
    b. Struggling for recognition as a parent
    c. Desire to be seen as relevant to the childbearing process

36. a. Age: including whether they are still working and whether they believe they are "old enough" to be grandparents
    b. Other grandchildren: excitement about the first grandchild but less enthusiasm for subsequent grandchildren
    c. Perception of their role as grandparents: a source of information and support, or are professionals the experts?

37. a. Make any changes in sleeping areas before the infant arrives; may feel displaced; prepare others for feelings of resentment and jealousy
    b. May look forward to a brother or sister and how the baby is born and grows but have little

perception of how small and helpless the infant will be; need assurance of parents' love
    c. Enjoy preparing for the baby, want information about growth and changes in the fetus; enjoy time alone with parents
    d. May be embarrassed by their parents' obvious sexuality, preoccupied with their own issues, and/or look forward to the infant; involve them to the extent for which they are comfortable

38. a. Has difficulty putting aside her own desires for the well-being of an infant; must give of herself before developmentally prepared to do so
    b. May be poor and have late prenatal care; must enlist others to provide support that a partner would provide
    c. May grieve for the exclusive relationship with the first child; concern about having enough time and energy to spread around; concern about the acceptance of new infant by another child or children

39. a. Extreme modesty, do not want male health care providers; may consult curanderas
    b. Avoid tying knots to prevent complications with the umbilical cord
    c. Strong belief in fate so may not seek prenatal care
    d. Modesty dictates female care providers; may need permission from husband for any treatment
    e. Avoid optimism about pregnancy; do not buy clothes or equipment until baby is born healthy

40. a. Low-income women may not be able to pay for classes. They may enter prenatal care late or have none and may miss opportunities even for free classes.
    b. Some want education so that they can fully participate in all decisions related to childbearing.
    c. Some want to obtain the skills to help them cope with the pain and demands of birth.

41. a. Dealing with discomforts common during early pregnancy, what to expect, the value of prenatal care, avoiding hazards
    b. Body mechanics, working during pregnancy, childbirth choices, the postbirth needs of the mother and infant

42. a. Do warm-up exercises.
    b. Ensure low-impact activities.
    c. Avoid excessive heart rate elevation.

43. Indications, options, surgical procedure, postoperative course

Critical Thinking Exercises

Answers for Critical Thinking Exercises will vary.

Case Studies

1. gravida 5, para 3, abortions; T = 2; P = 1; A = 1; L = 4
2. January 10

3. 19 weeks
4. Katherine's fundal height at the umbilicus is expected at 20 weeks and her gestation is 19 weeks by dates. It is possible that her pregnancy is more advanced than the dates would indicate, she may have hydramnios, or she could be carrying twins again.
5. The demands of her children are a probable cause for the delay in seeking prenatal care. In addition, she may feel that she knows from experience and does not feel the need for earlier prenatal care. She may feel that because pregnancy is not an illness, it does not demand special care.
6. Hemoglobin and hematocrit (H&H) or complete blood count; blood typing and Rh factor with an antibody screen; rubella titer; urinalysis (or just a screen ["dipstick"] for protein, glucose, and ketones). Other tests may be performed, based on Katherine's ethnicity (such as for sickle cell trait), risk factors, and her medical and obstetric history.
7. Inadequate financial resources may have been the chief reason Sara delayed prenatal care because she has limited income of her own and may be unable to depend on her parents for money. In addition, she has no partner support and apparently feels isolated. Embarrassment and fear of her family's response, especially because she has five siblings, may also play a part. Because she did not know what to do, she may have simply done nothing.
8. Altered health maintenance and body image disturbance are the priority nursing diagnoses this situation suggests. Other nursing diagnoses might include altered family processes and knowledge deficits because they contribute to the priority nursing diagnoses.
9. Potential conflicts include Sara's probable late entry into prenatal care, erratic clinic visits, and noncompliance with professionals' recommendations.
10. Financial assistance, nutritional consultation and assistance, transportation, and other social services
11. Sara is more likely to be poor because she ended her education early. She is likely to have more children in her lifetime, and her children also have a greater likelihood of ending their education early and being poor. Although Sara has a higher risk for these problems, they do not have to occur.

Review Questions

1. b	5. d	9. a	13. c
2. b	6. a	10. d	
3. d	7. b	11. d	
4. b	8. c	12. a	

CHAPTER 14: NUTRITION FOR CHILDBEARING

Matching Key Terms

1. d	4. i	7. a	10. h
2. e	5. k	8. f	11. g
3. b	6. j	9. c	

Key Concepts

1. Low birth weight, preterm birth, small for gestational age infants, failure to initiate breastfeeding
2. Macrosomia, cesarean birth, postpartum weight retention, low Apgar scores, hypoglycemia, overweight for children
3. a. Gain 25 to 35 pounds.
   b. Gain 28 to 40 pounds.
   c. Gain 15 to 25 pounds.
   d. Gain at least 11 pounds.
4. 0.5 to 2 kg; 1.1 to 4.4 pounds; 0.35 to 0.5 kg; 0.8 to 1 pounds
5. a. 4
   b. 4
   c. 9
6. 340
7. 46; 71
8. A; D; E; K
9. Legumes, nuts, dark-green leafy vegetables, broccoli
10. Excessive amounts of one vitamin or mineral may reduce the absorption of others; high doses of some vitamins (such as vitamin A) are toxic; a false sense of security may develop that causes the woman to eat a less healthy diet.
11. 8 to 10; limit fluids low in nutrients, such as carbonated drinks, coffee, tea, and high-sugar "juice" drinks
12. a. 7 to 9 ounces
    b. 3 vegetables, 2 fruits
    c. 3
    d. 71 g/day, or 6 to 8 ounces
    e. 6 to 8 teaspoons unsaturated fat; consume the rest only sparingly
13. Yin (cold) and yang (hot) applies to foods and conditions in many cultures, influencing what the woman eats during her pregnancy. She will balance a "hot" condition such as pregnancy by eating "cold" foods and vice versa.
14. a. Sour foods, fruits, noodles, spinach, and mung beans
    b. Fish, excessively salty or spicy foods, alcohol, rice, and unfamiliar foods
    c. "Hot" foods, such as rice with fish sauce, broth, salty meats, fish, chicken, eggs, and hot drinks
    d. May be deficient in calories, calcium, iron, zinc, magnesium, vitamins B_6 and D; high in sodium
    e. Increase in dark-green leafy vegetables increases calcium, iron, magnesium, and folic acid; tofu or broth from vinegar-soaked pork or chicken bones increases calcium and iron; increase in meat or poultry intake increases vitamin B_6 and zinc.
15. a. Pregnancy is considered "hot" and the postpartum period is considered "cold," so the diet is adjusted to balance.
    b. Foods include dried beans, rice, beef, pork, chicken, corn, chili peppers, tomatoes, and tortillas.
    c. Diet is high in fiber and complex carbohydrates but also high in fat and calories (overweight is a problem); low in vitamins A and D, iron, and calcium

16. Income lower than 185% of the federal poverty level; eligible throughout pregnancy and for 6 months postpartum if formula feeding or 1 year if breastfeeding

17. Vitamins C and A, folic acid, calcium, iron, zinc, magnesium, and B_6

18. Focus only on necessary changes; ask for the teenager's input; help her make changes that still keep her diet similar to that of her peers.

19. a. Combine vegetable foods that have complementary amino acids or eat small amounts of complete protein foods (such as cheese) with vegetables.
    b. Calcium-fortified soy products or supplement
    c. Vitamin B_{12}-fortified foods, such as cereal, or supplement

20. Have frequent small meals; reduce fatty foods; drink liquids between meals; eat a protein snack at bedtime; eat carbohydrate food before getting out of bed in the morning.

21. May begin pregnancy with a nutritional deficit if she has had several pregnancies (usually more than five), especially if they are closely spaced. Meeting the nutritional and other needs of her family may take priority over her own needs.

22. She needs to eat enough to supply all of the fetuses, as well as meet her own needs. Supplementation with calcium, iron, folic acid, magnesium, and zinc may be needed.

23. a. Obtaining substance is more important than eating well. Nutritional needs in pregnant women who abuse substances need to be fully explored.
    b. Metabolic rate increases and appetite decreases. Decreases the availability of some vitamins and minerals
    c. Deficient use of B_{12}, folic acid, niacin, B_6, magnesium, and zinc; impaired metabolism; alcohol may replace food in the diet. Vitamin–mineral supplement may be needed

24. a. Increases appetite, but women may not take in foods of good quality
    b. Alters the metabolism and may cause the woman to be malnourished
    c. Suppresses appetite; tendency to drink more alcohol or caffeine-containing beverages
    d. Depresses appetite

25. a. Pregnancy could deplete her own stores; could interfere with the recovery process and establishing a milk supply; she should not take appetite suppressants
    b. Adolescents may be deficient in many nutrients; they may lack iron and vitamin A and vitamin C.
    c. The woman may have inadequate B_{12}, D, or calcium levels.
    d. Prolonged lactation may result in the removal of calcium from the bones; must have adequate intake and/or supplementation

26. a. An occasional single glass of an alcoholic beverage may not be harmful; larger amounts may reduce the milk-ejection reflex and be harmful to the infant.
    b. Limit the intake to the equivalent of two cups of coffee; excess can make the infant irritable.

c. Drink 8 to 10 glasses or more according to thirst (excluding caffeinated beverages).

Case Study

1. Low hemoglobin (10.5 g/dL)
2. Anemia (hemoglobin of 10 g/dL or less) is a possibility because of Carmen's low hemoglobin at her initial visit and the close spacing of her children. Inadequate calcium intake is another concern because she may be lactose intolerant. Excess weight gain may occur because her current weight gain is approximately 8½ pounds more than would be expected at this point in her pregnancy. Refer to the text for food sources of iron and nondairy calcium.
3. In addition to discussing her likes and dislikes, the nurse should consider common low-cost foods. The nurse should also consider whether Carmen adheres to "hot" and "cold" foods during childbearing. If Carmen does not speak or read English, a fluent Spanish-speaking professional is ideal to help her understand her nutritional needs.

Review Questions

1. c	4. d	7. a
2. b	5. c	8. c
3. a	6. b	9. d

CHAPTER 15: PRENATAL DIAGNOSTIC TESTS

Matching Key Terms

1. h	3. d	5. f	7. b
2. g	4. e	6. c	8. a

Key Concepts

1. a. Confirm pregnancy, its location, and gestational age and determine whether it is multifetal; confirm fetal viability; adjunct to chorionic villus sampling
   b. Determine fetal viability, evaluate fetal anatomy, estimate gestational age, locate the placenta, determine fetal presentation, evaluate amniotic fluid volume and fetal movement, adjunct to amniocentesis
2. Transabdominal; it elevates the uterus and displaces the gas-filled intestines
3. An accurate gestational age is needed for accurate maternal serum alpha-fetoprotein (AFP) evaluation to identify intrauterine growth restriction or if there is a question regarding the expected date of delivery. It is most accurately assessed by measuring the crown-rump length at 6 weeks of gestation. During the last half of pregnancy, it is assessed by several measurements, including the biparietal diameter, femur length, and abdominal circumference. From 12 to 20 weeks, the biparietal diameter is the most accurate (±7 days).
4. a. Chromosomal abnormalities
   b. Open defects such as open neural tube defect
5. Multiple-marker screening includes maternal serum alpha-fetoprotein, human chorionic gonadotropin, and unconjugated estriol; it increases the detection of trisomies 18 and 21. Follow-up may include amniocentesis with karyotyping.

6. 10
7. a. Pregnancy loss
   b. Infection
   c. Limb-reduction defects
   d. Rh sensitization
8. a. To detect fetal genetic abnormalities, to detect AFP levels, to evaluate fetal conditions with Rh incompatibility
   b. To evaluate fetal lung maturity and identify fetal hemolytic disease
9. Ratio of 2:1; diabetes mellitus
10. Presence of these substances in the amniotic fluid confirms fetal lung maturity.
11. Two or more
12. A vibroacoustic stimulation test (VST) identifies whether fetal heart rate accelerations occur in response to sound stimulation; it shortens the nonstress test (NST) or confirms a nonreactive NST.
13. Fetal heart rate; uterine contractions
14. a. Breast self-stimulation
    b. Oxytocin infusion
15. Negative—normal (no late or significant variable decelerations); positive—abnormal (late decelerations following 50% or more of the contractions); suspicious or equivocal—intermittent late or variable decelerations; equivocal hyperstimulation—late decelerations with excessive contractions; unsatisfactory—fewer than three contractions in 10 minutes or poor-quality tracing
16. a. NST
    b. Fetal breathing movements
    c. Gross fetal movements
    d. Fetal tone
    e. Amniotic fluid volume
17. During fetal hypoxemia, blood is shunted away from the kidneys and lungs and toward the brain, resulting in a lower amniotic fluid volume.

Critical Thinking Exercises

Figure 15-9, A:
   a. 125 to 130 beats per minute (bpm)
   b. 10 minutes
   c. Seven total, four occurring with significant fetal movement (FM)
   d. None
   e. 25 to 30 bpm; 20 to 30 seconds
   f. Probably reactive: In this 10-minute period, there are at least two accelerations of at least 15 bpm that have a duration of at least 15 seconds.

Figure 15-9, B:
   a. 140 to 145 bpm
   b. 10 minutes
   c. None
   d. None
   e. No accelerations to analyze
   f. The test is incomplete because less than 20 minutes has elapsed. However, if there are still no accelerations during the next 30 minutes, the test will be nonreactive.

Note that the variability in both strips is only 5 bpm. If this low variability continues throughout the remainder of the testing period, the test illustrated in Figure 15-9, A, will be equivocal. It is also possible that these strips were obtained while the fetus was in a sleep cycle.

Case Studies

1. a. Pregnancy-induced hypertension may reduce placental perfusion, and the delivery of the baby is its only real cure. The amniocentesis is most likely being performed to assess the fetal lung maturity. If the lungs are mature, induction of labor is likely.
   b. Care before amniocentesis: displacement of the uterus with a rolled towel under the right hip; assessment of maternal blood pressure and fetal heart rates; ultrasound location of the fetus, placenta, and largest pockets of amniotic fluid. Care after amniocentesis: maternal rest for 30 to 60 minutes with electronic fetal monitoring; caution to avoid strenuous activity for a day or two; teach to report uterine contractions, vaginal bleeding, leaking amniotic fluid, fever
2. a. Diabetes is a disorder involving the blood vessels, and there is a possibility that the placental function is impaired because of this maternal condition.
   b. Findings that suggest normal placental function through the nonstress test include a normal baseline fetal heart rate (FHR) with a long-term variability of at least 10 bpm and two or more FHR accelerations of at least 15 bpm for at least 15 seconds in a 20-minute period.
   c. The test will probably be repeated at least weekly.

Review Questions

1. a	3. a	5. b
2. d	4. c	

CHAPTER 16: GIVING BIRTH

Matching Key Terms

1. g	3. h	5. c	7. f
2. e	4. b	6. d	8. a

Key Concepts

1. a. Contractions must be stronger in the upper uterus than in the lower uterus to propel the fetus toward the outside.
   b. Women cannot consciously cause labor to start or stop. Otherwise, many infants would be born early as the woman became tired of being pregnant or labor might be suspended when it became too intense.
   c. Intervals between contractions allow for the resumption of blood flow to the placenta to supply oxygen and remove waste for the fetus.
2. The upper uterus actively contracts to push the fetus downward, while the lower uterus is more passive to reduce resistance to fetal passage. Any other pattern would be ineffective at pushing the fetus out.

349

3. A full bladder increases pain and interferes with fetal descent.

4. Any maternal condition that reduces perfusion of the placenta, such as diabetes or hypertension, or fetal anemia, which reduces oxygen-carrying capacity, can reduce tolerance even for normal labor contractions.

5. In pregnancy, the decreased production of fetal lung fluid and fluid absorption into the interstitium of the lungs increase. During labor, the absorption of the lung fluid intensifies and compression of head and thorax causes the expulsion of additional fluid. After birth, the remainder is absorbed into pulmonary and lymphatic circulation.

6. Uterine contractions: first stage; uterine contractions and maternal pushing: second stage

7. They allow molding to adapt the fetal head to the size and shape of the maternal pelvis.

8. a. Longitudinal (common) or transverse (rare)
   b. Flexion (common) or extension (uncommon)
   c. Cephalic (common), breech, or shoulder (rare, <0.2%)

9. Refer to Figure 16-9 to complete this exercise. Frank breech is the most common.

10. a. Occiput
    b. Chin (mentum)
    c. Sacrum

11. They promote relaxation and the ability to work with her body's efforts rather than working against the natural forces.

12. a. Increased fetal glucocorticoid and androgens reduce placental progesterone production (which relaxes the uterus) and increase prostaglandin production (which stimulates the uterus).
    b. Higher estrogen levels make the uterus more sensitive to substances that stimulate it to contract, while lower progesterone levels allow it to be more easily stimulated.

13. *Braxton Hicks contractions:* irregular, mild contractions intensify near term; more noticeable in parous women; *lightening:* descent of the fetus toward the pelvic inlet increases pressure on bladder but allows easier breathing; more noticeable in nulliparas; *increased vaginal secretions* with the congestion of the vaginal mucosa caused by fetal pressure; *bloody show:* a mixture of cervical mucus and blood as the mucous plug is released; seen earlier and in greater quantity in nulliparas; *energy spurt; weight loss* of one to three pounds

14. Refer to Figure 16-12 to complete this exercise.

15. After the fetal head is born, the fetal shoulders are transverse (crosswise) in the pelvis and must rotate to pass under the pubic arch.

16. Latent phase: up to 3 cm dilation; active phase: 4 to 7 cm; transition phase: 8 to 10 cm

17. First stage: nullipara: 8 to 10 hours (range, 6 to 18 hours); parous woman: 6 to 7 hours (range, 2 to 10 hours). Second stage: nullipara: 50 minutes; parous: 20 minutes

18. Uterus has spherical shape; uterus rises upward in the abdomen; cord descends farther from the vagina; gush of blood

19. Firm uterine contraction compresses the bleeding vessels at the placental site to prevent hemorrhage.

20. Refer to Table 16-1 in your textbook to complete this exercise.

21. Condition of the mother and fetus; to establish a therapeutic relationship

22. Vaginal examination should *not* be performed if the woman is actively bleeding (not bloody show) because the examination may increase bleeding.

23. Time of rupture; whether rupture was spontaneous or artificial; quantity; fetal heart rate (FHR) for at least 1 minute; color (clear, possibly with bits of vernix, is normal; green indicates fetal meconium passage; yellow suggests infection); other characteristics (cloudy appearance suggests infection); odor (foul or strong odor suggests infection)

24. To prevent supine hypotension from aortocaval compression by the heavy uterus

25. a. Blood pressure higher than 140/90 mm Hg
    b. Temperature of 38°C (100.4°F) or higher

26. Use soft, indirect lighting. Keep the temperature comfortable with a fan or damp, cool washcloths. Have the woman wear socks for cold feet. Keep the woman reasonably clean by changing her disposable underpad as often as needed. Offer ice chips or a wet washcloth to wet her lips. Remind her to empty her bladder at least every 2 hours. Encourage her to frequently change positions, assuming the position of comfort (except the supine position). Offer a shower, whirlpool, or other water therapy.

27. Cardiopulmonary; thermoregulatory; identification bands

28. Hemorrhage; discomfort

29. A full bladder interferes with the contraction of the uterus.

Critical Thinking Exercises

1. Cervical dilation is 4 cm; effacement is 75%; presentation is cephalic; membranes are ruptured; fluid is normal. The woman is beginning the active phase of first stage labor.

Case Study

1. Regular contractions that have increased in duration, intensity, and frequency suggest true labor. Irregular contractions and those that do not intensify suggest false labor. In addition, discomfort is usually felt in her back or sweeping around to her lower abdomen. Erin should be instructed to come to the birth center if she thinks her membranes may have ruptured, even if she is not having contractions.

2. Priorities are to (a) assess the fetal heart rate and the color, odor, and character of the amniotic fluid; (b) assess Erin's vital signs; and (c) determine the nearness to birth by evaluating contractions and cervical dilation.

3. Either the nitrazine paper or the fern test or both may be used to evaluate whether the membranes have ruptured.
4. Active phase of first stage labor
5. The FHR is normal for a term fetus, and it is reassuring that the FHR accelerates with fetal movement.
6. Except for the greenish color, the amniotic fluid is normal. The amniotic fluid is green because the fetus passed meconium before birth.
7. Cephalic; right occiput posterior (ROP)
8. Assuming any of several upright positions and leaning forward during contractions; hands and knees; firm sacral pressure
9. Erin should avoid prolonged breath holding. She can be taught to take a deep breath and exhale it, then take another deep breath and push for 4 to 6 seconds at a time while exhaling. A final breath at the end of the contraction helps her relax.
10. The exact time to position Erin for birth will depend on how fast she has labored thus far. In general, a woman having her first baby is positioned for the birth when the fetal head crowns and remains visible between contractions.
11. The 1-minute Apgar score will be 9, with 1 point deducted for the baby's bluish hands and feet.
12. a. Suction to remove excess secretions; position on one side on a flat surface.
    b. Dry the baby quickly, particularly the head; place in a prewarmed radiant warmer or in skin-to-skin contact with a parent. Use a cap on the baby's dry head to reduce heat loss from that area when not in the radiant warmer.
13. The first 1 to 4 hours after the placenta delivers is the fourth stage of labor.
14. Firmness, height, and position of the uterine fundus; vital signs; amount of lochia. Observing and intervening for a full bladder helps prevent hemorrhage caused by the bladder's interference with uterine contraction.
15. Cold packs to the perineal area; analgesics; a warm blanket to limit the common postbirth chill

Review Questions

1. b	6. c	11. d	16. a
2. d	7. a	12. a	17. b
3. c	8. a	13. c	18. d
4. b	9. d	14. d	
5. b	10. b	15. b	

CHAPTER 17: INTRAPARTUM FETAL SURVEILLANCE

Matching Key Terms

1. e	3. b	5. g	7. a
2. c	4. d	6. f	

Key Concepts

1. Adequacy of maternal blood volume and flow to the placenta; normal maternal blood oxygen saturation; adequate exchange of oxygen and carbon dioxide in the placenta; open circulatory path between the placenta and fetus through umbilical cord vessels; normal fetal circulatory and oxygen-carrying functions
2. a. Sympathetic stimulation increases the heart rate and strengthens the heart contractions to increase cardiac output by releasing epinephrine and norepinephrine.
   b. Baroreceptors sense blood pressure changes in the carotid arch and major arteries to slow the heart and reduce the blood pressure, thus reducing cardiac output.
   c. Chemoreceptors in the medulla oblongata, aortic arch, and carotid bodies sense changes in oxygen, carbon dioxide, and pH to increase the heart rate.
   d. The adrenal glands secrete epinephrine and norepinephrine in response to stress and release aldosterone to cause retention of sodium and water, thus increasing the blood volume.
   e. The fetal cerebral cortex causes the fetal heart rate to increase during fetal movement and decrease during fetal sleep. The hypothalamus coordinates the branches of the autonomic nervous system. The medulla oblongata maintains the balance between forces that speed and slow the fetal heart rate.
3. Refer to text, "Pathologic Influences on Fetal Oxygenation," to complete this exercise.
4. Refer to text, "Auscultation and Palpation" and "Electronic Fetal Monitoring," to complete this exercise.
5. The pressures of a solid intrauterine pressure catheter are slightly higher than those of the fluid-filled catheter. The fluid-filled catheter is sensitive to the height of the catheter tip in relation to the transducer.
6. a. 110 to 160 beats per minute (bpm)
   b. A rate less than 110 bpm that persists for at least 10 minutes
   c. A rate greater than 160 bpm that persists for at least 10 minutes
   d. Fluctuations in the fetal heart rate
7. Narcotics or sedatives; fetal sleep; tachycardia; prematurity; decreased central nervous system oxygenation; abnormalities of the central nervous system, heart, or both
8. Variability reflects the normal function of the autonomic nervous system, which helps the fetus adapt to the stress of labor.
9. Refer to text, "Periodic Patterns in FHR," and Table 17-1 and Figures 17-8, 17-9, and 17-10 to complete this exercise.
10. Fetal scalp stimulation, vibroacoustic stimulation, fetal scalp blood sampling, fetal oxygen saturation monitoring, umbilical cord blood gases and pH immediately after birth
11. 7.25; 7.35
12. a. Check blood pressure to identify hypotension or hypertension, contractions to identify uterine hyperactivity, and recent maternal medications to identify sedative effects; perform a vaginal examination to identify prolapsed cord; initiate internal monitoring to provide more accuracy.

b. Change the position to displace the uterus and decrease aortocaval compression; discontinue oxytocin and/or administer tocolytics to reduce uterine activity.

c. Administer oxygen at 8 to 10 L/min through a snug facemask.

d. Reposition or perform amnioinfusion to reduce umbilical cord compression.

13. a. Add fluid to create a cushion around the umbilical cord.

b. Dilute thick meconium to reduce the effects of possible aspiration at birth.

Review Questions

1. c	3. a	5. a
2. b	4. b	6. d

CHAPTER 18: PAIN MANAGEMENT FOR CHILDBIRTH

Matching Key Terms

1. e	3. b	5. f
2. d	4. a	6. c

Key Concepts

1. Childbirth pain is a normal process; the woman has several months to prepare; labor pain has a foreseeable end; labor pain is not constant; labor pain ends with the birth.

2. Excessive pain can result in fear and anxiety, which stimulate the sympathetic nervous system to release substances that simultaneously cause vasoconstriction and the pooling of maternal blood in her vascular system, plus a higher uterine muscle tone with the reduction of effective contractions. The net effect is that blood flow to and from the placenta decreases and labor contractions are less effective, thus prolonging labor.

3. The fetal occiput is pushed against the woman's sacral promontory with each contraction, causing intense back pain. In addition, the fetus must usually rotate into the occiput anterior position to be born, so labor is often longer.

4. Relaxation, cutaneous stimulation, mental stimulation, breathing

5. Direct: The fetal heart rate (FHR) has a decreased variability. Indirect: Maternal hypotension will decrease the fetal blood flow.

6. The test dose is administered to identify an inadvertent subarachnoid or intravascular injection of the drug. Evidence of these problems includes a rapid and intense motor and sensory block (subarachnoid injection) or numbness of the tongue and lips, lightheadedness, dizziness, and tinnitus (intravascular injection).

7. a. Inadvertent dural puncture may allow spinal fluid to leak, causing intense headache that is worse when sitting or standing. A blood patch may give prompt relief. Lying flat and adding hydration help rebuild the spinal fluid.

b. Prehydration with warmed intravenous solution (500 to 1000 mL or more) and avoiding aortocaval compression reduce any hypotensive effects.

c. Regularly assess the bladder and have the woman void at least every 2 hours; may need to catheterize the patient

d. Coach the woman to push with contractions if she cannot feel them. Forceps or vacuum extraction may be necessary.

8. The subarachnoid block punctures the dura and arachnoid membranes, entering the space that contains cerebrospinal fluid, which confirms the correct location for an injection of the anesthetic drug for this block.

9. Consult your text, "Pharmacologic Pain Management," to complete this exercise.

10. Bed rest with oral or intravenous hydration; blood patch

11. These drugs have combined opioid agonist–antagonist effects and should not be administered to a woman who has had a recent dose of a pure opioid agonist (may reverse the effectiveness of the first drug) or to a woman who is addicted to opiates such as heroin (may precipitate acute withdrawal).

Case Study

1. The nurse must be careful to avoid assumptions, such as the pregnancy was unplanned, that Alice did not have prenatal care and that she and her husband cannot learn nonpharmacologic pain management methods. You can probably think of other assumptions that nurses should avoid.

2. Initial interventions are to tell Alice and her husband kindly that her labor pattern is normal right now and show them data that indicate that the mother and fetus are doing well. The nurse should speak calmly and in a soothing voice, conveying to Alice and her husband that they can have confidence in their caregivers and that Alice is capable of giving birth.

3. The nurse should teach Alice simple breathing and relaxation techniques between the contractions. Say something like, "I'm going to teach you how to breathe so that you can cope with labor better" in a positive manner that conveys the expectation that the techniques *will work,* rather than doing the teaching in a tentative manner. Give liberal positive feedback when Alice uses the techniques that are taught and give her husband positive feedback for his coaching.

4. It would be better for Alice to delay taking medication until her labor is in the active phase. Administration of analgesics too early can slow labor progress. However, this fact must be balanced against the adverse effects of excessive pain and anxiety.

5. At this point, Alice could probably receive either an opioid analgesic or an epidural block.

6. The nurse must prehydrate Alice with 500 to 1000 mL of a warmed intravenous solution, check her blood pressure frequently to detect hypotension, and observe the FHR for signs of reduced placental perfusion that can occur with maternal hypotension. The nurse must also observe for bladder distention related

to a loss of sensation and high volumes of intravenous fluids. Alice may need coaching to push during the second stage if she cannot feel the urge. In addition, the nurse must be alert for signs of catheter migration.

7. The nurse must continue to observe for bladder distention, which can result in poor uterine contraction and a postpartum hemorrhage. Return of sensation must be documented. The nurse must assist Alice to the bathroom at first in case she still has reduced sensation or hypotension that could result in a fall.

Review Questions

1. b   3. c   5. d
2. d   4. b   6. c

CHAPTER 19: NURSING CARE DURING OBSTETRIC PROCEDURES

Matching Key Terms

1. a   3. d
2. c   4. b

Key Concepts

1. Prolapse of the umbilical cord, infection, and placental abruption
2. Obtain the baseline fetal heart rate (FHR) before and compare FHR after procedure; assess the temperature every 2 hours; keep the woman clean and dry.
3. Observe the FHR for changes that may occur with uterine contractions. Assess for excessive contractions that can reduce fetal oxygen supply (see Chapters 16 and 17).
4. Assess the FHR every 15 minutes during first-stage labor and every 5 minutes during second-stage labor. Problems include tachycardia (>150 to 160 beats per minute [bpm]), bradycardia (<110 to 120 bpm), late decelerations, and reduced FHR variability. Assess uterine activity for contractions that are too frequent or too long or a uterus that does not relax for at least 60 seconds between contractions. The blood pressure and pulse identify changes from the baseline; temperature assessment identifies an infection that may occur with ruptured membranes. Intake and output, assessment for headache, blurred vision, behavioral changes, increased blood pressure and respirations, decreased pulse, rales, wheezing, and coughing identify possible water intoxication. A postpartum hemorrhage may occur if an overstimulated uterus cannot effectively contract.
5. In addition to identifying the true cause of the nonreassuring assessments, interventions may include discontinuing the oxytocin infusion, increasing the rate of the nonadditive infusion, positioning to avoid aortocaval compression, and administering oxygen through a facemask. Internal monitoring may be initiated if not already in place. The physician may also order a tocolytic drug if uterine hyperactivity is the problem.

6. a. A nonstress test evaluates placental function and apparent fetal health to avoid stressing a fetus that may already be compromised.
   b. Ultrasound guides the version and helps monitor the FHR. It will also confirm the fetal age, presentation, and adequacy of amniotic fluid.
   c. A tocolytic drug relaxes the uterus to make the version easier to perform.
   d. Administering Rh immune globulin destroys fetal Rh-positive red blood cells (RBCs) that might stimulate anti-Rh antibodies in the Rh-negative woman. These may enter the mother's bloodstream because of tiny placental disruptions during the version.
   e. FHR monitoring evaluates how the fetus is tolerating the version and when the fetal condition returns to baseline afterward.
   f. Uterine activity monitoring identifies persistent contractions that may herald the onset of labor.
7. Add a catheter to the delivery table to empty the mother's bladder, making more room for the instrument-assisted birth. Postpartum, observe for trauma, usually lacerations (bright red bleeding with a firm fundus) or hematoma (pain, edema, and discoloration). Cold packs to the perineal area limit bruising and edema. Observe for reddening, mild bruising, or small lacerations where the forceps were applied. A chignon is typical if a vacuum extractor is used. Explain that these minor problems usually quickly resolve. Facial asymmetry, usually seen when crying, suggests nerve damage that resolves more slowly.
8. An upright position with pushing, delayed pushing until the urge is felt, use of an open-glottis technique with pushing; daily perineal massage during the last 3 weeks of pregnancy
9. The infant may be born preterm if a cesarean birth is scheduled. Absorption of lung fluid may be delayed, resulting in transient tachypnea. Injury can occur, such as lacerations or bruising.
10. a. To reduce gastric secretions
    b. A wedge under the hip avoids aortocaval compression by the heavy uterus.
    c. These tests identify the reserve to tolerate blood loss, risk for poor blood clotting to control a hemorrhage, and blood type for possible transfusion and enables caregivers to prepare blood to be immediately ready if the need for a transfusion arises.
    d. Reduces the risk for postpartum infection
    e. Keeps the bladder out of the way of the uterine incision

Case Study

1. Post-term gestation is the probable reason for induction.
2. Tests for fetal lung maturity, such as the lecithin/sphingomyelin (L/S) ratio, and for presence of phosphatidylglycerol (PG) and phosphatidylinositol (PI) may be performed. Although Linda is 42 weeks pregnant, incorrect dates could mean that her fetus is actually younger.

3. Set up as a secondary infusion, regulated by a pump, start and increase the rate slowly, and add to the primary infusion line at the lowest possible port. This technique ensures that the oxytocin can be quickly discontinued if the need arises. The pump precisely controls the infusion. Observe the FHR and uterine activity for nonreassuring signs or uterine hyperstimulation.

4. Before the amniotomy, obtain baseline information about the FHR. Place absorbent underpads under Linda's hips. After the amniotomy, assess the FHR for at least 1 minute and report nonreassuring signs or significant changes from baseline; observe and chart the quantity, color, clarity, and odor of the amniotic fluid.

5. No changes in the oxytocin are needed at this time, although amniotomy may increase contractions enough to allow a dosage reduction.

6. The oxytocin infusion should be discontinued because some contractions have only a 30-second resting interval. This could exhaust the fetal oxygen reserve and lead to distress. In addition, labor is now well established and dilation is progressing, so stimulation does not appear to be warranted.

7. Actual care depends on how quickly the surgery must occur. Provide emotional support to reduce anxiety. Keep the partners together as much as possible. Provide preoperative teaching, abbreviated as necessary for the actual situation. Perform preoperative procedures, such as an indwelling catheter and abdominal shave. Explain who will be present at the birth and their responsibilities. Explain the recovery room care. Pad bony prominences. Secure the legs with a safety strap. Tilt the table or place a wedge under one hip to avoid aortocaval compression. Apply the grounding pad and other monitors. Clean the incision line and apply a sterile dressing.

8. Take vital signs every 15 minutes for 1 to 2 hours. Observe the uterus for firmness and position, lochia, urine output, intravenous infusion, abdominal dressing, and pain relief needs. Observe for the return of motion and sensation (for regional block anesthesia) or the level of consciousness (for general anesthesia or if sedative drugs were administered).

Review Questions

1. b	5. d	9. c
2. d	6. a	10. d
3. a	7. c	
4. c	8. b	

CHAPTER 20: POSTPARTUM ADAPTATIONS

Matching Key Terms

1. h	6. i	11. e
2. k	7. l	12. d
3. c	8. b	13. g
4. j	9. f	
5. m	10. a	

Key Concepts

1. a. Stretched uterine muscle fibers contract and gradually regain their former size and contour.
   b. The number of uterine muscle cells remains the same, but each cell decreases in size through catabolism.
   c. The outer area of the endometrium (decidua) is expelled with the placenta. The remaining decidua separates into two layers: The superficial layer is shed in the lochia and the basal layer regenerates new endothelium.

2. Lochia rubra contains blood, mucus, and bits of decidua; is red in color; and has a duration of approximately 3 days. Lochia serosa contains serous exudate, erythrocytes, leukocytes, and cervical mucus; it is a pinkish color; and its duration is from the 4th to the 10th day. Lochia alba contains leukocytes, decidual cells, epithelial cells, fat, cervical mucus, and bacteria; it is white or colorless; its duration varies from the 11th day until the 3rd to 6th week.

3. The blood volume and cardiac output increase as the blood from the uteroplacental unit returns to the central circulation and as excess extracellular fluid enters the vascular compartment for excretion. Because the stroke volume increases, the pulse decreases.

4. Pregnant and postpartum women have higher fibrinogen levels, which increase the ability to form clots; however, factors that lyse clots are decreased. Some women have another risk in addition to this baseline risk: those who have varicose veins, a history of thrombophlebitis, or a cesarean birth.

5. A full bladder interferes with the ability of the uterus to firmly contract and can occlude open vessels at the placental site. This allows them to freely bleed.

6. a. and b. Estrogen and progesterone prepare the breasts for lactation.
   c. Prolactin initiates milk production in the alveoli.
   d. Oxytocin causes milk ejection from the alveoli into the lactiferous ducts.

7. Rho(D)—mother is Rh−, newborn is Rh+; rubella vaccine—if her prenatal rubella antibody screening shows she is nonimmune.

8. Refer to text, "Procedure: Assessing the Uterine Fundus," to complete this exercise.

9. Refer to text, "Focused Assessments After Vaginal Birth," to complete this exercise.

10. The answers to this exercise should be in your own words and should fit the women you care for in your clinical setting.

11. a. Observe the respiratory rate and depth (every 30 minutes to 1 hour if epidural narcotics were used); monitor for apnea for epidural narcotic administration; auscultate breath sounds for retained secretions; assist the mother to turn, cough, and deep-breathe; use incentive spirometer.
    b. Assess for the return of peristalsis by auscultating bowel sounds; observe for abdominal distention; observe surgical dressing for intactness and drainage; observe the incision line after dressing

removal for signs of infection (REEDA); gently palpate the fundus.

    c. Monitor the intravenous (IV) line for the rate of flow and site condition; observe the urine for the amount, color, and clarity.

12. Progressively increase activity, drink adequate fluids (at least eight glasses of water daily), and add dietary fiber (found in fruits and vegetables and whole-grain cereals, bread, and pasta) to prevent constipation. Prunes are a natural laxative.

13. Fever; localized area of redness, swelling, or pain in the breasts that is unrelieved by support or analgesics; persistent abdominal tenderness or feelings of pelvic fullness or pelvic pressure; persistent perineal pain; frequency, urgency, or burning when urinating; change in the lochia character (increased amount, return to red color, passage of clots, or foul odor); localized tenderness, redness, or warmth of the legs

14. Bonding describes the initial, rapid attraction felt by parents toward their newborn infant. It is a one-way process, from the parent to the infant. Attachment describes a longer-term, two-way process that binds the parents and infant. Attachment is facilitated by positive feedback from the infant and by mutually satisfying experiences.

15. Maternal touch progression is from fingertipping to palm touch to enfolding the infant and bringing him or her close to the body.

16. The mother progresses from calling the infant "it" to referring to the infant as "he" or "she" to using the infant's given name.

17. Refer to text, "The Process of Maternal Role Adaptation," to complete this exercise.

18. "Postpartum blues" describes a mild, transient depression that affects more than 70% of American women. It has an onset within the first week after birth and is characterized by fatigue, weeping, mood instability, and anxiety. The mother may not be able to define why she is upset. The primary nursing care is to give the woman empathy and support and let her know that the condition is usually self-limiting.

19. The nurse should involve the father in infant care teaching and decisions. Fathers may not know what to expect from newborns and benefit from information about growth and development. A review of any prenatal teaching is helpful as well.

20. The nurse should help the parent or parents acknowledge their feelings and deal with them to facilitate their attachment with the child.

21. The nurse should help parents individually interact with each twin rather than interacting with them as a "package." It is important to individually point out essential qualities and characteristics of each infant.

22. Avoidance cues include looking away, splaying the fingers, arching the back, and fussiness. These are clues that the infant needs some quiet time.

Case Study

1. Nita's fundus is not well contracted probably because of a full bladder as it is positioned to the right of the umbilicus. Her multifetal birth and multiparity increase the risk for postpartum hemorrhage.

2. Massage the uterus to cause it to firmly contract and control bleeding. The next intervention should be to assist Nita to empty her bladder or catheterize her if she is unable to void. Otherwise, the uterus will relax again.

3. You should immediately teach Nita how to assess her uterus for firmness and the relationship between a full bladder, her multiparity, and her multifetal birth to uterine contraction.

4. No interventions are needed. Bradycardia and a slight elevation in temperature are common at this time.

5. The best nursing response is to reassure Nita that the afterpains are typically short term and that analgesics can ease them. In addition, teach her that a full bladder will worsen afterpains.

6. Two factors that increase afterpains in Nita's case: multiparity and the uterine overdistention with two fetuses.

7. Analgesics taken at least 30 minutes before the expected time of breastfeeding can decrease afterpains. Lying in a prone position with a small pillow or folded blanket under the abdomen often helps.

8. Teach Nita to gradually increase her ambulation, drink additional fluids (at least eight glasses of water daily), and increase dietary fiber. Prunes are a natural laxative, and she can consult her birth attendant for recommended laxatives if natural remedies do not work.

9. RhoGAM is administered to the Rh-negative mother if her infant is Rh positive and if she has not previously built up anti-Rh antibodies. The rubella vaccine is administered to the nonimmune postpartum woman because it is highly unlikely that she will get pregnant soon.

10. Nita should be cautioned to avoid another pregnancy for at least 3 months.

11. Nita's fundus is slightly higher than usual, but this is explained by her multiparity and delivery of twins.

12. Lochia flow should be rubra (possibly changing to serosa), scant, and free of foul odor or clots.

13. Slight reddening is typical of normal healing at this early stage. Close approximation of the edges and lack of drainage confirm that the healing seems to normally occur. Proper perineal cleansing and pad application should be reinforced. The nurse should also review the signs and symptoms of infection to report.

Review Questions

1. a	6. b	11. a
2. b	7. d	12. d
3. c	8. a	13. a
4. d	9. c	14. c
5. a	10. d	

Matching Key Terms

1. f   4. e   7. g
2. h   5. d   8. a
3. b   6. c
9. *b
10. d (females)
11. c (*abnormal if present before 24 hours)
12. i   14. a   16. *f   18. g
13. *h   15. *j   17. *d (males)19. a
20. c (*suggests the infant is preterm if excessive)
21. b
22. d (females)
23. *j   24. *k   25. *e   26. *g
27. *d (males)
28. c (*suggests the infant is preterm if excessive)

Key Concepts

1. a. Decreased blood oxygen level and pH and an increased blood carbon dioxide level stimulate the respiratory center in the medulla. Occlusion of the umbilical cord vessels may terminate the flow of a placental substance that inhibits respiration.
   b. The sudden change in the environmental temperature at birth stimulates skin sensors, subsequently stimulating the brain's respiratory center.
   c. Fetal chest compression during vaginal birth forces additional lung fluid from the chest. Added stimuli for breathing include suctioning, drying, holding, sounds, and light.
   d. Tactile stimuli that occur during birth stimulate the skin sensors. Placing infants skin-to-skin with their mothers further stimulates these skin sensors.
2. Residual air in the lungs allows the alveoli to remain partially expanded after exhalation. This reduces the work necessary to expand the alveoli with subsequent breaths.
3. a. 4   e. 1
   b. 2   f. 3
   c. 8   g. 7
   d. 6   h. 5
4. Thin skin; blood vessels near the surface; little insulating subcutaneous fat; heat readily transferred from the internal organs to the skin; a greater ratio of surface area to body mass
5. Evaporation occurs when wet surfaces are exposed to air and dry conditions. Conduction occurs when the infant is exposed to direct contact with a cool surface. Convection refers to heat loss by air currents near the infant. Radiation refers to heat loss when the infant is near a cold surface. All methods except evaporation can also be a source of heat gain, such as contact with warm blankets, warmed air currents near the infant, or warm incubator walls.
6. Brown fat is metabolized to generate heat, which is transferred to the blood vessels running through it and then circulated to the rest of the body. Infants who may have inadequate brown fat include preterm infants, those with intrauterine growth restriction, and those exposed to prolonged cold stress.
7. Heat production requires oxygen for metabolism, which can exceed the infant's capacity to supply oxygen. Glucose use is accelerated when the metabolic rate increases to produce heat, possibly depleting these stores and resulting in hypoglycemia. Metabolism of glucose and brown fat without adequate oxygen causes increased production of acids. These acids interfere with the transport of bilirubin to the liver, where it can be conjugated and excreted, thus causing jaundice.
8. Values for all three are higher in the newborn than in older infants or adults. The fetus needs these higher levels to supply adequate oxygen to the tissues. Fetal hemoglobin (hemoglobin F) carries more oxygen than adult hemoglobin.
9. Vitamin K is produced in the intestines by the normal intestinal flora. Newborns cannot produce this flora until a few days after starting to eat. Vitamin K is necessary to activate the clotting factors.
10. Refer to the text, "Stools," to complete this exercise.
11. Glucose lower than 40 mg/dL
12. Preterm or small-for-gestational-age infants are at risk because adequate glycogen and possibly fat may not have accumulated. Post-term infants may have used up their stores of glycogen before birth as a result of deteriorating placenta function. Large-for-gestational-age infants may produce excessive insulin that quickly consumes their glucose; this is particularly true if the mother is diabetic. In addition, stress or hypothermia may consume all available glucose.
13. a. Newborns have more erythrocytes for their size, and these break down faster than adult erythrocytes, producing a greater quantity of bilirubin to be excreted.
   b. The liver is immature and does not immediately produce enough glucuronyl transferase to conjugate bilirubin as quickly as it is produced.
   c. Lack of normal intestinal flora prevents the reduction of conjugated bilirubin to urobilinogen for excretion. Large amounts of β-glucuronidase in the intestines convert conjugated bilirubin back into the unconjugated form.
   d. Feeding helps establish normal intestinal flora.
   e. Birth trauma may cause added hemolysis of erythrocytes, adding to the bilirubin load.
   f. Metabolism of brown fat for heat production and asphyxia, which results in anaerobic metabolism, both of which produce fatty acids. The fatty acids bind more readily to albumin than to bilirubin, resulting in more unconjugated and unbound bilirubin in the circulation. Prevention of cold stress and asphyxia and the time of first feeding may be altered by nursing interventions.
   g. Newborns have fewer albumin binding sites and decreased albumin-binding capacity compared with adults and older children.

   h. Rh, ABO, or others

   i. Preterm and late preterm infants have immature conjugation abilities.

   j. Asian, Native American, or Eskimo infants, or having a sibling who had jaundice

14. Pathologic jaundice has any of these characteristics: appears before 24 hours of age; direct bilirubin level higher than 2 mg/dL; rate of bilirubin increase greater than 5 mg/dL/day; bilirubin level higher than 12 mg/dL in a term infant or 10 to 14 mg/dL in a preterm infant; jaundice that persists after the second week of life.

15. a. Inadequate intake of colostrum causes the retention of meconium, which is high in bilirubin. High levels of beta-glucuronidase in the intestine deconjugate bilirubin in the meconium, adding to the load on the liver. Poor intake reduces the milk supply, worsening the problem. Nursing measures and teaching to stimulate the infant to nurse better, and thus increase milk production, are appropriate treatments.

   b. True breast milk jaundice is characterized by increasing bilirubin levels after the first 3 to 5 days of life; levels peak at 5 to 10 mg/dL at 2 weeks after birth, and it takes several months to reach normal levels. Treatment may include phototherapy, temporarily discontinuing breastfeeding for 24 to 48 hours, or both.

16. Infants have more fluid for their size than adults, with a larger proportion located outside the cells.

17. a. A newborn's kidneys are not well equipped to handle a large load of fluid, possibly resulting in fluid overload.

   b. Newborns have half of an adult's ability to concentrate urine and thus cannot efficiently conserve fluid.

18. Leukocytes slowly respond to the site of infection and are inefficient in destroying invading organisms. The usual inflammatory response and fever are often not present because of the immature hypothalamus.

19. a. IgG is received from the mother to provide passive antibodies to viruses and bacteria to which the mother has immunity. It also protects against bacterial toxins. The infant increases significant production of his or her own IgG beginning at 6 months of age.

   b. IgM is produced by the infant to protect against gram-negative bacteria.

   c. IgA is produced by the infant and is received in colostrum and breast milk to protect against infections of the respiratory and gastrointestinal systems.

20. Newborns during the first period of reactivity are wide awake and active. Respirations may be as high as 80 breaths/min, and the heart rate may be as high as 180 beats/min (bpm). Respiratory assessments show nasal flaring, crackles, retractions, and increased mucous secretions. This is an ideal time to facilitate parent–infant acquaintance because both are highly interested

in each other. After the first sleep period following the first period of reactivity, infants are alert, interested in feeding, and often pass meconium. The pulse and respiratory rates may increase, and some infants may have cyanosis or periods of apnea. Mucous secretions increase. The nurse must be alert for respiratory complications during this stage.

21. Refer to text, "Behavioral States," to complete this exercise.

22. Cardiorespiratory problems; obvious anomalies

23. Caput: cause—pressure against the mother's cervix during labor; features—crosses suture line; teaching—disappears within 12 hours to several days Cephalhematoma: cause—pressure during birth; features—does not cross suture line; teaching—may take weeks to months to resolve, may be higher risk for jaundice

24. a. Associated with other anomalies; carefully assess infants

   b. Single palmar crease that often occurs in infants who have chromosomal abnormalities such as Down syndrome

   c. May indicate spina bifida occulta or failure of the vertebra to fully close

   d. Associated with chromosomal disorders

   e. Indicates facial nerve injury with paralysis during birth

25. Refer to Table 21-2 to complete this exercise.

26. Refer to Procedure 21-1 and Table 21-2 to complete this exercise.

27. Tachypnea (sustained); retractions that continue after the first hour; nasal flaring after the first hour; cyanosis involving the lips, tongue, and trunk (central cyanosis); grunting; seesaw respirations; asymmetry of chest expansion

28. Jitteriness, poor muscle tone, sweating, respiratory signs (dyspnea, apnea, and cyanosis), hypothermia, high-pitched cry, lethargy, seizures, eventually coma; some show no signs of hypoglycemia

29. Female: labia majora darker than surrounding skin and completely cover the clitoris and labia minora; white mucous discharge or pseudomenstruation; hymenal or vaginal tags; patent urinary meatus and the vagina. Male: pendulous scrotum that is darker than surrounding skin and covered with rugae; testes palpable in the scrotal sac; meatus centered at the tip of the glans penis; prepuce covering the glans and adherent to it

30. a. Suggests polycythemia; may contribute to higher bilirubin levels as the excessive erythrocytes break down, so observe for more severe jaundice and emphasize to parents

   b. Indicates meconium passage *in utero;* observe infant for associated respiratory difficulties

   c. Erythema toxicum; differentiate from infection; teach parents that the rash is self-limiting

   d. Mongolian spots; more common in dark-skinned infants; most disappear during early childhood; teach parents who are unfamiliar with these

357

e. Nevus flammeus (port-wine stain); large or obvious ones can later be removed by laser surgery

f. Café-au-lait spots; more than six spots or spots larger than 1.5 cm are associated with neurofibromatosis and should be reported to the physician

31. Bruises on the face or upper body are often present when the infant had a nuchal cord at birth.

Critical Thinking Exercises

Answers to Critical Thinking Exercises will vary.

Case Studies

1. Total maturity score is 43.
2. The infant's maturity rating is between 40 and 42 weeks (approximately 41 weeks).
3. Weight is 3005 g; length is 48 cm; head circumference is 33 cm. The infant is appropriate-for-gestational-age (AGA) in all measurements.
4. All measurements fall near the 25th percentile, which means that 75% of infants of this gestational age are larger and 24% are smaller. The nurse would not anticipate the need for additional care or expanded assessments or care based on the gestational age assessment alone.

Review Questions

1. b	7. c	13. d	19. b
2. d	8. d	14. a	20. a
3. a	9. b	15. d	21. d
4. b	10. d	16. a	
5. d	11. c	17. d	
6. a	12. c	18. b	

CHAPTER 22: THE NORMAL NEWBORN: NURSING CARE

Key Concepts

1. Suction the mouth first and then the nose (if needed). The infant might gasp when the nose is suctioned, drawing any secretions that are in the mouth into the airway.
2. The head is approximately one-fourth of the newborn's total body surface area and thus is a large surface for heat loss. Damp hair presents a continuing source of evaporative heat loss.
3. If the infant's temperature has significantly decreased, the nurse may wish to confirm it with a rectal temperature. Look for and correct sources of heat loss, such as wet clothing or exposed skin. Wrap the flexed infant snugly in warm blankets. A radiant warmer, regulated by a skin probe, may be needed for very low temperatures. Teach parents about maintaining the infant's temperature, particularly if their actions have contributed to the low temperature.
4. a. Conduction
   b. Conduction
   c. Radiation
5. Base your answer on the following: When blood glucose levels decrease, permanent brain damage may occur. Feeding the infant will help maintain appropriate glucose levels. Repeating the glucose level screenings will confirm that appropriate blood levels are being maintained to prevent brain damage.
6. When the temperature is stable
7. For bleeding and urination
8. Notify physician if there is no urinary output within 6 to 8 hours, bleeding more than a few drops with the first diaper changes, or displacement of the Plasti-Bell. Apply pressure if any bleeding occurs. Report signs of infection, such as redness, edema, tenderness, and discharge (a yellow exudate that dries is normal). Apply petrolatum gauze to the site of a Gomco circumcision.
9. Signs of infection include redness at the cord base, exudate or failure to dry, and odor. Keep the cord area dry by keeping the diaper low.
10. Identification is accomplished by matching the imprinted numbers on the adult's wristband with the infant's identification band. The numbers should be matched every time the infant is reunited with the parent. The nurse should visually match the numbers or have a parent read the imprinted numbers from his or her band.
11. Low or elevated temperature; signs of localized infection, such as redness, edema, discharge, foul odor drainage; lethargy; poor feeding; periods of apnea without an obvious cause; any unexplained changes in behavior
12. a. Vitamin K, which is necessary for normal blood coagulation, is administered because the infant's gastrointestinal tract is sterile at birth and temporarily lacks the microorganisms that will synthesize vitamin K.
    b. Erythromycin ointment is used to prevent eye infections acquired in the mother's birth canal, such as gonorrhea.
    c. Hepatitis B immunization is administered to promote the infant's manufacture of antibodies against this viral infection of the liver.
13. Mothers who are positive for hepatitis B (carriers) may transmit the organism to their infant at birth. A dose of hepatitis B immune globulin within 12 hours of birth, in addition to the vaccine, provides passive antibody protection until the infant manufactures his or her own active antibodies to the virus.
14. Refer to text, "Follow-Up Care," to complete this exercise.

Critical Thinking Exercises

Answers to Critical Thinking Exercises will vary.

Review Questions

1. c	3. a	5. d
2. b	4. b	6. a

CHAPTER 23: NEWBORN FEEDING

Matching Key Terms

1. c	2. d	3. b	4. a

Key Concepts

1. 8 lb × 45–50 kcal/day = 360–400 cal/day; 20 kcal/oz = 18–20 oz/day; 18–20 oz × 30 mL = 540–600 mL of fluid per day

2. Colostrum, which is produced during the first week, is a thick, yellow substance rich in immunoglobulins, especially immunoglobulin A (IgA). It has laxative effects and is high in protein, fat-soluble vitamins, and minerals. It is low in carbohydrates, fat, and lactose. Transitional milk begins 7 to 10 days after lactation begins; immunoglobulins and proteins decrease; lactose, fat, and calories increase. Mature milk begins 2 weeks after the onset of lactation; it has a bluish color and provides 20 cal/oz.

3. Refer to text, "Breast Milk and Formula Composition," to complete this exercise.

4. Prolactin stimulates the breasts to produce milk. It is enhanced by suckling and removing the milk from the breasts, and it is inhibited by estrogen, progesterone, and placental lactogen during pregnancy and by inadequate removal of milk after nursing begins. Oxytocin stimulates the milk-ejection reflex. It is enhanced by comfort, thinking about the infant, and the stimulation of suckling. It is inhibited by discomfort or inadequate suckling.

5. Breast shells used in late pregnancy can draw nipples out. In addition, using a breast pump for a few minutes before feeding might help draw out the nipples.

6. a. Feel like a cheek
   b. Slightly firmer than a cheek
   c. Hard, shiny, taut tissue

7. a. The mother cups the breast in a "C" position, with her thumb on top and the fingers underneath. This is preferred because her fingers are less likely to slip toward the nipple than with the scissors position.
   b. In the V hold, the mother guides her nipple by securing it between her index and middle finger.

8. Nutritive suckling is evidenced by smooth, continuous movements with only occasional pauses to rest. Swallowing may follow each suck or after two or three sucks. Nonnutritive suckling produces fluttery or choppy motions without the sound of swallowing. Infant swallowing has a soft "ka" or "ah" sound.

9. Break suction before removing the infant from the breast by inserting a finger between the infant's gums or indenting the breast tissue near the infant's mouth.

10. 1.5; 3; 8–12

11. Frequent nursing stimulates peristalsis, which increases the rate of excretion of bilirubin in the stools.

12. After a feeding or at night

13. Serious infections such as tuberculosis, human immunodeficiency virus (HIV) infection, maternal cancer, maternal substance abuse

14. a. Use rigid polypropylene plastic containers with a tight cap.
    b. Milk may be stored in the refrigerator for 48 hours (preferred) or in the refrigerator's freezer for 1 month; it can be kept in a deep freeze at 0°F for 6 months.
    c. Do not microwave. Thaw in the refrigerator or by holding under running water.

15. a. Wash the top of the can and the can opener just before opening and pouring into washed bottles and capping. Refrigerate an open can and discard any remaining milk after 48 hours.
    b. Dilute the concentrated liquid with an equal part of water. Do not overdilute or underdilute. Fill clean bottles with diluted formula as in ready-to-feed.
    c. Dilute the formula in a clean bottle exactly as directed, usually one scoop per two ounces of water. As in concentrated liquid formula, do not overdilute or underdilute.

16. a. Feed the infant every 3 to 4 hours, but do not adhere to a rigid schedule.
    b. Do not prop the bottle. To do so may cause aspiration of formula. Bottle propping is associated with dental caries when the primary teeth erupt and with ear infections.
    c. Do not microwave formula because it may have "hot spots" that would burn the infant.
    d. Discard all remaining formula after 1 hour of use.

Case Study

1. A good initial action would be to help Margaret calm her fussy baby so that the infant will be more likely to nurse. This action accomplishes two goals: (1) it helps Margaret learn the skill of comforting her infant and (2) it increases the likelihood that the infant will nurse well when correctly positioned at the breast.

2. After the infant is calmer, suggest positions that Margaret can use to begin nursing. Support her arm in the chosen position with pillows or blankets. Explain the basics of helping her infant latch on to the breast: stimulating the infant's mouth until it opens wide, then drawing the infant close; inserting the nipple and areola well back into the mouth; checking to see that the lips are flared on the breast tissue. Describe and have Margaret observe for typical patterns that indicate nutritive suckling: smooth rhythmic suckling, interrupted by swallowing with a soft "ka" or "ah" sound.

3. Teach Margaret that the milk-ejection reflex may take as long as 5 minutes to occur and that nursing periods that are too short will provide only the foremilk, which has a lower fat content, is less satisfying, and does not promote the infant's growth. If the infant receives only the foremilk regularly, she will want to nurse often and will be less satisfied. Engorgement is also more likely. Teach her to break the suction before removing the infant from the breast. Positioning the infant to avoid pulling on the nipple and ensuring that the areola is well into the infant's mouth will help reduce nipple soreness, although it will not totally prevent it.

4. Infants usually feed every 2 to 3 hours and should not sleep longer than 5 hours without nursing. Teach the mother to plan on nursing 8 to 12 times in each 24-hour period. Duration is generally approximately 10 to 15 minutes on each breast. The infant should nurse on the first breast until nonnutritive suckling

begins; then the mother should change to the other breast. Switching back and forth between breasts several times during feedings reduces the amount of hindmilk secreted.

5. Wear a well-fitting bra day and night. Avoid creams, ointments, or soaps on the breasts. Clean with plain water. Express colostrum and rub it into the breasts. Wear absorbent pads in the bra if breasts are leaking, but do not allow the wet pad to have prolonged contact with the breast. Leave bra flaps down after nursing. See also Nursing Care Plan 24-3 and "Mothers Want to Know: Solutions to Common Breastfeeding Problems" in your textbook.

6. Refer to text, "Mothers Want to Know: Is My Baby Getting Enough Milk?" in your textbook.

Review Questions

1. b	3. d	5. c
2. a	4. a	6. b

CHAPTER 24: THE CHILDBEARING FAMILY WITH SPECIAL NEEDS

Matching Key Terms

1. e	3. c	5. d
2. a	4. f	6. b

Key Concepts

1. a. Development of independence from parents is interrupted. The teenage girl usually becomes more dependent on them, rather than becoming more independent of her family home.
   b. Education is often interrupted and may never be completed. Overall, the educational level is lower.
   c. Reliance on the welfare system is more likely because of an incomplete education and limited job skills.

2. Anemia, labor dystocia, preeclampsia, preterm birth, victims of violence during pregnancy

3. a. There is a higher incidence of chromosome abnormalities such as Down syndrome.
   b. Older women are more likely to have underlying chronic medical conditions that complicate pregnancy such as diabetes or hypertension.
   c. There is a higher incidence of multifetal gestation, preterm delivery, dysfunctional labor, preeclampsia, gestational diabetes, spontaneous abortion, placenta previa, abruption placentae, and cesarean birth. Infants are more likely to be a low birth weight.

4. a. She may have less energy to cope with the demands of an infant plus the day-to-day activities of living.
   b. She may have less peer support because most other women her age have teenagers or young adults.

5. Most substances ingested by the mother cross the placenta and enter the fetal circulation. The fetus cannot metabolize the substance as quickly, so the substance lingers for a prolonged time in the fetal body.

6. Refer to textbook, Table 24-1, to complete this exercise.

7. Cocaine directly stimulates uterine contractions. Preterm labor contractions are rarely abrupt and intense at their onset. The fetus or neonate may have problems related to the maternal cocaine, such as abruptio placentae, premature rupture of the membranes, precipitous birth, stillbirth, tachycardia, irritability, muscular rigidity, hypertension, and an exaggerated startle reflex.

8. Withdrawal of heroin can be fatal for the fetus. The mother can be put on methadone during the pregnancy, but the neonate will need to withdraw from that medication after birth.

9. a. Late prenatal care, failing to keep appointments, not following recommendations
   b. Poor grooming, inadequate weight gain, weight gain pattern that does not conform to that expected for the gestational age
   c. Spontaneous abortions, premature births, abruptio placentae, stillbirths
   d. Anger or apathy toward pregnancy, particularly if these are evident at a time when the normal ambivalence of early pregnancy should be resolved

10. a. Profuse sweating, hypertension, irregular respirations, lethargic response to labor, lack of interest in interventions, dilated pupils, increased body temperature, sudden onset of severely painful contractions, emotional lability and paranoia, fetal tachycardia, and fetal hyperactivity
    b. Withdrawal symptoms, such as yawning, diaphoresis, rhinorrhea, restlessness, excessive tearing, nausea, vomiting, and abdominal cramps

11. Facial abnormalities cause parental concerns about how others will accept their child because the defect is obvious. Genital defects cause ambiguity and anxiety about the child's identity: Is the baby a boy or girl? How should the baby be dressed? How should we respond to questions about the infant's gender?

12. Parents must grieve for the expected normal child before they can detach from this fantasy and move on to accepting the child they have.

13. The father, as well as the mother, must be assisted to deal with the shock and sadness, rather than all the attention being focused on the mother's grief. Only when the father deals with his emotions can he support his partner and explain the loss to the couple's family and friends.

14. Woman: multiple injury sites; late entry into prenatal care; increased risk for low maternal weight gain and anemia; more substance abuse, increased STDs and risk for postpartum depression. Fetus: prematurity, low birth weight, and neonatal death

15. Tension building: when threats and angry behavior escalate; increased use of alcohol and drugs; the woman tries to avoid or placate her abuser.
Battering: with hitting, burning, beating, or raping the woman. The woman often simply endures the abuse.

Honeymoon phase: when the abuser is overly solicitous and tries to make up with his partner. He often insists on having intercourse to prove that she forgives him. The woman wants to believe that he will never abuse her again.

Review Questions

1. c   3. b   5. a
2. d   4. c

CHAPTER 25: PREGNANCY-RELATED COMPLICATIONS

Matching Key Terms

1. c   2. a   3. b

Key Concepts

1. Termination of a pregnancy without action taken by the woman or any other person.
2. Refer to the text, "Spontaneous Abortion," to complete this exercise.
3. Fibrinogen and platelets—decreased; prothrombin and partial thromboplastin time—prolonged; fibrin degradation products—increased; D-dimer–positive
4. The nurse can explain that most spontaneous abortions occur because of factors or abnormalities that could not be avoided. In addition, allow the patient the opportunity to express her feelings.
5. Abrupt onset of shoulder pain may occur with a ruptured ectopic pregnancy because blood accumulating in the abdomen irritates the diaphragm.
6. Explain the side effects such as nausea and vomiting. Teach the woman to refrain from consuming alcohol, ingesting vitamins containing folic acid, or having sexual intercourse until human chorionic gonadotropin (hCG) is not detectable in the serum (usually 2 to 4 weeks).
7. Elevated hCG levels; vaginal bleeding that varies in amount and color; uterine enlargement greater than expected for the gestation; nondetectable fetal heart activity; excessive nausea and vomiting; early onset of preeclampsia
8. Most molar tissue is benign, but choriocarcinoma is a possibility. Serum hCG levels will be evaluated every 1 to 2 weeks. Pregnancy must be avoided until normal prepregnancy hCG levels are attained.
9. Foods high in iron should be emphasized to aid in restoring hemoglobin levels. These include liver, red meat, spinach, egg yolks, carrots, and raisins. She should also include vitamin C foods, which increase the utilization of iron. Use the information in the text to formulate your explanation.
10. Refer to the text, "Hemorrhagic Conditions of Late Pregnancy," to complete this chart.
11. The woman and her family should be taught to assess the vaginal discharge, fetal movement counts, and uterine activity. She should be given guidelines for what to report. Curtailment of sexual intercourse should be discussed.

12. Cocaine is a vasoconstrictor, including the constriction of the uterine endometrial arteries, which leads to premature placental separation.
13. Much or all of the blood may be trapped by the placenta, which may remain attached at the edges.
14. Early signs: tachycardia, diminished peripheral pulses, normal or slightly decreased blood pressure, tachypnea, pallor and coolness of the skin and mucous membranes. Late signs: decreasing blood pressure, pallor, skin that is cold and clammy, urine output less than 30 mL/hr, restlessness, agitation, and decreased mentation
15. Lateral positioning with the head flat to increase cardiac return and enhance circulation to the placenta and vital organs; restricted maternal movement to reduce the demand for oxygen; provide explanations, reassurance, and emotional support to reduce anxiety that would increase the demand for oxygen
16. a. Reduced blood flow causes a reduced glomerular filtration rate, which causes an increase in blood urea nitrogen (BUN), creatinine, and uric acid levels. Glomerular damage, resulting from reduced perfusion, allows protein to leak across the glomerular membrane, resulting in interstitial fluid accumulation, hypovolemia, and increased blood viscosity and hematocrit (hemoconcentration) value. Angiotensin II and aldosterone are secreted in response to hypovolemia, further increasing the blood pressure.
    b. Reduced perfusion decreases liver function. Hepatic edema and subcapsular hemorrhage may occur. The serum may have elevated liver enzyme levels.
    c. Vasoconstriction leads to pressure-induced rupture of the small capillaries, resulting in small cerebral hemorrhages. Symptoms, such as headache and visual disturbances, may result.
    d. Reduced colloid oncotic pressure may result in pulmonary edema.
    e. Reduced perfusion may cause infarctions or abruptio placentae. The risk for HELLP syndrome is also higher. The fetus may have a growth restriction and persistent hypoxemia.
17. Edema of preeclampsia typically occurs above the waist: in the face and fingers. A sudden weight gain often precedes visible edema.
18. Epigastric pain occurs with liver capsule distention, which often heralds an imminent convulsion.
19. Central nervous system depression results in diminished deep tendon reflexes and respiratory depression, pulse ox reading of <95%. Reduced urinary output can cause magnesium to accumulate to unsafe levels.
20. Calcium gluconate
21. Chronic hypertension is present before 20 weeks of gestation.
22. a. The woman must have Rh-negative blood because she will not make anti-Rh antibodies if she is also Rh positive.

b. The newborn must have Rh-positive blood because Rh-negative blood cannot induce the development of anti-Rh antibodies in the woman.

c. An indirect Coombs test should be negative, indicating that the woman has not made anti-Rh antibodies (become sensitized) to Rh-positive blood during the pregnancy.

d. The direct Coombs test identifies maternal antibodies in the newborn's blood and should be negative.

23. ABO incompatibility may occur if a type O mother has a fetus who is type A, B, or AB because these blood types contain an antigen that is not present on type O erythrocytes. Many type O people have developed high levels of antibodies to blood types A, B, or AB, and the antibodies can cross the placenta and damage fetal erythrocytes that are one of these types. The effects are usually less severe than an Rh incompatibility.

Case Study

1. The main objective of the nurse's assessment is to identify why Patricia had a sudden excessive weight gain. Pregnancy-induced hypertension (PIH) is a likely suspect, but the nurse must assess for other possible causes such as a substantially increased food intake.

2. The staff must determine whether Patricia's weight gain is the result of PIH and take steps to treat it.

3. The nurse should assess for other signs and symptoms of PIH: hypertension; urine protein; edema, particularly of the face and fingers; epigastric pain; visual disturbances, such as spots or blurring; severe and unrelenting headache; dyspnea.

4. A dipstick test to identify proteinuria should be performed to identify excessive levels in the urine. Reduced kidney perfusion causes glomerular damage, causing the protein to be lost.

5. The nurse needs Patricia's past pattern of weight gain and her previous vital signs to evaluate today's information more accurately.

6. The nurse should ask Patricia whether her rings are tight (finger edema); whether she sees spots in front of her eyes, has blurring of vision, or has had severe headaches (cerebral edema); whether she has upper abdominal pain or nausea (distended liver capsule); and whether she has difficulty breathing (pulmonary edema).

7. Refer to Table 25-3 to complete this exercise.

8. Patricia's PIH is mild, and the fetal signs are favorable. Since the fetus is 34 weeks, delay of birth would be favorable unless the PIH worsens. In that case, poor placental perfusion is likely to cause the fetus more problems, including possible fetal demise, than preterm delivery.

9. Teaching involves activity restrictions, including how to achieve them, and the assessment of fetal activity, maternal blood pressure, weight, and urine protein. The woman and family must be taught what signs and symptoms to report and when to return for fetal surveillance studies and regular prenatal visits.

1. b	4. d	7. d	10. d
2. d	5. c	8. b	11. c
3. a	6. b	9. a	

CHAPTER 26: CONCURRENT DISORDERS DURING PREGNANCY

Matching Key Terms

1. b	2. d	3. a	4. c

Key Concepts

1. a. Polydipsia (excess thirst)
   b. Polyuria (excess urine output)
   c. Polyphagia (excess appetite)
   d. Weight loss

2. Hypoglycemia and hyperglycemia are associated with more spontaneous abortions and congenital malformations.

3. With no vascular impairment, hyperglycemia can lead to macrosomia. Vascular impairment limits glucose and oxygen transport to the fetus and may result in intrauterine growth restriction.

4. a. They decrease in the first trimester because of reduced maternal food intake and uptake of glucose by the embryo/fetus.
   b. They increase in the second and third trimesters because of maternal insulin resistance and greater food intake.
   c. They usually decrease during labor because of exertion and the lack of food intake. Euglycemia is maintained with an intravenous (IV) infusion of insulin and glucose.
   d. They decrease in the postpartum period because of the loss of hormones from the placenta, which causes insulin resistance.

5. If her glucose challenge test (a screening test) is 140 mg/dL or higher, she needs to undergo the diagnostic 3-hour oral glucose tolerance test.

6. To increase her sense of control and the likelihood that she will adhere to the therapeutic recommendations

7. Releasing the tissue after the needle insertion; injection over 2 to 4 seconds; quick needle withdrawal

8. These sugars quickly increase the blood glucose levels to high levels and alter glucose control for many hours, resulting in wide swings between high and low levels.

9. Rales, dyspnea on exertion, cough, hemoptysis, progressive edema, heart palpitations, and orthopnea

10. Class III

11. Heparin is the anticoagulant of choice because it does not cross the placenta.

12. Each labor contraction causes up to 500 mL of blood to be shifted from the uterus and placenta to the central circulation. Approximately 500 mL of blood returns to the central circulation when the placenta delivers. The added blood volume increases the diseased heart's workload and can result in congestive heart failure.

13. Her excess weight gain may be caused by excess food, fluid retention from cardiac decompensation or excess salt intake, or preeclampsia (see Chapter 24). Thus, you must assess her diet and other signs and symptoms of cardiac decompensation and preeclampsia.

14. Folic acid is needed for cell duplication and the growth of the fetus and placenta. Folic acid deficiency is associated with a higher incidence of neural tube defects. It is difficult to get the required pregnancy amount by diet alone, and folic acid is often destroyed by cooking.

15. Placental infarctions occur that decrease the exchange surface of the placenta.

16. Pain (abdomen, chest, vertebrae, joints, extremities); pallor; signs of cardiac failure

17. Fetal loss, prematurity, preeclampsia, renal complications, preterm rupture of membranes, miscarriage, and fetal death in the first trimester

18. Many anticonvulsants are associated with teratogenic effects, such as significant fetal abnormalities. Yet, without the drugs, grand mal seizures are more likely to occur, which can cause fetal hypoxia, acidosis, and death.

19. Early, acute stage: flu-like symptoms for a few weeks, followed by seroconversion a few weeks or months later
Middle, asymptomatic period: low-level viral replication and loss of CD4 cells
Transitional period: symptomatic disease
Late, crisis period: symptomatic disease

20. Use the information on pp. 563-569 to complete this table.

21. AIDS is said to occur when the immune system does not protect the person and opportunistic infections occur.

22. Zidovudine (AZT)

23. Support grieving and retention of patient control; promote wellness (nutrition, rest, activity, avoidance of crowds and poor sanitary conditions, skin care); teach that breastfeeding is contraindicated; reinforce medication information.

24. Use the information on pp. 568-569 to complete this table.

Case Study

1. During early pregnancy, fetal demand for glucose tends to cause maternal hypoglycemia. Debra is near the beginning of her second trimester, so increasing resistance to insulin in her cells and the rapid breakdown of insulin occur to make more glucose available to her fetus.

2. Debra will probably need increasing amounts of insulin as her pregnancy progresses. In addition, the goal is to maintain her blood glucose level as near to normal as possible; thus, she will need to test her blood glucose as many as five to seven times each day and may take more frequent insulin doses (regular and intermediate acting). Her diet should have approximately 2200 to 2400 cal/day distributed among three meals and two to four snacks.

3. Routine prenatal visit testing includes vital signs and the fetal heart rate; an assessment of her blood glucose levels (including her daily logs); and urinalysis for protein, glucose, and ketones. Glycosylated hemoglobin testing is performed as needed.

4. Tests needed as pregnancy progresses are designed to evaluate placental function and fetal health and maturity. These include maternal serum α-fetoprotein, ultrasound, fetal echocardiography, "kick counts," nonstress or contraction stress test, biophysical profile, amniotic fluid index, or amniocentesis to evaluate fetal lung maturity. Doppler velocimetry may also be performed.

5. Possible fetal effects include congenital defects, large or small fetal size, and persistent fetal hypoxia.

6. Labor may be induced or a cesarean delivery performed if the fetus shows signs of decreased placental perfusion with hypoxia. While in labor, Debra will have hourly blood glucose evaluations to determine her need for insulin. Tight glucose control during labor minimizes newborn hypoglycemia.

7. The neonatal nurse should anticipate possible newborn hypoglycemia if the newborn was exposed to high maternal blood glucose *in utero*, with high fetal insulin secretion to metabolize the glucose. After birth, the glucose supply is cut off, while the pancreas continues to secrete large quantities of insulin temporarily.

8. The newborn will need frequent blood glucose monitoring for the first few hours after birth. See Chapter 30 for more information about caring for the infant of a diabetic mother.

Review Questions

1. b	4. d	7. b
2. b	5. a	8. c
3. a	6. c	9. b

CHAPTER 27: THE WOMAN WITH AN INTRAPARTUM COMPLICATION

Matching Key Terms

1. b	3. d	5. e
2. c	4. a	

Key Concepts

1. Uterine contractions must be coordinated, strong enough, and numerous enough to propel the fetus through the woman's pelvis.

2. Use Table 27-1 in the text to complete this exercise.

3. Amniotomy; oxytocin augmentation

4. All nursing actions focus on helping the woman make each push most effective by correcting or identifying causes contributing to ineffective pushing.

5. They add the force of gravity to maternal pushes.

6. a. Help the woman understand that her tissues can distend to accommodate the fetus; apply warm compresses to the perineum.
   b. Teach the woman to push only when she feels the urge or with every other contraction; administer fluids as ordered; offer reassurance.
7. Upright positions favor fetal descent (gravity), and with that descent, fetal head rotation.
8. Uterine overdistention with hypotonic dysfunction; abnormal fetal presentation(s); fetal hypoxia; postpartum hemorrhage resulting from uterine overdistention
9. a. Dilation of at least 1.2 cm/hr; descent of at least 1.0 cm/hr
   b. Dilation of at least 1.5 cm/hr; descent of at least 2.0 cm/hr
10. For the mother: promotion of comfort, conservation of energy, emotional support, position changes that favor normal progress, and assessments of infection For the fetus: observation for signs of intrauterine infection and compromised fetal oxygenation
11. a. Place her in a side-lying position, administer oxygen, maintain blood volume with nonoxytocin IV fluids, stop oxytocin if in use, administer terbutaline or other tocolytic drug that may be ordered.
    b. Help the woman focus on nonpharmacologic pain control methods if analgesia is not possible; remain with the woman.
12. Urinary incontinence, increased vaginal discharge, loss of the mucous plug
13. Points to include are avoid sexual activity, take temperature four times a day, and report if higher than 100°F (37.8°C), report contractions
14. Side effects of β-adrenergic drugs include maternal and fetal tachycardia, decreased blood pressure, wide pulse pressure, dysrhythmias, myocardial ischemia, chest pain, pulmonary edema, hyperglycemia and hypokalemia, tremors, and restlessness. Propranolol (Inderal), a β-blocking drug, should be available to reverse the effects.
15. a. Prostaglandin synthesis inhibitors block the action of prostaglandins, which stimulate uterine contractions; an example is indomethacin.
    b. Calcium antagonists block the action of calcium, which is necessary for muscle contraction; an example is nifedipine.
16. In addition to studying the text, refer also to a drug reference manual.
    a. Observe the maternal blood pressure, pulse, respirations, and fetal heart rate to identify tachycardia or hypotension; assess lung sounds; assess for the presence of dyspnea or chest pain to identify pulmonary edema or myocardial ischemia; obtain ordered glucose and potassium levels; have propranolol available.
    b. Observe for a urine output of at least 30 mL/hr, the presence of deep tendon reflexes, and a respiration of at least 12 breaths/min; assess heart and lung sounds; observe bowel sounds and assess for constipation; have calcium gluconate available.
    c. Observe for nausea, vomiting, heartburn, rash, and abnormal bleeding; check the fundal height; have the woman do kick counts to identify fetal movements.
    d. Teach about flushing of the skin and headache; observe the maternal pulse [report if higher than 110 beats/min (bpm)], fetal heart rates, and maternal blood pressure; warn of postural hypotension; and teach to assume a sitting or standing position gradually after lying down.
    e. Assess lung sounds; teach the woman to report chest pain or heaviness, as well as any difficulty breathing. Patients should also be made aware of the possible side effects of nervousness and insomnia.
17. Complete: The cord is visible at the vaginal opening. Occult prolapsed cord cannot be seen or felt on vaginal examination but is suspected based on the fetal heart rate. The cord may slip into the vagina, where it can be felt as a pulsating mass. It may slip outside the vagina, where it is visible.
18. Relieve the pressure on the cord with position changes; increase fetal oxygenation.
19. Complete rupture—open communication between the uterine and peritoneal cavities; incomplete rupture—rupture into the peritoneum or broad ligament but not into the peritoneal cavity; dehiscence—the partial separation of a previous uterine scar
20. Amniotic fluid is rich in thromboplastin, initiating uncontrolled clotting that consumes normal clotting factors.
21. If the mother's condition deteriorates, the fetal condition will inevitably also deteriorate because the fetus is completely dependent on the woman for oxygen, nutrients, and waste removal.
22. Despite stable maternal and fetal vital signs, an enlarging uterus following trauma suggests abruptio placentae. Promptly notify the physician.

Case Studies

1. The nurse must (a) attempt to verify whether Ann's membranes have ruptured but without performing a vaginal examination; (b) determine when they ruptured; (c) assess the maternal vital signs and fetal heart rate, looking specifically for signs of infection; (d) assess for contractions that may indicate preterm labor, as well as a preterm premature rupture of membranes (PROM).
2. Fluid draining from the vagina; positive nitrazine and fern tests; cloudy fluid; fetal tachycardia; occasional contractions
3. The vaginal fluid drainage and the positive nitrazine and fern tests suggest that Ann's membranes have ruptured. Infection is suggested by the cloudy fluid and fetal tachycardia. Contractions suggest preterm labor.
4. A vaginal examination is not advised because the vaginal discharge is typical of amniotic fluid (meaning that the membranes are truly ruptured), there already appears to be an infection, Ann's gestation is preterm, and

she is already having contractions. Little information is likely to be gained from the examination, and it might introduce more microorganisms into the uterus.

5. Initiating intravenous fluids should be the top priority because (a) hydration with fluids may stop the preterm labor contractions and (b) venous access may be quickly needed for emergency procedures.

6. A side-lying position with the head of the bed kept low increases the placental blood flow and reduces pressure of the fetal presenting part on the cervix. Bed rest may reduce uterine activity.

7. Urine output of at least 30 mL/hr, the presence of deep tendon reflexes, and a respiratory rate of at least 12 breaths/min suggest that the magnesium level is within safe limits. Serum drug levels will also be ordered (see Chapter 26 for additional information).

8. Teach her the importance of maintaining even spacing of the drug; set her alarm clock to take the terbutaline during the night; expect side effects such as palpitations, tremors, restlessness, weakness, or headache. Report a heart rate higher than 110 bpm, chest pain, or dyspnea.

9. Explain the activity restrictions her doctor recommends and explore with her how she can maintain them. Teach her the signs and symptoms of recurrent preterm labor, and tell her to return to the hospital if they occur. Teach her the relationship of hydration and uterine irritability, and tell her to drink at least eight full glasses of water each day. Teach her the signs of a urinary tract infection to report urgency, increased frequency, and pain.

Review Questions

1. c	5. c	9. d	13. a
2. b	6. a	10. b	
3. d	7. d	11. c	
4. a	8. b	12. d	

CHAPTER 28: THE WOMAN WITH A POSTPARTUM COMPLICATION

Matching Key Terms

1. c	3. e	5. f
2. b	4. d	6. a

Key Concepts

1. Early postpartum hemorrhage occurs within 24 hours of birth; late hemorrhage occurs after this time. More than 500 mL of blood after vaginal birth or more than 1000 mL of blood after a cesarean birth constitutes a postpartum hemorrhage.

2. Uterine atony occurs when the figure-eight muscle fibers of the uterus do not firmly contract to compress the bleeding endometrial vessels at the placental site.

3. The uterus is difficult to locate, and when found, it is soft rather than firm and higher than the expected level near the umbilicus. It may become firm with massaging but fails to remain firm. One *saturated* pad per 15 min represents an excessive blood loss.

4. Support the lower uterus with one hand while gently but firmly massaging the fundus until it contracts. Push on the fundus *after the uterus is firm* to express clots that have accumulated in the uterine cavity and could interfere with continued uterine contraction. Check for a distended bladder, often indicated when the uterus is displaced to one side (usually the right). Have her urinate or catheterize her if necessary. Drugs, such as oxytocin or methylergonovine, may be needed to maintain uterine contractions. Maintain intravenous access.

5. Excess, usually brighter red, bleeding in the presence of a firmly contracted uterus that is in the expected location suggests a laceration.

6. Pain is the greatest distinction because confined bleeding exerts pressure on the sensory nerves. The uterus is firm, thereby excluding uterine atony as the cause. Lochia is normal because the bleeding is concealed, excluding a bleeding laceration. An increasing pulse and respiratory rate and decreasing blood pressure are signs of hypovolemia that may occur with any type of hemorrhage.

7. a. Stimulation of baroreceptors and the release of catecholamines result in the vasoconstriction of peripheral blood vessels and an increasing heart rate and blood pressure. Gradual tachycardia is typically the earliest sign of hypovolemia. Respiration increases as the woman attempts to increase her intake of oxygen. The skin is pale and cool, and the capillary refill is prolonged.

   b. Inadequate perfusion results in a buildup of lactic acid and metabolic acidosis, resulting in vasodilation, which accelerates blood loss. The skin becomes cold and clammy. Urine output decreases or even ceases as the circulation to the kidneys is reduced. When the blood volume is inadequate to perfuse the brain and heart, death results.

8. Women should be told the normal sequence, amount, and duration of lochia. They should be taught the assessment and expected descent of the fundus. Guidelines should be provided for reporting deviations from the normal amount of fluid.

9. They have higher levels of clotting factors (fibrinogen; factors III, VIII, and X) and the suppression of factors that prevent clot formation (plasminogen activator and antithrombin III). In addition, venous stasis occurs during pregnancy and blood vessel injuries can occur during birth.

10. Refer to "Thromboembolic Disorders" in the text to complete this chart.

11. Heparin: activated partial thromboplastin time (aPTT). Warfarin: prothrombin time and international normalized ratio (INR). NOTE: aPTT and PTT are not specifically mentioned in the chapter. Only INR is specifically mentioned for warfarin therapy.

12. Teach the heparin injection technique to the patient and a family member, as appropriate. Teach the patient to report any unusual bruising or petechiae, nosebleeds, bloody urine, bleeding gums, or increased

vaginal bleeding; use a soft toothbrush; and do not go barefoot. Teach the side effects of the specific antico-agulant. Caution regarding drugs or alcohol, which should not be taken with the specific anticoagulant. Teach when to return for laboratory studies.

13. Signs and symptoms vary according to the degree of pulmonary blood flow obstruction but include sudden sharp chest pain, abdominal pain, low grade fever, tachycardia, dyspnea, tachypnea pulmonary rales, cough, hemoptysis, decreased partial pressure of oxygen (arterial blood gases), as well as atelectasis and pleural effusion seen on X-ray studies.

14. A temperature of 38°C (100.4°F) or higher after the first 24 hours, occurring on at least 2 days during the first 10 days following birth

15. All of the parts of the female reproductive tract are connected to each other and to the peritoneal cavity. The area is richly supplied with blood vessels and lymphatics, providing a well-nourished, dark, warm environment that favors bacterial growth.

16. Amniotic fluid, blood, and lochia make the normally acidic vagina more alkaline, fostering the growth of organisms. The necrotic endometrial lining with lochia promotes the growth of anaerobic organisms. Small areas of trauma allow microorganisms to enter the tissues. However, granulocytes in the endometrium and lochia help prevent infection. Aseptic technique and careful handwashing help prevent the transfer of organisms to the mother.

17. These signs suggest a paralytic ileus caused by the spread of the infection into the peritoneal cavity. The nurse should assess bowel sounds and report all findings to the physician.

18. Edema, warmth, redness, pain, tenderness, separation of the edges, and seropurulent drainage

19. Apricot, plum, prune, and cranberry juices help to acidify the urine, which makes the urine less favorable to microorganisms.

20. Stasis of milk promotes the growth of infecting microorganisms, possibly leading to the formation of an abscess.

21. Septic thrombophlebitis also involves an infection and usually affects the pelvic venous system. It requires antibiotic and anticoagulant treatment.

22. Postpartum depression symptoms include the *persistent* loss of interest in surroundings and the loss of loving or pleasurable feelings; *persistent* fatigue, complaints of ill health, and difficulty concentrating; *persistent* loss of interest in food; and *persistent* sleep disturbances. It is the persistence of these behaviors and feelings that marks the difference.

23. Bipolar disorder is characterized by both manic episodes (with irritability, hyperactivity, euphoria, grandiosity, little sleep, and poor judgment) and depressive episodes (characterized by tearfulness, preoccupations of guilt, feelings of worthlessness, sleep and appetite disturbances, and inordinate concern with the baby's health or delusions about the baby's being dead or defective). Major depression

has only the depression features and not the manic characteristics.

Case Study

1. The medication could be taking longer than usual to exert its analgesic properties, it could be outdated, Jana's pain tolerance at this time could be very low, or other birth trauma may have occurred. In addition, although Jana's fundal height is appropriate, she may need to urinate because it has been 1.5 hours since the birth and her bladder may be fuller than it appears.

2. The nurse needs more information about the pain: location, intensity on a 1 to 10 scale (comparing its present level with the level before she took the analgesic), character, and whether anything worsens or improves it. In addition, the nurse must look at Jana's perineal area for evidence of a hematoma.

3. If Jana still has not voided, the nurse should carefully assess her bladder and place her on the bedpan to void. However, Jana's symptoms suggest a concealed hemorrhage with early hypovolemia: unrelieved pain and a rising pulse in the presence of a firm fundus and normal lochia. Unrelieved pain is not typical of a full bladder, although it may worsen the pain of a hematoma. Therefore, Jana should not ambulate to the bathroom because of the higher risk of fainting. If she does not promptly void, it would be appropriate to catheterize her (assuming there is an order), both to see whether emptying her bladder relieves the pain and to determine her urine output, which is a significant indicator of her fluid volume status. The physician or nurse-midwife should be promptly notified of all assessments and interventions.

Review Questions

1. c	4. d	7. c	10. c
2. a	5. b	8. d	
3. b	6. a	9. a	

CHAPTER 29: THE HIGH-RISK NEWBORN: PROBLEMS RELATED TO GESTATIONAL AGE AND DEVELOPMENT

Matching Key Terms

1. d	3. c	5. a
2. e	4. b	

6. a	11. c	16. a or c	21. b or c
7. b or c	12. a	17. b or c	22. a
8. c	13. c	18. a	23. b or c
9. b or c	14. b or c	19. c	
10. a	15. c	20. a	

Key Concepts

1. a. Born before the 38th week of gestation begins
   b. Birth weight of 2500 g (5 pounds 8 ounces) or less
   c. Birth weight of 1500 g (3 pounds 5 ounces) or less
   d. Birth weight of 1000 g (2 pounds 3 ounces) or less
   e. Birth weight of less than expected for the duration of gestation

2. Periodic breathing is the cessation of breathing for 5 to 10 seconds without other changes; apneic spells that last more than 20 seconds and/or are accompanied by cyanosis and bradycardia

3. The prone position is associated with an increased incidence of sudden infant death syndrome (SIDS). However, the prone position allows the immature preterm infant to use respiratory muscles more efficiently, reduces respiratory effort, and increases oxygenation and lung compliance.

4. Hydration keeps secretions thin, so they are more easily removed.

5. a. Thin skin with little insulating fat
   b. Less heat-producing brown fat accumulation
   c. Extended extremities increase exposure to the air for heat loss.
   d. Immature temperature control center in the brain

6. Radiant warmers, incubators, warmed oxygen, measures to reduce air currents, transparent plastic blanket over the radiant warmer bed, keeping portholes of incubators closed as much as possible, heated blankets and hats when out of the incubator or radiant warmer, padding surfaces with warmed blankets when the procedures are performed

7. Greater water loss through the thin, permeable skin; non-flexed positioning that increases insensible losses; drying effects of outside heat sources; rapid respiratory rate and use of oxygen; poor ability of the kidneys to concentrate or dilute urine before 35 weeks of gestation; poor ability of the kidneys to regulate electrolytes

8. Monitoring intake and output, weighing diapers to determine the difference between the dry and the wet weight, collecting urine with cotton balls at the perineum to check the specific gravity, weighing the unclothed infant daily or twice daily on the same scale at the same time of the day

9. Dehydration: decreased urine output; increased weight loss; increased urine specific gravity; dry skin or mucous membranes; sunken anterior fontanel; poor tissue turgor; increased blood sodium, protein, and hematocrit. Overhydration: increased urine output with below-normal specific gravity; edema; too-rapid of a weight gain; bulging fontanel; decreased blood sodium, protein, and hematocrit; moist breath sounds

10. Maternal infection, incomplete passive antibody transfer from the mother during the third trimester, immature immune response, therapeutic procedures that are often invasive and damage their delicate skin

11. Poor suckling, swallowing, and breathing coordination; immature gag reflex; high expenditure of energy for sucking related to the nutrients ingested

12. a. Aspirate of the residual from the previous feeding
    b. Measure the abdominal circumference to identify distention.
    c. Test stool for reducing substance, indicating malabsorption of carbohydrates.
    d. Test for occult blood in the stool.

13. Association of the comfort of fullness with sucking; preparation for nipple feeding

14. Breast milk has immunologic benefits; it is more easily digested; it provides enzymes, hormones, and growth factors; it causes less stress because the baby can better regulate respirations and suckling; the mother's body keeps the baby warm.

15. Tachypnea, nasal flaring, retractions, cyanosis, grunting on expiration, decreased or wet breath sounds, acidosis with hypoxemia; chest X-ray film showing "ground-glass" appearance or atelectasis

16. Bronchopulmonary dysplasia and retinopathy of prematurity

17. Placental deterioration with chronic hypoxia, weight loss, oligohydramnios, and meconium passage into the amniotic fluid; continued placental function with continued growth that increases the risk for birth injury or cesarean birth

18. a. Rapid use of glycogen stores
    b. Little insulating subcutaneous fat
    c. Polycythemia secondary to hypoxia before birth, with more erythrocyte breakdown after birth

19. Symmetric: the infant is smaller than normal for gestation but the head, chest, length, and weight are proportionate; the problem began early in pregnancy. Asymmetric: head, chest, and length are normal but the weight is decreased; the problem began during second half of pregnancy. Infants who have a symmetric growth restriction are more likely to have long-term consequences.

20. Fractures of the clavicle, damage to the brachial plexus or facial nerve, cephalhematoma, and bruising, shoulder dystocia

Case Study

1. The most likely nursing diagnoses are an ineffective infant feeding pattern related to fatigue when nursing; the risk for an ineffective thermoregulation related to the immaturity of temperature regulation and minimal body fat; and a knowledge deficit (parents) related to the special needs of the preterm infant.

2. Point out how Kaylee has begun to gain weight. Emphasize the benefits of the mother's breast milk for a preterm infant, even if some must be given by gavage. Encourage the parents to hold and stroke Kaylee to the limits of her tolerance, and point out when she positively responds to them. Involve the parents in her care. Gradually, have the parents take over more of her care while unobtrusively observing. Place her name on the incubator to personalize it. Note her individual responses to care, such as her likes and dislikes or amusing habits. Provide visual stimulation (as tolerated) as you would for other newborns. Give parents the telephone number to the nursery and encourage them to call at any time. If available, refer them to a parental support group.

Review Questions

1. b   5. b
2. c   6. a
3. a   7. c
4. d

CHAPTER 30: THE HIGH-RISK NEWBORN: ACQUIRED AND CONGENITAL CONDITIONS

Matching Key Terms

1. c   3. e   5. d
2. a   4. b

Key Concepts

1. In primary apnea, the infant may respond to stimulation when respiration ceases. In secondary apnea, the infant does not respond to stimulation and loses consciousness. Secondary apnea is more ominous because stimulation is not enough to reverse it, blood oxygen levels decrease further, and the infant loses consciousness.
2. Refer to the text, under each of the titles, to complete this exercise.
3. Bilirubin is the waste products of excess erythrocyte breakdown after birth. Jaundice is the staining of the skin and sclerae by bilirubin. Kernicterus occurs when the bilirubin levels are high enough to stain the brain tissue. Bilirubin encephalopathy is an extension of kernicterus that includes damage to brain tissue by bilirubin staining.
4. Bilirubin encephalopathy is more likely to occur at lower bilirubin levels in the preterm infant than in the term infant.
5. Refer to the text, "Nursing Care Plan: The Infant with Jaundice," to formulate your explanation.
6. Exchange transfusion replaces the infant's blood that has high bilirubin levels, low erythrocytes, and many sensitized erythrocytes with blood that has normal levels of these components. In addition, the blood that replaces the infant's blood is not sensitive to the circulating antibodies from the mother that have destroyed the infant's own erythrocytes.
7. a. Hepatitis B, rubella
   b. Candidiasis, which may also occur in an infant with AIDS
   c. Cytomegalovirus, herpes (with disseminated infection), rubella, toxoplasmosis
   d. Group B streptococcal infection
   e. Gonorrhea, chlamydia
   f. Human immunodeficiency virus/AIDS
8. Immune system immaturity, with a slower reaction to invading organisms; poor localization of an infection that allows a more extensive spread of infection; less effective blood–brain barrier
9. Early onset sepsis is related to the prolonged rupture of membranes, prolonged labor, or chorioamnionitis; it begins within 24 hours of birth and rapidly progresses. Mortality is 5% to 20%. It often involves the respiratory system or central nervous system.

Late-onset sepsis develops after 1 week and is caused by exposure to organisms after birth. It usually involves the central nervous system. Mortality is 5%, often with long-term effects.
10. Signs of infection are often subtle. They include temperature instability, respiratory problems, and changes in feeding habits or behavior. Septic shock can quickly develop.
11. The blood is analyzed at the highest (peak) and lowest (trough) levels to provide a basis for any changes needed in the dosage and to prevent toxic effects on body tissues.
12. If a diabetic woman has vascular changes, placental blood flow may be reduced, interfering with fetal growth. If a diabetic woman does not have vascular changes and her glucose levels are poorly controlled, she transfers large amounts of nutrients to the fetus. The fetus secretes large amounts of insulin to metabolize these nutrients, resulting in macrosomia.
13. a. High fetal insulin levels interfere with surfactant production.
   b. Maternal glucose supply ends, but the infant temporarily continues a high level of insulin production.
   c. Parathyroid hormone production is reduced.
   d. Poor oxygenation requires that the fetus produce more erythrocytes.
14. Length and head circumference are usually normal for the gestational age. The face is round and red, body is obese, and muscle tone is poor. The infant is irritable and may have tremors when disturbed.
15. Signs include jitteriness, tremors, diaphoresis, rapid respirations, low temperature, and poor muscle tone.
16. To prevent sluggish blood flow and ischemia to vital organs
17. Infants appear hungry, but sucking and swallowing are poorly coordinated; frequent regurgitation, vomiting, and diarrhea; signs typical of hypoglycemia but with a normal blood glucose level; restlessness; failure to gain weight
18. The infant has poor coordination of sucking and swallowing, reducing the actual milk intake. At the same time, energy expenditure is high because of excess activity.
19. Intellectual impairment

Case Study

1. The positive Coombs test performed on the cord blood obtained at birth indicates that antibodies from the mother have attached to the infant's red blood cells.
2. Monitoring of Steven's bilirubin level and skin color for jaundice are essential related assessments.
3. Phototherapy is the appropriate treatment at this time. The light causes bilirubin in the skin to change into a water-soluble form that can be excreted.
4. Nursing interventions related to phototherapy include the following:
   ■ Cover the infant's closed eyes with patches to prevent light damage. Check the placement of the

patches hourly. Cover the reproductive organs with a diaper or another covering.

- Change the infant's position every 2 hours to distribute light exposure evenly over the skin surface. Check the fiberoptic blanket at the same intervals to ensure maximum exposure of the skin surface.
- Check the infant's axillary temperature every 2 to 4 hours. Place a skin probe on the infant if he or she is in an incubator.
- Monitor the intake and output. Weighing diapers is the most accurate output measurement.
- Remove the infant from the lights as little as possible, such as for feeding or other care. This will not be necessary if a phototherapy blanket is used.

5. Side effects may include frequent loose, green stools; a tanned appearance in dark-skinned infants; skin rash; or temporary lactose intolerance.
6. High bilirubin levels may cause kernicterus, with possible bilirubin encephalopathy as bilirubin deposits can cause staining of the brain. Bilirubin encephalopathy has a high mortality, and survivors may suffer from cerebral palsy, mental retardation, hearing loss, or other neurologic and developmental problems.
7. Steven should have an exchange transfusion to replace the blood that has a high bilirubin level because of the massive erythrocyte destruction with blood that is not affected by the maternal antibodies in Steven's system. It is essential to prevent kernicterus and possible encephalopathy.
8. Type O Rh-negative blood that is cross-matched to be compatible with the mother's is transfused. The transfused blood is not affected by the maternal antibodies circulating in Steven's system.
9. The exchange transfusion is performed by removing small portions of Steven's blood and replacing it with an equal amount of donor blood. This process is continued until approximately twice his blood volume has been exchanged.
10. The expected results are that approximately 85% of Steven's erythrocytes will be replaced, and the bilirubin will be reduced to approximately 50% of the pre-exchange level.
11. Complications of exchange transfusion may include infection, acid–base imbalances, necrotizing enterocolitis, hemorrhage, thrombosis, thrombocytopenia, cardiac dysrhythmias, and hypocalcemia.
12. The nurse's role in the procedure is to prepare the equipment and blood, assess the infant during and after the procedure, and keep accurate records of the blood withdrawn and infused. The transfusion is performed under a radiant warmer with a cardiac monitor in place.

Review Questions

1. b	3. a	5. b	7. d
2. d	4. d	6. b	

CHAPTER 31: MANAGEMENT OF FERTILITY AND INFERTILITY

Matching Key Terms

1. d	3. f	5. g	7. b
2. c	4. e	6. a	

Key Concepts

1. The typical failure rate reflects the way real people use a contraceptive and includes mistakes or inconsistencies in use. It is most meaningful when counseling patients.
2. Menstrual irregularities, breast tenderness, weight gain, headaches, depression, hair loss, and decreased bone density
3. Pregnancy is rare after the age of 50 years or if menstruation has ceased for at least 1 year.
4. Sperm may be in the ductal system, distal to the ligation of the vas deferens, and able to impregnate a woman.
5. They cause thickening of the cervical mucus, which helps prevent penetration by sperm and makes the endometrial lining unfavorable for implantation. They prevent ovulation for 14 weeks.
6. They suppress estrogen and prevent secretion of follicle-stimulating and luteinizing hormones, thus preventing ovulation; they also make the cervical mucus too thick for sperm to penetrate and the endometrium less hospitable for implantation.
7. They thicken the cervical mucus to inhibit sperm penetration and make the endometrium less hospitable.
8. a. Have a back-up method readily available for side effects with discontinuance or missed doses.
   b. Take at the same time of day to maintain constant blood levels, maximize effectiveness, and reduce breakthrough bleeding.
   c. Stop pills and use a backup if pregnancy is suspected; get a sensitive pregnancy test.
   d. Combination pills reduce milk production, and small amounts are transferred to the milk; use after lactation is well established.
   e. Interactions may alter the effectiveness of each medication; inform the health care provider of all medications.
9. Check blood pressure; evaluation for side effects or adverse reactions
10. High doses of an oral contraceptive within 72 hours of unprotected intercourse; high doses of progestin-only contraceptives; insertion of the copper intrauterine device within five days; mifepristone, Plan B One Step, and Next Choice; Ulipristal acetate (Ella)
11. Pelvic infections associated with the IUD are usually caused by sexually transmitted diseases (STDs). If the woman and her partner are mutually monogamous, the risk for STDs is low, thus reducing the risk for an IUD-associated infection.
12. Check for the tail weekly for 4 weeks, then monthly after the menstrual period and if you have signs of expulsion (cramping or unexpected bleeding). Visit

your health care provider if the strings are longer or shorter than before. Report signs of infection or pregnancy.

13. Avoidance of systemic hormones, protection from STDs

14. The spermicide adds a chemical barrier to the mechanical barrier of the condom and lubricates the condom to reduce tearing.

15. Avoid douching for at least 6 hours to avoid washing the protection away.

16. Natural membrane condoms do not protect from STDs, including HIV.

17. It is less effective (typical failure rate of 21%), and many women do not like its appearance.

18. She should have it checked yearly, after a weight gain or loss of more than 10 pounds, or after any pregnancy or abortion.

19. Any error in predicting ovulation or safe times for intercourse may result in pregnancy.

20. Complete this table as you read the text in this chapter.

21. Abnormal hormone stimulation, acute or chronic illness, infections of the genital tract, anatomic abnormalities, exposure to toxins, therapeutic treatments for cancer or other illness, excessive alcohol intake, illicit drug ingestion, elevated scrotal temperature, antibodies produced by the man or the woman that alter the function

22. Disorders of the central or autonomic nervous system, spinal cord disorders, peripheral vascular disease, and drugs

23. Diabetes, neurologic disorders, surgery that affects sympathetic nerve function, drugs (therapeutic or illicit), some spinal cord injuries, anatomic abnormalities, excessive alcohol intake, and psychologic factors

24. Obstruction, inflammation, or infection in the genital tract

25. Cranial tumors, stress, obesity, anorexia, systemic disease, and ovarian or endocrine abnormalities

26. Dysfunction in the hypothalamus or pituitary gland, failure of the ovaries to respond to FSH and LH stimulation, cancer chemotherapy, excessive alcohol intake, and cigarette smoking

27. Infections, endometriosis, or surgery that causes adhesions or scarring, congenital anomalies, or an obstruction

28. Polyps or cervical damage from surgical procedures, hormonal imbalances

29. Abnormalities in the fetus or placenta; maternal factors, such as structural abnormalities or autoimmune diseases

30. Refer to Table 31-5 in your textbook to complete this exercise.

31. a. The risk for multifetal pregnancies increases because multiple ova may be released and thus fertilized.

　　b. Ovarian hyperstimulation syndrome may cause an exudation of fluid into the woman's peritoneal and pleural cavities.

32. Low sperm count, genetic defect carried by the male, woman's desire for a biologic child without having a male partner.

33. A personal and family health history is taken; questions are asked about social habits and personality. Other tests include a physical examination and laboratory studies, including those for genetic defects. The donor sperm is frozen and held for 6 months before use.

34. Refer to the text, "Assisted Reproductive Techniques," to complete this exercise.

Review Questions

1. b	5. b	9. b	13. c
2. d	6. a	10. b	14. b
3. a	7. c	11. d	
4. c	8. d	12. a	

CHAPTER 32: WOMEN'S HEALTH CARE

Matching Key Terms

1. f	3. b	5. d
2. a	4. e	6. c

Key Concepts

1. Obesity, inactivity, smoking

2. Monthly by all women older than 20 years; 1 week after the menstrual period begins or on a specific day of the month if she is not menstruating

3. Yearly starting with women at the age of 40 years. Earlier screenings may be recommended for women at high risk for breast cancer.

4. Monthly for women older than 18 years and by those younger than 18 years if sexually active

5. Schedule the examination approximately 2 weeks after her menstrual period; do not douche or have sexual intercourse for at least 48 hours before the examination; do not use vaginal medications, sprays, or deodorants.

6. a. Firm, hard, freely mobile nodules that may or may not be tender and do not change during the menstrual cycle; observation with possible excision and pathologic analysis

　　b. Thickening or multiple smooth, well-delineated nodules; tenderness and pain noticeable during the latter half of the menstrual cycle; fine needle aspiration with possible open biopsy if fluid is bloody; drugs not usually prescribed; nonsteroidal anti-inflammatory drugs (NSAIDS) may provide adequate pain relief

　　c. Firm, irregular mass with enlarged axillary nodes, nipple retraction, pain, and discharge; surgical biopsy; no treatment if ductal ectasia is confirmed

　　d. Serous or serosanguineous discharge from the nipple; excision of mass and duct with analysis of discharge to rule out malignancy

7. Surgical therapy removes a part or all of the breast. Adjuvant therapy may include radiotherapy, chemotherapy, immunotherapy, and hormone therapy. Breast reconstruction assists in the psychologic recovery.

8. a. Absence of menses by the normal age of menstruation. Causes: Turner's syndrome (single X chromosome), exposure to diethylstilbestrol, abnormal reproductive tract development, hormonal imbalances, systemic disease, hypothalamic–pituitary abnormalities, excessive exercising, or eating disorders
   b. Cessation of menses for 6 months in a woman who has established menstruation. Causes: systemic disease, hormonal imbalances, strenuous aerobic exercise, poor nutrition, hormonal contraceptives, and ovarian tumors
9. Complications of an unrecognized pregnancy, such as spontaneous abortion, anatomic lesions (benign or malignant), drug-induced bleeding, systemic disorders, failure to ovulate, uterine cancer
10. Urge the woman to seek medical help. Help the woman record bleeding episodes and associated symptoms. Teach about needed lifestyle changes, such as adequate nutrition and the discouragement of rigorous dieting.
11. a. Mild analgesics and reassurance about the cause of the discomfort
    b. Oral contraceptives and prostaglandin-inhibiting drugs, such as NSAIDs
    c. Medications to suppress endometrial tissue proliferation; medication to suppress ovarian hormones; hysterectomy with bilateral salpingo-oophorectomy; lysis of adhesions and laser vaporization of the lesions
12. Urge the woman to seek a thorough examination to diagnose her problem properly. Teach dietary changes, exercises, stress management, and techniques to promote sleep and rest (refer to "Women Want to Know: How to Relieve Symptoms of PMS").
13. Refer to "Elective Termination of Pregnancy" in your textbook to complete this exercise.
14. Postmenopausal bleeding suggests endometrial cancer.
15. Estrogen alone would cause endometrial hyperplasia if the woman has her uterus.
16. Breast cancer, heart disease
17. Initially, no signs occur. When they appear, they include the loss of height, back pain, the "dowager's hump," disappearance of the waistline, and abdominal protrusion. Fractures of the hip, vertebrae, and wrist are the most common osteoporosis-associated breaks.
18. Periodic pelvic examinations, Pap tests, ultrasonography, and tests for tumor markers
19. Refer to "Infectious Disorders of the Reproductive Tract" in your textbook to complete this exercise.
20. Bacteria, often *Chlamydia trachomatis* and *Neisseria gonorrhoeae*, ascend through the cervix into the upper reproductive tract and pelvic cavity. Here the organisms cause a chronic inflammatory response that causes scarring of the fallopian tubes and adhesions near the tubes. Infertility is a common result.

Review Questions

1. c	3. a	5. b	7. d
2. d	4. c	6. a	8. c

CHAPTER 33: PHYSICAL ASSESSMENT OF CHILDREN

Matching Key Terms

1. g	5. j	9. h	13. b
2. d	6. a	10. k	
3. i	7. m	11. c	
4. l	8. e	12. f	

General Approaches to Physical Assessment

1. T	3. F	5. T
2. T	4. F	6. T

Techniques for Physical Examination

1. Indirect
2. Fingertips
3. Back of the hand
4. Dull
5. Bell

6. b	8. c	10. T	12. T
7. a	9. T	11. F	13. T

14. Use a measuring board or use a tape measure with the child lying down.
15. It provides some indication of nutritional status and may detect tumor growth or an abnormal rate of development.
16. Balanced
17. Nipple line
18. Muscle mass; fat
19. 22 (120.5 × 703/3844)
20. a. Age; sex
    b. Horizontal
    c. Vertical
    d. Intersect
    e. Percentile
21. Non–insulin-dependent diabetes mellitus
22. Abdomen; upper arm
23. Alopecia; hirsutism
24. Hair
25. 1 to 2
26. V (trigeminal); VII (facial)
27. Allergies
28. Notch between the nose and upper lip
29. Ask the child to stick out his or her tongue as though licking a lollipop.

30. X	32. e	34. a	36. c
31. b	33. d	35. f	37. F
38. T	40. T	42. T	
39. F	41. F	43. F	

44. When they have reached menarche
45. 5
46. At a site away from the tenderness, place the hand perpendicular to the abdomen, press down slowly, then lift the hand.
47. Explain the procedures, be honest and direct, and use a matter-of-fact approach.
48. To screen for testicular cancer, which has a high incidence in young men

49. b	53. c	57. F	61. F
50. a	54. T	58. T	
51. d	55. F	59. T	
52. e	56. T	60. T	

Review Questions

1. d	4. a	7. d	10. a
2. c	5. b	8. a	
3. b	6. d	9. b	

CHAPTER 34: EMERGENCY CARE OF THE CHILD

Matching Key Terms

1. j	5. c	9. h	13. g
2. b	6. d	10. a	
3. e	7. f	11. k	
4. i	8. m	12. l	

General Guidelines for Emergency Nursing Care

1. Communicate an attitude of calm confidence; establish a trusting relationship with the child and family; try to avoid separating the child and parents; designate one staff member as the caretaker of the child and liaison to the parents; tell the truth; provide incentives and rewards; and assess the child's unspoken thoughts and feelings.
2. Encourage the family members to move to a quiet place; encourage them to talk about their feelings; use reflective statements; avoid defensiveness and justification of your own or others' behaviors; speak in simple sentences.

3. f	5. d	7. c	9. e
4. f	6. g	8. a	

Growth and Development Issues in Emergency Care

1. c	3. e	5. d
2. b	4. a	

The Family of a Child in Emergency Care

1. Fear; anxiety
2. Fear that their child will die

Emergency Assessment of Infants and Children

1. The triage nurse performs the initial observation in the emergency setting and decides the level of care needed for the child.
2. Respiratory rate and effort; skin color; response to the environment
3. A: airway assessment; B: breathing assessment; C: cardiovascular assessment; D: disability (neurologic assessment); E: exposure

4. T	6. F	8. F
5. T	7. T	

9. F: full set of vital signs; G: give comfort/assess for pain; H: history and head-to-toe assessment; I: inspect back and isolate
10. Respiratory rate, pulse, temperature, and blood pressure

11. S: signs and symptoms; A: allergies; M: medications taken/immunization history; P: prior illness or injuries; L: last meal/eating habits; E: events leading up to this illness or injury
12. Complete blood count with differential count, serum electrolytes, glucose, and urinalysis
13. All medication dosages and fluid amounts are calculated according to the child's weight in kilograms.

Cardiopulmonary Resuscitation of the Child

1. Shock; respiratory failure
2. 12 to 20/min; 3 to 5
3. Perform the Heimlich maneuver.
4. Perform abdominal thrusts. The lay rescuer should use cardiopulmonary resuscitation (CPR).
5. A blind finger sweep is not performed because of the risk of forcing the object farther down into the airway.
6. Place the infant in downward-slanting position and administer five back blows, alternating with five chest thrusts.
7. Brachial artery; carotid or femoral artery
8. 100 compressions/min
9. 5

The Child in Shock

1. H	4. D	7. H	10. F
2. C	5. C	8. F	11. F
3. D	6. C	9. F	

Pediatric Trauma

1. T	2. T	3. F	4. F
5. T			

6. Assess and manage any life-threatening injuries.
7. A: assessment and management of airway; B: breathing; C: circulation; D: disability (neurologic deficits)
8. Assess for pain; inspect and document any and all signs of injury by performing a head-to-toe assessment; and obtain a history of the injury.
9. Motor vehicle: Was the child wearing a seatbelt or sitting in a child's car safety seat? What type of seatbelt? What was the speed of the vehicle? With what did the vehicle collide? Where on the motor vehicle was the location of the impact? Where was the victim seated in the vehicle? How much damage was done to the vehicle?
   Fall: How far did the child fall? How did the child land? On what type of ground did the child land? Did any objects "break" the child's fall?
   Penetrating injury: How long and wide was the blade of the knife? How far away was the gun when it was fired? What type of gun was used? What was the caliber of the gun?
10. Indicators: a history inconsistent with physical findings; activity leading to the trauma is inconsistent with the child's age and condition; delay in seeking treatment for the trauma; history of other emergency visits. Physical findings: bruises and fractures in various stages of healing; injuries that are unusual for children; patterns of injury indicating a specific object caused the injury

11. Continuous assessment of the child's respiratory, circulatory, and neurologic status

Ingestions and Poisonings

1. Oral ingestion
2. a. Removing the toxic substance
   b. Diluting the toxin
   c. Performing gastric lavage
   d. Administering activated charcoal
   e. Giving a specific antidote for the toxic substance
3. It does not completely remove the toxin; vomiting is uncomfortable for the child; it may interfere with subsequent interventions; it can be misused by others in the household.

4. F   7. T   10. F
5. T   8. T   11. F
6. T   9. F   12. T

13. What substance was ingested? How much was ingested? What was the approximate time of the ingestion? Has the child's condition changed from the time of ingestion? What treatment was administered at home?

Environmental Emergencies

1. Bite marks that look like fangs; burning at the site; ecchymosis and erythema; pain or numbness; edema
2. Wound irrigation and débridement; tetanus prophylaxis if not current; antibiotics if there is a high probability of infection; rabies treatment may be necessary

Submersion Injuries

1. Hypoxia
2. The diving reflex is stimulated when the face is submerged under cold water. As a result, blood is shunted away from the periphery, which increases the blood flow to the brain and heart.
3. Neurologic system

Heat-Related Emergencies

1. Move the child to a cool place and start additional cooling measures.
2. Move the child to a cool place; start additional cooling measures such as loosening/removing wet clothes and applying cool, dry clothes. Offer oral fluids if there is no alteration in mental status or vomiting.
3. Hot, dry, red skin; change in level of consciousness or coma; rapid, weak pulse; rapid, shallow breathing; elevated core body temperature ($>105°F$)

Dental Emergencies

1. F
2. T

Review Questions

1. c   5. b   9. a   13. c
2. c   6. c   10. a   14. c
3. d   7. d   11. c   15. a
4. a   8. d   12. a

CHAPTER 35: THE ILL CHILD IN THE HOSPITAL AND OTHER CARE SETTINGS

Matching Key Terms

1. e   3. f   5. a
2. d   4. c   6. b

Settings of Care

1. a. Hospital (including 24-hour observation, emergency hospitalization, outpatient/day facilities, medical-surgical units, intensive care units, and rehabilitative care)
   b. School-based clinics
   c. Community clinics
   d. Home care

2. T   4. F   6. T   8. T
3. T   5. F   7. T   9. T

Stressors Associated with Illness and Hospitalization

1. The child's age; cognitive development; preparation; coping skills; culture; previous experiences with the health care system; parents' reactions to the illness
2. Infant; toddler
3. Protest: Child is agitated, resists caregivers, cries, and is inconsolable.
   Despair: Child is hopeless, quiet, withdrawn, and apathetic.
   Detachment: The child may ignore the parents but is interested in environment, plays, and seems to form relationships with caregivers and other children.
4. The nurse needs to explain to parents that regression in this situation is normal and encourage parents to reinforce appropriate behavior while allowing the regressive behavior to occur.
5. The nurse should ask the parents about the toddler's home routines (e.g., feeding, bathing, and bedtime) and try to adapt the hospital routines to what the toddler is accustomed.
6. Because preschoolers lack an understanding of body integrity, they fear mutilation and are afraid of bodily harm from invasive procedures.
7. The nurse can encourage the child to participate in his or her care. This may promote a sense of control. Examples include making menu selections and assisting with his or her treatments when appropriate. The nurse can encourage the child's independence when appropriate.
8. Because peer groups are so important during adolescence, adolescents experience anxiety when separated from their peers. Meeting other hospitalized adolescents can help with this issue.
9. Regression in toileting or self-feeding skills; temper tantrums; clinging; crying

Factors Affecting a Child's Response to Illness and Hospitalization

1. Child's age; child's level of cognitive development; parents' response to illness or hospitalization; child's preparation for the experience; child's coping skills

2. Blowing bubbles or singing to promote relaxed breathing; using imagery for the older child; using distraction techniques such as singing, playing games, or listening to music. Teaching coping mechanisms and having the child practice them before undergoing a procedure can help a child feel more in control and more relaxed.

3. Increased self-confidence; mastery of self-care skills; learning new information and new coping skills

Playrooms in Health Care Settings

1. Therapeutic play is guided by health team members to help meet the physical and psychologic needs of the child.

2. During an emotional outlet or dramatic play, the child acts out or dramatizes real-life stressors.

3. The playroom should have no association with unpleasant experiences, so the child should not receive any treatments (including medications) in the playroom.

4. A reward system can be used in which the child receives a reward when a previously set goal is met. Rewards can be stickers, trading cards, small toys, and the like. Another example is allowing the child to blow bubbles as a fun way to do deep-breathing exercises.

Admitting the Child to a Hospital Setting

1. Admission should not be a series of questions directed at the child and family but a time of collaboration between nurse and family. The nurse should be aware of the child's and family's needs and should structure the admission process to meet those needs.

2. The immediate physiologic needs of the child; the emotional needs of the child and family

The Ill Child's Family

1. Even parents who believe they are in control of their child before admission find themselves in an unfamiliar environment in the hospital. Parents may be confused about what they can and cannot do.

2. Siblings may experience jealousy, insecurity, resentment, confusion, and anxiety.

Developmental Approaches to the Hospitalized Child

1. c	3. d	5. e	7. a
2. f	4. d	6. b	

Review Questions

1. b	4. d	7. d	10. d
2. c	5. a	8. c	
3. d	6. c	9. d	

CHAPTER 36: THE CHILD WITH A CHRONIC CONDITION OR TERMINAL ILLNESS

Matching Key Terms

1. e	3. h	5. c	7. b
2. g	4. d	6. a	8. f

9. Children with a chronic illness are living longer. Advances in medicine have led to children living with illnesses that were previously fatal. Both the quality of life and longevity have been enhanced by improvements in diagnostic testing and treatment.

10. Children with special health care needs are those who have, or are at risk for, a chronic physical, developmental, behavioral, or emotional condition and who also require health care and related services of a type and amount beyond that generally required for children.

The Family of the Child with Special Health Care Needs

1. A situational crisis is an unexpected crisis for which the family's usual problem-solving abilities are not adequate.

2. Family cohesiveness

3. Establishing and accessing internal and external sources of support; reframing a situation to highlight positive rather than negative aspects; successfully coping; maintaining high-quality communication patterns; being flexible; maintaining social ties; preserving family boundaries

4. F

5. T

The Grieving Process

1. Not only the child but also the entire family

2. a. Denial
   b. Anger and resentment
   c. Bargaining
   d. Sadness or depression
   e. Acceptance

3. F

4. T

The Child with Special Health Care Needs

1. Age at the onset of the condition; growth, and development

2. Self-esteem; autonomy

3. T

4. F

The Child with a Chronic Illness

1. To achieve and maintain the highest level of physical, emotional, and psychosocial health and function possible

2. To remain intact; to achieve and maintain normalization; to maximize function

3. The child's physical condition

4. Increase the parents' confidence; acknowledge the parent as a person and as the expert on the child; provide the parent with information about the child's condition and how to manage it; provide the parent with easy ways to access the child's health care providers for when questions and problems arise; in words and actions, demonstrate that you see the child as valuable and unique; help the parents recognize the child's

potential and abilities; help the parents understand and meet the child's growth and development needs.

5. F   6. T   7. T   8. F

The Terminally Ill or Dying Child

1. c   3. b   5. T   7. T
2. a   4. d   6. T

Caring for the Dying Child

1. a. Meeting with the agency's pastoral care team or personal spiritual counselor
   b. Attending nursing support groups mediated by a pastor, social worker, or counselor
   c. Participating in patient care conferences or ethics committee meetings
2. Whether or not to inform the child of the prognosis
3. T   6. F   9. F   12. F
4. F   7. T   10. T
5. T   8. F   11. T

Review Questions

1. a   3. a   5. b   7. d
2. b   4. a   6. c   8. a

CHAPTER 37: PRINCIPLES AND PROCEDURES FOR NURSING CARE OF CHILDREN

Matching Key Terms

1. c   3. b   5. a
2. f   4. d   6. e

Preparing Children for Procedures

1. The child's age; developmental level; personality; present level of knowledge and understanding; past experiences; coping skills; family situation
2. T   4. T   6. F   8. F
3. T   5. F   7. T

Transporting Infants and Children

1. a. Age and development of the child
   b. Physical condition
   c. Destination
   d. Safety

Using Restraints

1. T   3. T
2. T   4. F

Infection Control

1. a. Blood
   b. All body fluids, secretions, and excretions except sweat
   c. Nonintact skin
   d. Mucous membranes
2. Transmission-based precautions
3. If the hands are contaminated with blood or body fluids or are visibly soiled, clean hands with soap and water.
   - If the hands are clean, use an alcohol-based hand rub before and after touching potentially contaminated surfaces near the patient, before and after patient contact, before putting on gloves for a procedure, and after removing the gloves.
   - Put alcohol-based hand rub on the hands, rub over all surfaces of hands and fingers, and allow to thoroughly dry (total time, approximately 20 seconds).

Bathing Infants and Children

1. 100°F
2. Testing the water temperature on the inside of the wrist or elbow
3. 3
4. Inhalation of powder into the lungs can cause severe respiratory consequences. If the powder becomes moist, it provides a growth medium for microorganisms.

Oral Hygiene

1. T   2. F   3. F

Feeding

1. There is a risk for aspiration when an infant drinks from a propped bottle.
2. a. Allow the child to sit at a table.
   b. Allow him to feed himself.
   c. Have the parents bring his own utensils from home.

Vital Signs

1. Take an axillary temperature if the child is younger than 4 to 6 years or if the child has had oral surgery or is uncooperative, immunosuppressed, or neurologically impaired.
2. The measurement may be inaccurate if liquids were consumed within 30 minutes of measurement, if the child is crying, or if the child is undergoing oxygen therapy or nebulization treatments.
3. F   5. T   7. F   9. T
4. F   6. T   8. F

Fever-Reducing Measures

1. Removing blankets and heavy clothing; lowering the room temperature; using a mechanical cooling blanket
2. Acetaminophen; ibuprofen

Specimen Collection

1. Standard
2. Nasal washing
3. Latex
4. Posterior iliac crest

Gavage and Gastrostomy

1. Tube placement is verified when the tube is inserted, any time the feeding is interrupted, before each bolus feeding, and every 4 to 8 hours during continuous feedings.
2. Aspiration of enteral fluid and pH measurement of the aspirate (should have a pH of 5 or lower)
3. F   4. F   5. T   6. F

Enemas

1. 360 to 480 mL; 3 inches

375

Care of Ostomies

1. T
2. T

Oxygen Therapy

1. An oxygen hood can be used for infants. Toddlers and preschoolers can use a nasal cannula, blow-by, or facemask. Older children prefer the non-rebreather masks.

Assessing Oxygenation

1. Adequate oxygen saturation
2. Report it to the physician, because the child may require oxygen therapy.

Chest Physiotherapy

1. Percussion is rhythmic clapping with a cupped hand over the affected part of the lung or the simulation of this movement with a percussion cup or mechanical percussor.
2. Postural drainage is the positioning of the patient to promote gravity-assisted drainage of the lungs.
3. Before meals or 1 to 1.5 hours after meals

Tracheostomy Care

1. a. Assessing the stoma area for signs of an infection and skin breakdown
   b. Changing tracheostomy ties
   c. Cleaning the tracheostomy site and inner cannula
   d. Changing the tracheostomy tube
   e. Suctioning
2. At least every 8 hours
3. Five seconds
4. Turned off

Surgical Procedures

1. Two hours before the time of arrival at the hospital
2. Auscultate the lungs to identify any abnormal breath sounds or areas of diminished or absent sounds. Encourage early ambulation, deep breathing, and coughing. Incentive spirometers can increase respiratory movement. To facilitate air exchange, the nurse can engage the child in games such as blowing cotton, a windmill, or bubbles.
3. a. Anxiety and fear related to separation from family, as well as an unfamiliar environment and personnel
   b. Acute pain related to surgical incision
   c. Deficient knowledge related to unfamiliarity with procedures and expected outcomes
   d. Interrupted family processes related to surgical procedure
   e. Risk for deficient fluid volume related to NPO status before and after surgery, as well as nausea and vomiting

Review Questions

1. b	4. b	7. a	10. a
2. a	5. c	8. d	11. d
3. b	6. b	9. c	12. b

CHAPTER 38: MEDICATION ADMINISTRATION AND SAFETY FOR INFANTS AND CHILDREN

Matching Key Terms

1. c	3. d	5. e
2. b	4. f	6. a

Pharmacokinetics in Children

1. a. Gastric acidity
   b. Gastric emptying
   c. Gastrointestinal motility
   d. Enzyme activity
2. T
3. F
4. F
5. The renal system is immature at birth. The newborn's glomerular filtration rate is approximately 30% to 50% that of an adult, and the renal tubules function less efficiently. Infants and young children cannot concentrate urine as well as older children or adults can. Because of this renal immaturity, medications may not be excreted.
6. When certain medications are used, the peak and trough serum levels are measured to monitor medication concentration.
7. Trough

Psychologic and Developmental Differences

1. a. Nurses should ask the parents about medication allergies, child's ability to take medications (e.g., liquid versus solid), and special techniques they use to administer medicines.
   b. Allow the parents to administer certain medications (e.g., oral, otic, and ophthalmic) if the child will cooperate.
   c. Ask the parents to report if a medication does not seem to be effective.
2. Toddler: Give explanations through play; allow the child to see and handle the equipment first; allow him to help squirt liquid preparations into his mouth. Allow the parent to give the medication if the child prefers. Use as little restraints as possible because the child will resist the restraint. Offer praise when the child takes the medication. Rewards, such as stickers, are useful.
   Preschooler: Offer a choice about what to drink after taking oral medication (limit to two choices). Offer a Band-Aid (preferably a colorful one) after an injection.
   School-age child: Offer a choice of drinks when possible (as with preschooler). The child may need a source of distraction to cooperate with painful procedures such as venipuncture or injection. Praise for cooperation and use rewards such as stickers.

Calculating Dosages

1. F	2. F	3. F

Medication Administration Procedures

1. a. Use the six rights of medication administration.
   b. Double-check the medication calculations before administering; double-check the pharmacy

calculations of unit dose medications before administering.

   c. Have two nurses check the following medications: insulin, oral hypoglycemics, sedatives, narcotics, chemotherapy, digoxin, anticoagulants, K^1 and Ca^{21} salts, and dextrose solutions .20% dextrose.

2. When admitting children to a hospital unit, the nurse obtains a list of all prescription and over-the-counter medications or herbal preparations a child is taking at home and assesses parents' knowledge of the medications. This includes the name of the medication, the dose, number of times a day the child is taking the medication, the parent's knowledge of side effects, any allergic reactions the child might have experienced, and the time the medication was last administered. To ensure patient safety, the nurse compares the listed medications and allergies with medications the admitting physician has ordered.

3. The nurse can check to see whether the medication is available as a liquid. If not, the medications (except those that are enteric-coated or sustained-release) can be crushed and mixed with a nonessential food such as apple sauce.

4. Because medications can alter the flavor of the food, the child may associate that food with the undesirable flavor and refuse it in the future, even without the medication added. Thus, only foods not essential to the child's diet should be used for mixing with medications.

5. F   6. F   7. T   8. T

9. The nurse places the child on his or her lap with the child's right arm behind the nurse's back and with the nurse's left hand holding the child's left hand. The nurse supports the child's head with the nurse's left arm and secures it between his or her arm and body. The nurse secures the child's legs between the nurse's legs. (Reverse sides if the nurse is left handed.)

10. Notify the physician and report what medication was vomited and how much time has elapsed since administration.

11. Verify that the tube is properly positioned before administering medication. Flush the tube with water after the medication is administered.

Administering Injections

1. Explanations should be tailored to the child's level. Explain the reason for the injection and describe the sensations that the child can expect to feel. The child may need to be assured that the injection is not a punishment for any misbehavior.

2. Ice can be applied to the injection site for several minutes before the injection to numb the area. Children can be taught how to use guided imagery, deep breathing, or distraction to cope with the discomfort. Topical anesthetics such as EMLA cream are effective in reducing any injection pain.

3. b   5. a   7. F   9. F
4. c   6. T   8. T

Administering Subcutaneous Injections

1. Circulation
2. a. Fat pads above the iliac crests
   b. Hips
   c. Lateral upper arms
   d. Anterior thighs
3. T   4. F   5. F

Intradermal Injections

1. Testing [such as allergy testing or purified protein derivative (PPD)]
2. Inner aspect of the forearm or upper back
3. Insert needle bevel up at a 15-degree angle. The needle will barely penetrate the skin, and when the medication is injected, it will form a wheal.

Rectal and Vaginal Administration

1. T   2. F   3. T

Ophthalmic and Otic Administration

1. F   2. T   3. F

Inhalation Therapy

1. Spacer
2. Whistle
3. 10 seconds

Intravenous Therapy

1. Consider the rate and type of fluid to be administered, the projected length of time the IV will be needed, availability of veins, and the child's developmental level. The child's dominant hand should be avoided as a site for injection.

2. Use guided imagery, for example, putting on a "magic" glove. Try distraction with music, toys, seek-and-find books.

3. Clean the area well and place a liberal amount of EMLA cream on the site. Cover with a transparent occlusive dressing and leave in place for 1 to 2 hours to anesthetize the area.

4. To prevent inadvertent fluid overload

5. At least every hour

6. Assess for signs of infiltration (edema, erythema, pain, blanching, and coolness) and phlebitis (streaking on the skin above the vein). Discontinue the IV if any of these signs are present.

7. 0 to 10 kg: 100 ml/kg; 10 to 20 kg: 1000 ml plus 50 ml/kg/day for each kg between 10 and 20 kg; more than 20 kg: 1500 ml plus 20 ml/kg/day for each kg more than 20 kg

8. 1800 mL; 1300 mL

9. These medications are not diluted and are injected (pushed) directly into the IV catheter using the port closest to the patient.

10. The needle is placed into the injection port nearest the child, and the medication is injected away from the child into the tubing above the port.

11. To complete the delivery of the medication from the IV tubing into the patient

12. Every 6 to 12 hours (to maintain patency)
13. To administer medications, blood products, IV fluids, and parenteral nutrition long-term to chronically ill children
14. An implanted venous access device consists of a catheter that is connected to a port or reservoir. The catheter tip rests at the junction of the superior vena cava and right atrium. The port is under the skin and is accessed with a noncoring needle placed through the skin into the port.
15. Phlebitis, infection, and thrombosis

Administering Blood or Blood Products

1. F 3. T 5. F
2. T 4. T

Child and Family Education

1. The name of the medication; reason it is to be administered; action of the medication; expected side effects and what to do if they occur; when to notify the health care provider; any dietary restrictions; how to take the medication; how to measure the dosage correctly; how to use droppers or syringes

Review Questions

1. a 3. a 5. b 7. d
2. c 4. d 6. c

CHAPTER 39: PAIN MANAGEMENT FOR CHILDREN

Matching Key Terms

1. d 4. a 7. g
2. h 5. c 8. b
3. f 6. e 9. i

Definitions and Theories of Pain

1. Whatever the experiencing person says it is, existing whenever the person says it does
2. An unpleasant sensation and emotional experience associated with actual or potential damage
3. T 5. F 7. F
4. F 6. T

Research on Pain in Children

1. F 2. F

Myths About Pain and Pain Management in Children

1. T 3. F 5. T
2. F 4. T

Assessment of Pain in Children

1. Behavioral; physiologic
2. More purposeful
3. Hunger, discomfort, and stress
4. Restlessness
5. Punishment
6. a. They fear bodily harm.
   b. They have an awareness of death.

7. They may not report pain, believing that the nurse must already be aware of it.
8. To provide an objective measure of the pain experience; to provide children with an effective tool to communicate about their pain
9. 3
10. The Oucher

Nonpharmacologic and Pharmacologic Pain Interventions

1. They provide a focus for distraction, and they produce relaxation.
2. Children who are distracted may be able to ignore or "forget" the pain, but the pain still exists.
3. Relaxation; focused concentration; rhythmic breathing
4. A technique that allows a person to notice body states not usually noticed and to bring them under control
5. Relaxation, decreased anxiety, decreased pain
6. A form of focused or narrowed attention, an altered state of consciousness accompanied by relaxation
7. Transmission of pain signals
8. Naloxone (Narcan)
9. Cardiac arrest
10. F 12. T 14. F 16. T
11. T 13. T 15. T 17. T

Review Questions

1. a 4. d 7. c 10. d
2. d 5. a 8. b
3. b 6. c 9. d

CHAPTER 40: THE CHILD WITH A FLUID AND ELECTROLYTE ALTERATION

Matching Key Terms

1. a 4. g 7. d 10. k
2. c 5. b 8. h 11. j
3. e 6. f 9. i

Review of Fluid and Electrolyte Imbalances in Children

1. F 2. T 3. F 4. F
5. T
6. Extracellular
7. Water; solutes
8. Sodium; potassium; magnesium
9. 7.35; 7.45
10. a. Chemical and cellular buffers
    b. Respiratory system
    c. The kidneys
11. Bicarbonate; proteins
12. Increase
13. Hydrogen ions; bicarbonate
14. b 17. e 20. a 23. b
15. f 18. c 21. d
16. a 19. d 22. c

Dehydration

1. T	3. T	5. F	7. F
2. F	4. T	6. T	

Diarrhea

1. An increase in the frequency, fluidity, and the volume of stools
2. Gastroenteritis
3. Food intolerance; medications; malabsorption; colon disease; obstruction; irritable bowel syndrome; stress; infectious diseases elsewhere in the body
4. The high carbohydrate content of these drinks may worsen diarrhea. In addition, they do not replace the electrolytes lost through diarrhea.
5. To prevent dehydration, to reduce the stool frequency and volume, and to reduce the duration of diarrhea
6. Choose from complex carbohydrates (rice, bread, cereals, noodles, potatoes, and crackers), yogurt, cooked vegetables, and lean meats. Avoid fatty foods and simple sugars.
7. Change diapers immediately after each bowel movement, wash skin with mild soap and pat dry, apply "barrier" ointment (e.g., A & D), and avoid using commercial baby wipes. Reposition at least every 2 hours.

Vomiting

1. T	2. T	3. F	4. F

Review Questions

1. d	4. d	7. b	10. a
2. b	5. a	8. c	
3. b	6. a	9. b	

CHAPTER 41: THE CHILD WITH AN INFECTIOUS DISEASE

Matching Key Terms

1. l	4. i	7. k	10. a
2. e	5. f	8. g	11. h
3. c	6. b	9. j	12. d

13. Epidemiology is the study of the distribution of health and illness within a population and the factors that determine the health status of that population. Recently, epidemiologic efforts have focused on identifying health-promoting factors not just on disease prevention.

Review of Disease Transmission

1. d	3. b	5. a
2. e	4. c	

Infection and Host Defenses

1. Skin; intact mucous membranes

Immunity

1. c	3. a	5. b
2. e	4. d	

Viral Infections

1. f	4. h	7. b	10. d
2. c	5. a	8. j	11. k
3. i	6. e	9. g	

12. The oral polio vaccine (OPV) can cause vaccine-associated paralytic poliomyelitis (VAPP) because it is a live vaccine.

Bacterial, Rickettsial, Borrelia, Helminth, and Fungal Infections

1. T	3. T	5. T	7. F
2. T	4. T	6. F	8. T

Sexually Transmitted Diseases (STDs)

1. d, h	4. a	7. e	10. F
2. f	5. g	8. T	11. T
3. b, h	6. a, c	9. T	

Review Questions

1. b	3. b	5. c	7. c
2. b	4. d	6. c	8. d

CHAPTER 42: THE CHILD WITH AN IMMUNOLOGIC ALTERATION

Matching Key Terms

1. d	5. b	9. a	13. l
2. f	6. k	10. g	
3. j	7. h	11. m	
4. i	8. e	12. c	

Review of the Immune System

1. c	5. g	9. a	13. F
2. f	6. b	10. F	
3. i	7. h	11. F	
4. d	8. e	12. T	

Human Immunodeficiency Virus (HIV) Infection

1. a. Via the placenta
   b. During delivery
   c. Through breastfeeding
2. Zidovudine (ZDV)
3. The administration of trimethoprim-sulfamethoxazole to infants exposed to HIV from approximately 4 to 6 months of age to 12 months or when the infant is found to be HIV negative
4. a. Maximize viral suppression.
   b. Preserve immune function.
   c. Decrease disease progression.
   d. Delay medication resistance.

Corticosteroid Therapy

1. They decrease monocyte and macrophage differentiation and lymphokine production, leading to T-cell inhibition.
2. The child may develop an acute adrenal insufficiency.
3. Adrenocorticotropic hormone (ACTH)
4. Every other day
5. To minimize the risk for gastrointestinal (GI) bleeding, administer corticosteroids with food or milk. To

379

deal with an increased appetite, offer low-calorie, low-salt snacks throughout the day.

Immune Complex and Autoimmune Disorders

1. a. Kawasaki disease
   b. Post-streptococcal glomerulonephritis
2. Antibodies that act against the body's own cells, tissues, and organs
3. T   5. T   7. T
4. F   6. T   8. F

Allergic Reactions and Anaphylaxis

1. An immune response to an antigen (allergen) that causes a hypersensitivity reaction in various body systems
2. b   3. a   4. d   5. c
6. Laryngospasm, edema, cyanosis, shock, vascular collapse, and cardiac arrest
7. A preloaded, automatic delivery system of injectable epinephrine available in 0.3-mg (EpiPen)® and 0.15-mg (EpiPen Jr.)® doses
8. A biphasic reaction is a reaction that follows an initial anaphylactic reaction. Manifestations can be as severe as the initial reaction and can occur within hours or days of the first episode. Prompt treatment of the initial reaction with epinephrine seems to decrease the risk for biphasic reactions.
9. Food allergies

Review Questions

1. b   4. d   7. b
2. c   5. b   8. a
3. a   6. c   9. b

CHAPTER 43: THE CHILD WITH A GASTROINTESTINAL ALTERATION

Matching Key Terms

1. f   5. g   9. c   13. b
2. j   6. d   10. m   14. n
3. a   7. h   11. e
4. l   8. k   12. i

Review of the Gastrointestinal System

1. To ingest food and fluids, begin digestion, and propel food into the intestines
2. To digest and absorb nutrients, detoxify and eliminate waste, and maintain fluid and electrolyte balance
3. Phagocytosis, bile production, detoxification, glycogen storage and breakdown, and vitamin storage
4. Via the placenta

Disorders of Prenatal Development

1. T   3. F   5. T
2. T   4. T
6. Polyhydramnios
7. Aspiration
8. Coughing; cyanosis; choking with feedings
9. Parenterally

10. Cover the stoma with gauze, change the gauze often, clean daily with half-strength hydrogen peroxide, and use skin barriers.
11. c   13. b   15. d
12. e   14. a   16. f

Motility Disorders

1. Small, frequent feedings of predigested formula, such as Pregestimil or Nutramigen, will reduce the amount of formula in the stomach, decrease distention, and minimize reflux. More frequent feedings with frequent burping are usually the first line of treatment.
2. a. H_2-receptor antagonists, such as cimetidine and ranitidine
   b. Prokinetic agents, such as metoclopramide
   c. Mucosal protectants, such as sucralfate
   d. Proton pump inhibitors, such as omeprazole
3. Over time, the rectum enlarges because of the chronic retention of stool. This can result in the failure to control the external sphincter, leading to encopresis.
4. Stress
5. Diffuse abdominal pain, alternating constipation and diarrhea, undigested food and mucus in stool, normal growth

Inflammatory and Infectious Diseases

1. F   4. T   7. F
2. F   5. T   8. T
3. T   6. T   9. F
10. Crohn disease can affect any area of the gastrointestinal (GI) tract and all of its layers. It has periods of remission and exacerbations. Surgery may be required for complications, but it is not curative. Ulcerative colitis affects only the colon and mucosa and submucosa. It can be cured by a colectomy. See Table 43-4 in your text.
11. a. Anti-inflammatory agents
    b. Antibacterials
    c. Antibiotics
    d. Immunosuppressive agents

Obstructive Disorders

1. Progressive, projectile, non-bilious
2. Stools with bloody mucus, sausage-shaped abdominal mass
3. With a barium or air enema or with an ultrasound-guided water enema
4. Volvulus
5. Delayed passage or the absence of meconium stool
6. Enterocolitis

Malabsorption Disorders

1. T   2. F   3. F   4. T

Hepatic Disorders

1. Fecal-oral route, contaminated food and water
2. Blood, secretions, sexual contact, and breast milk
3. Blood and blood products
4. Blood

5. Fecal-oral route
6. Parenteral transmission, sexual contact
7. a. Anorexia, nausea and vomiting, right upper quadrant (RUQ) pain, fever, malaise, irritability, and depression
   b. Jaundice, urticaria, dark urine, and light-colored stools
   c. Bleeding, encephalopathy, ascites, and acute hepatic failure
8. Hepatitis A (HAV); hepatitis B (HBV)
9. T   11. F   13. T   15. T
10. F   12. F   14. T
16. Ascites; varices; encephalopathy
17. Liver transplantation

Review Questions

1. d	5. b	9. b	13. d
2. b	6. c	10. a	14. c
3. b	7. d	11. b	
4. d	8. a	12. b	

CHAPTER 44: THE CHILD WITH A GENITOURINARY ALTERATION

Matching Key Terms

1. f	4. e	7. h	10. a
2. d	5. j	8. g	
3. i	6. b	9. c	

Review of the Genitourinary System

1. Abdominal
2. Urinary tract infections
3. Nephron
4. 10
5. 4.6; 8.0

Enuresis

1. F	3. F	5. T
2. T	4. T	

Urinary Tract Infections (UTIs)

1. b	2. c	3. d	4. a

5. Urine culture
6. Suprapubic aspiration
7. Vesicoureteral reflux, bladder emptying problems, and urethral problems
8. Intravenous
9. Pyelonephritis
10. Keep the foreskin of boys clean; cleanse the perineal area in girls from front to back; encourage children to urinate at least four times/day; offer fluids throughout the day; avoid bubble baths; use cotton, not synthetic, underwear.

Cryptorchidism

1. T	2. F	3. T	4. T

Hypospadias and Epispadias

1. Circumcised
2. Epispadias; hypospadias

3. Chordee
4. Urethral stents

Miscellaneous Disorders and Anomalies of the Genitourinary Tract

1. c	3. e	5. b
2. a	4. d	

Acute Post-Streptococcal Glomerulonephritis

1. Hematuria, proteinuria (0 to 2+), edema, renal insufficiency, hypertension
2. They travel through the circulation and get trapped in the glomeruli, creating an inflammatory response and damaging the glomeruli. This decreases the glomerular filtration rate, which leads to renal insufficiency.
3. Increase
4. Diuresis

Nephrotic Syndrome

1. Proteinuria (3+ to 4+), hypoalbuminemia, edema, anorexia, fatigue, respiratory infection, weight gain, and hyperlipidemia
2. Prednisone
3. When the urine protein level is zero to trace for 5 to 7 consecutive days

Acute Renal Failure

1. b	4. b	7. c	10. T
2. b	5. a	8. T	11. F
3. a	6. c	9. F	

Chronic Renal Failure and End-Stage Renal Disease (ESRD)

1. Waste products; excess body fluids; electrolytes; minerals
2. Arteriovenous fistula or graft
3. Infection of the peritoneal cavity
4. Fluid and electrolyte imbalances, acid–base imbalances, osteodystrophy, anemia, poor growth, hypertension, fatigue, decreased appetite, nausea and vomiting, and neurologic changes
5. Kidney transplantation
6. Rejection
7. The need to take immunosuppressive drugs

Review Questions

1. b	4. a	7. c	10. d
2. d	5. d	8. a	
3. b	6. b	9. b	

CHAPTER 45: THE CHILD WITH A RESPIRATORY ALTERATION

Matching Key Terms

1. h	6. f	11. q	16. d
2. m	7. l	12. g	17. i
3. p	8. o	13. a	
4. k	9. n	14. j	
5. b	10. e	15. c	

Review of the Respiratory System and Diagnostic Tests

1. T	3. T	5. F
2. F	4. T	6. T

Allergic Rhinitis

1. Two years
2. Rhinorrhea; itching eyes, nose, ears, and palate; paroxysmal sneezing; dark circles under eyes; rubbing nose upward with the palm of hand
3. They can add ¼ teaspoon of table salt to 1 cup of warm water.

Sinusitis

1. Upper respiratory infection
2. Acute otitis media with effusion
3. Acetaminophen; warm, moist compresses

Otitis Media

1. T	2. F	3. T

Pharyngitis and Tonsillitis

1. F	2. T	3. F

Laryngomalacia

1. Inspiratory stridor with or without retractions

Croup

1. a	3. b	5. T	7. T
2. c	4. d	6. F	8. F

Epiglottitis

1. Sudden-onset high fever, sitting in tripod position, nasal flaring, retracting, tachycardia, drooling, dysphagia, and dysphonia
2. Tongue depressor

Bronchitis

1. Virus
2. Rest; humidification; increased fluid intake

Bronchiolitis

1. 50
2. It can live on the skin for up to 1 hour and on nonporous surfaces for up to 6 hours.
3. To prevent nosocomial transmission of the virus to other patients
4. Respiratory syncytial virus (RSV) monoclonal antibody (Synagis)

Pneumonia

1. Chest physiotherapy before meals and before bed; change position every 2 hours; elevate head of bed; assist older children to cough and deep breathe
2. 95

Foreign Body Aspiration

1. Nuts; grapes; hard candy; popcorn; hot dogs; raw carrots; large chunks of food
2. Aphonia; apnea

Pulmonary Noninfectious Irritation

1. Aspiration, trauma, drug ingestion, shock, massive transfusions
2. Passive smoking
3. Carbon monoxide

Apnea

1. b	2. a	3. c

4. The time and duration of the episode, skin color, heart rate, O_2 saturation, precipitating trigger, and any actions taken to stimulate breathing
5. Monitor use; cardiopulmonary resuscitation (CPR)

Sudden Infant Death Syndrome (SIDS)

1. T	2. F	3. T	4. T

Asthma

1. Increased
2. Expiration
3. Lowers
4. Dilate airway and/or relieve bronchospasm
5. Status asthmaticus
6. Swimming
7. Decrease inflammation
8. Peak flow meters
9. Exposure to triggers
10. Belly breathing; pursed lip breathing

Bronchopulmonary Dysplasia (BPD)/Chronic Lung Disease of Infancy (CLD)

1. T	2. T	3. F	4. F

Cystic Fibrosis (CF)

1. F	3. F	5. T	7. F
2. T	4. T	6. T	8. T

Tuberculosis (TB)

1. a	3. b	5. T	7. F
2. c	4. T	6. F	

Review Questions

1. b	4. b	7. b	10. b
2. a	5. c	8. c	11. c
3. b	6. c	9. c	12. a

CHAPTER 46: THE CHILD WITH A CARDIOVASCULAR ALTERATION

Matching Key Terms

1. f	4. k	7. i	10. b
2. h	5. g	8. l	11. a
3. c	6. j	9. e	12. d

More Definitions

1. T	3. T	5. T	7. F
2. F	4. T	6. F	8. T

Review of the Cardiovascular System

1. Placenta
2. Foramen ovale
3. Ductus arteriosus
4. Decreases; increases

Cardiovascular Assessment

1. T	3. T	5. T	7. F
2. F	4. T	6. F	8. T

Physiologic Consequences of Congenital Heart Disease

1. Resting tachycardia and difficulty in feeding

2. e	4. a	6. c
3. b	5. d	

7. Weighing daily
8. The apical heart rate; the dose with another nurse; for signs of digoxin toxicity
9. Chronic hypoxia
10. Calming the child; placing the child in the knee–chest position; administering oxygen and if necessary, morphine; and phenylephrine, a potent vasoconstrictor, may be necessary.

Left-to-Right Shunting Lesions and Obstructive Lesions

1. Patent ductus arteriosus
2. Coarctation of the aorta
3. Ventricular septal defect; atrial septal defect
4. Atrioventricular septal defect
5. Pulmonary stenosis
6. Aortic stenosis

Cyanotic Lesions with Altered Pulmonary Blood Flow

1. g	3. e	5. a	7. b
2. f	4. c	6. d	

Acquired Heart Disease

1. T	4. T	7. T	10. F
2. T	5. F	8. T	
3. T	6. T	9. F	

Cardiomyopathies

1. Hypertrophic cardiomyopathy
2. Dilated cardiomyopathy
3. β-Blockers; calcium channel

Dysrhythmias

1. Supraventricular tachycardia
2. Hypoxia
3. Asystole
4. Vagal
5. Epinephrine

High Cholesterol in Children and Adolescents

1. Tobacco use; increased low-density lipoprotein (LDL) and cholesterol; hypertension; decreased physical activity; obesity
2. 110 to 129; 130

Review Questions

1. a	4. c	7. c	10. d
2. b	5. d	8. d	11. a
3. a	6. d	9. b	12. a

CHAPTER 47: THE CHILD WITH A HEMATOLOGIC ALTERATION

Matching Key Terms

1. i	4. a	7. d	10. g
2. k	5. j	8. e	11. b
3. f	6. h	9. c	

Review of the Hematologic System

1. a. To transport oxygen to the tissues
   b. To destroy foreign cells
   c. To prevent blood loss
2. a. Decrease in the number of red blood cells (RBCs) or their hemoglobin content
   b. Increase in the number of RBCs
   c. Decrease in the production of white blood cells (WBCs)
   d. Source of platelets

Iron Deficiency Anemia (IDA)

1. Cow's milk, which is not iron fortified, replaces formula, which is. It may also irritate the immature bowel, which can lead to gastrointestinal (GI) blood loss.
2. They have compromised tissue oxygenation, resulting from decreased hemoglobin levels.
3. Adolescent growth spurt; poor dietary intake; menstruation in females
4. Cow's milk, formula, cereal

Sickle Cell Disease (SCD)

1. a. Low oxygen concentrations
   b. Acidosis
   c. Dehydration
2. Pain, tissue ischemia, infarcts, organ damage

3. g	5. d	7. e	9. b
4. f	6. a	8. c	

Beta-Thalassemia

1. Autosomal recessive
2. Hemosiderosis
3. Iron
4. Deferoxamine (Desferal)

Hemophilia

1. Her father has hemophilia; her mother is a carrier.
2. Factor VIII; factor IX
3. Swelling, pain, and stiffness
4. X

von Willebrand Disease (VWD)

1. F	2. T	3. F	4. T

Immune Thrombocytopenic Purpura (ITP)

1. T   3. T   5. T
2. T   4. F

Disseminated Intravascular Coagulation (DIC)

1. T   2. T   3. F

Aplastic Anemia

1. Granulocytes; erythrocytes; megakaryocytes
2. Petechiae, ecchymosis, pallor, epistaxis, fatigue, tachycardia, anorexia, infection
3. Colony-stimulating factor

ABO Incompatibility and Hemolytic Diseases of the Newborn

1. A; B
2. Negative; positive
3. Delivery, miscarriages, and abortions

Hyperbilirubinemia

1. T   3. F   5. F
2. F   4. T

Review Questions

1. c   4. c   7. d   10. b
2. b   5. c   8. d
3. c   6. d   9. b

CHAPTER 48: THE CHILD WITH CANCER

Matching Key Terms

1. f   4. g   7. i   10. e
2. a   5. j   8. d
3. h   6. c   9. b

Review of Cancer

1. Neoplasm
2. Invasion; metastasis
3. Staging describes the extent of the disease locally, regionally, and systemically and guides the therapy for most solid tumors. Each tumor has its own specific system of staging, which assists in determining treatment and prognosis.
4. T   5. F   6. F   7. T
8. The child should be positioned prone with a small pillow under the hips to facilitate access to the posterior iliac crest.

The Child with Cancer

1. a. Chemotherapy
   b. Radiotherapy
   c. Surgery
2. Antineoplastic drugs
3. a. Hematopoietic system
   b. Gastrointestinal tract
   c. Integumentary system
4. Nadir is the time of the greatest bone marrow suppression when blood counts will be the lowest and usually occurs 7 to 10 days after chemotherapy administration.

The greatest concern during the period of bone marrow suppression is infection.
5. Neutropenia
6. B   8. B   10. C
7. B   9. B   11. B
12. 5-HT3 serotonin antagonists
13. To obtain a small piece of the tumor for microscopic examination to confirm the tumor type and to guide therapy decisions
14. To provide easy IV access so that the child does not have to undergo frequent venipunctures for IV access
15. Dose; treatment site
16. 7 to 10
17. Erythema where the skin has been irradiated
18. Bone marrow transplant (BMT) uses bone marrow to reconstitute the immunologic function. Hematopoietic stem cell transplant (HSCT) uses a unique immature cell present in the peripheral circulation to restore immunologic function in a similar manner.
19. Any type of blood cell
20. h   22. d   24. b   26. g
21. f   23. a   25. c   27. e

Leukemia

1. Immature white blood cells (WBCs)
2. Fever; pallor; excessive bruising; bone or joint pain; malaise; lymphadenopathy; enlarged liver and spleen; abnormal (either high or low) WBC counts; anemia; thrombocytopenia
3. Bone marrow aspiration and biopsy
4. Combination chemotherapy
5. When immature blast cells in the bone marrow are reduced to less than 5%
6. As WBCs break down in response to chemotherapy, they release uric acid, which is poorly water soluble, into the serum, which can compromise kidney function. Allopurinol and IV fluids with sodium bicarbonate are administered to decrease the serum uric acid level and alkalinize the urine.
7. a. Central nervous system
   b. The testes
8. A rectal thermometer can damage delicate rectal tissues and cause abscesses.
9. 500 cells/mm^3
10. Use a soft-bristled toothbrush or Toothettes. Perform oral hygiene four times a day. If the platelet count is low, use a cotton-tipped applicator, finger cot, or washcloth wrapped around a finger instead of a toothbrush. Do not use mouthwash containing alcohol. Notify the physician at first sign of mouth ulcers.
11. Administer the varicella-zoster immunoglobulin to the child within 96 hours.
12. Limit any activity that could result in a head injury. Encourage the child to participate in quiet activities. No contact sports. Use soft-bristled toothbrushes, Toothettes, or gauze swab to clean the teeth. Give stool softeners to prevent straining with stools but do not use suppositories. Check the urine and stools for blood. Avoid sharp foods such as pretzels and chips. Teach the

384

child how to control nosebleeds and gently blow the nose. Evaluate menstrual flow in adolescent girls.

Brain Tumors

1. Tumor location; child's age and stage of development
2. a. Headache
   b. Vomiting in the morning after getting out of bed
3. Magnetic resonance imaging (MRI)
4. Surgery and chemotherapy

Other Childhood Cancers

1. F	4. T	7. T
2. F	5. T	8. T
3. F	6. F	9. T

Review Questions

1. a	5. d	9. c	13. a
2. d	6. a	10. b	14. b
3. c	7. c	11. a	
4. b	8. b	12. a	

CHAPTER 49: THE CHILD WITH AN ALTERATION IN TISSUE INTEGRITY

Matching Key Terms

1. k	4. h	7. j	10. c
2. d	5. e	8. f	11. g
3. i	6. b	9. a	

Review of the Integumentary System

1. a. Protects the deeper tissues from injury, drying, and foreign matter invasion
   b. Regulates temperature
   c. Aids in the excretion of wastes
   d. Produces vitamin D
   e. Initiates the sensations of touch, pain, heat, and cold

2. T	3. F	4. T	5. F

Impetigo

1. Bacterial
2. *Staphylococcus aureus;* group A beta-hemolytic streptococcus
3. Bullous impetigo presents as small vesicles, which can progress to bullae. The lesions are initially filled with serous fluid and later become pustular. The bullae rupture, leaving a shiny, lacquered-appearing lesion surrounded by a scaly rim. Crusted impetigo initially appears as a vesicle or pustule, which ruptures to become an erosion with an overlay of honey-colored crust. When the crusts are removed, the erosion easily bleeds.
4. Impetigo is treated with topical and oral antibiotics. Wash the lesions thrice a day with a warm, soapy washcloth. Then, apply topical antibiotics. Severe cases are treated with oral antibiotics.
5. Acute glomerulonephritis
6. Wash hands often and well, keep the child's nails short, do not share linens and eating utensils used by

the child, have the child sleep alone, and complete the full course of antibiotics.
7. Community-acquired methicillin-resistant *S. aureus* (MRSA)

Cellulitis

1. Cellulitis is a bacterial infection of the subcutaneous tissues and dermis.
2. Lower extremities, buccal, and periorbital regions
3. Affected areas will appear red, hot, swollen, and painful; lymphangitis will occur with red streaking of the surrounding area; edema and purple discoloration of eyelids appear with decreased eye movement if the periorbital area is affected; lymph node enlargement, fever, malaise, and headache occur.
4. Administer an initial intramuscular or intravenous dose of an antibiotic, then complete a 10-day course of antibiotics and warm compresses. Hospitalization and intravenous antibiotics are required if cellulitis affects a joint or the face. Incision and drainage of the affected area may be necessary.
5. Have the child rest in bed with the affected leg elevated. Warm moist soaks should be applied every four hours. Administer antibiotics as ordered. Give acetaminophen for fever or pain. Assess for signs of sepsis or spread of infection. In addition, of course, practice frequent handwashing!

Candidiasis

1. *Candida albicans*
2. White, curd-like plaques on the tongue, gums, or buccal membranes that are difficult to remove
3. Does she have vaginal itching or discharge? Does she have any tenderness or redness of the nipples? Ask about her methods of cleaning bottles, nipples, and pacifiers and about the infant's prior feeding patterns.
4. Nystatin oral suspension
5. Swab 1 mL of oral nystatin suspension onto the infant's gums and tongue every six hours until 1 to 2 weeks after symptoms have disappeared.

Tinea Infections

1. a. Scalp
   b. Trunk, face, and extremities
   c. Feet
2. a. Griseofulvin orally for 6 to 8 weeks
   b. Antifungal preparations such as clotrimazole (Lotrimin) or miconazole (Monistat) topically thrice a day to affected area until lesions are gone for 1 week
   c. Topical antifungal preparation applied twice daily to lesions and at least 1-inch beyond the lesion borders
   d. Topical antifungal agent such as clotrimazole (Lotrimin), miconazole (Monistat), or oxiconazole (Oxistat) applied twice daily until lesions have been cleared for 1 week

3. T	4. F	5. F

Herpes Simplex Virus (HSV) Infection

1. HSV 1 infection of the fingers that is transmitted during oral or tracheal care of a child with a herpes infection
2. Oral or topical acyclovir (Zovirax)
3. The mother can try to feed the child frozen ice pops, noncitrus juices, milk, or flat soda. Small, frequent meals of soft, bland foods may be tolerated.

Lice Infestations

1. F
2. F
3. Nits are visible silvery, grayish-white specks, resembling dandruff. that are firmly attached to the hair shafts near the scalp. Nits resemble dandruff but are more difficult to remove from the hair. They are commonly found ¼ to ½ inch from the scalp surface behind the ears and at the nape of the neck. An adult louse is a small gray speck that quickly crawls and is difficult to see.
4. Treatment involves an over-the-counter antilice product, such as permethrin 1% (Nix) cream rinse, which kills both lice and eggs with one application.
5. After the hair is treated with a pediculicide, all nits must be removed from the hair. The child should be rechecked in 7 to 10 days for an infestation. Parents should be advised to wash clothing, bedding, and linens in hot water and to dry at a hot dryer setting. Items that cannot be washed can be dry-cleaned or sealed in plastic bags for 3 weeks. Combs and brushes must be cleaned through boiling or soaking in an antilice shampoo or hot water for 15 minutes.

Mite Infestation (Scabies)

1. By close personal contact with infected individuals.
2. Intense itching, especially at night; papules, vesicles, and nodules on the wrists, finger webs, elbows, umbilicus, axillae, groin, and buttocks; presence of burrows (fine, grayish, threadlike lines) that are difficult to see because of inflammation and excoriation from scratching.
3. A topical application is applied to the body and head, avoiding the eyes and mouth. Lotion is kept on the body for the recommended period of time (usually 8 to 14 hours), and then the child is bathed.

Atopic Dermatitis

1. High levels of histamine trigger an inflammatory response resulting in erythema, edema, and intense pruritus. Scratching increases itching, leading to an "itch-scratch-itch" cycle.
2. It is scaly on the flexor surfaces of the wrists, ankles, knees, elbows, neck creases, eyelids, and dorsum of hands and feet. Chronic lichenification results from persistent scratching. Areas may be weeping and possibly infected.
3. Avoid trigger factors such as overheating, soaps, wool clothing, or any skin irritant. Apply moisturizer while the skin is damp to hydrate the skin. Use corticosteroid creams for inflamed or lichenified areas.

Oral antihistamines can be used to break the itch-scratch-itch cycle, particularly at night.

Seborrheic Dermatitis

1. Cradle cap
2. a. Nonpruritic oily yellow scales on the scalp, forehead, and eyebrows and behind the ears
   b. Confluent erythema in the diaper area and intertriginous areas and around the umbilicus
3. Remove scales daily by shampooing with a mild baby shampoo or an over-the-counter antiseborrheic shampoo containing sulfur and salicylic acid, selenium, or tar. Massage the scalp with warm mineral oil before shampooing to loosen the scales. Use a fine-toothed comb or clean soft-bristled toothbrush to loosen the scales.

Contact Dermatitis

1. An inflammatory reaction to irritants that results from prolonged contact with irritants or as a result of a delayed hypersensitivity response to an allergen
2. Cool compresses; antipruritic lotions; Aveeno baths; topical steroid creams; oral antihistamines
3. Rinse the child's skin with cool water immediately and wash clothing in hot, soapy water.
4. T   5. T   6. T

Acne Vulgaris

1. Sebaceous hair follicles on the face, neck, back, shoulders, and upper chest
2. When the sebaceous or sweat glands become blocked, a blackhead or a pimple is formed. If these rupture under the skin, inflammation occurs.
3. a. Use sunscreen to reduce photosensitivity; do not apply together with benzoyl peroxide.
   b. Avoid exposure to sunlight.
   c. If sexually active, use contraception because of the drug's teratogenic effect on the fetus.
4. Wash the face twice a day with an antibacterial soap and shampoo hair daily. Avoid vigorous scrubbing and picking or squeezing pimples. Use only water-based cosmetics. Get adequate rest and exercise and eat a balanced diet.

Miscellaneous Skin Disorders

1. Wear identification describing the allergy and stating the treatment. Keep an EpiPen with the child at all times when outdoors.
2. If the stinger is in the skin, it can be removed by carefully scraping it out horizontally. Do not squeeze the area because more venom will be released. Wash with soap and water. A meat tenderizer paste applied to the area may be soothing.
3. Because of the risk for toxic encephalopathy
4. Immediately cover the affected areas with warm hands and clothing. Do not massage the area. Rewarm by immersing in a warm water bath (90°F to 106°F) until all parts are thawed and the skin appears flushed.

5. The child should wear warm, layered clothing; hat; gloves; and two pairs of socks (one wool and one cotton). Teach children to warm their hands and feet when they begin to sting. Do not allow young children to play in extremely cold temperatures.

6. Remove with tweezers as close to the skin as possible, taking care to remove the head. If the mouth parts remain, remove with a sterile needle. Wash the area with soap and water.

7. d   8. a   9. b   10. c

Burn Injuries

1. b   3. b   5. c   7. b
2. a   4. c   6. a   8. c

9. Avoid sun exposure, especially between 10 A.M. and 3 P.M. during the summer. Apply ultraviolet A and B protective sunscreens with SPF of >15 to the child's skin. Apply frequently. Use a waterproof sunscreen if children are in and out of water. Wear a hat and shirt. Sunscreen is contraindicated for infants younger than 6 months of age. Infants should be kept in the shade away from reflecting sun rays.

10. a. Silver nitrate solution
    b. Mafenide acetate cream
    c. Silver sulfadiazine cream

11. A hypovolemic condition that develops after a burn injury that affects more than 15% to 20% of the total body surface area

12. a. Cardiac arrest or dysrhythmia
    b. Tissue damage
    c. Myoglobinuria
    d. Metabolic acidosis

Review Questions

1. b   4. c   7. d   10. c
2. a   5. d   8. b   11. d
3. c   6. b   9. b   12. a

CHAPTER 50: THE CHILD WITH A MUSCULOSKELETAL ALTERATION

Matching Key Terms

1. e   6. n   11. k
2. c   7. f   12. g
3. h   8. m   13. j
4. o   9. d   14. b
5. l   10. a   15. i

16. a. Adduction
    b. Inversion
    c. External rotation
    d. Internal fixation

17. T   19. F   21. F   23. T
18. F   20. T   22. T   24. F

Review of the Musculoskeletal System

1. a. Immovable joints
   b. Slightly movable joints
   c. Freely movable joints

2. a. In the internal organs
   b. Along the skeleton
   c. In the heart

Casts and Traction

1. a. Pain
   b. Paresthesia
   c. Pallor
   d. Pulselessness
   e. Paralysis
2. Osteomyelitis
3. Muscle and nerve irritation of the shoulder and upper arm
4. Skeletal
5. Extensive tissue damage
6. Skin
7. Russell
8. Separated

Limb Defects and Clubfoot

1. T   4. T   7. T
2. T   5. F   8. F
3. F   6. T   9. F

Developmental Dysplasia of the Hip

1. a. Femoral head that can be displaced with manipulation
   b. Asymmetric gluteal skin folds, limited abduction, and shorter-appearing femur on the affected side
   c. Gait variation with lurching toward the affected side
2. a. Abduction
   b. Flexion
   c. External rotation
3. Avascular necrosis
4. Mobility; transportation; skin integrity; toileting; constipation; clothing; comfort; safety; keeping cast clean and dry; inactivity; isolation

Legg–Calvé–Perthes Disease

1. T   2. T   3. F   4. F

Slipped Capital Femoral Epiphysis (SCFE)

1. Above
2. Knee, groin, or thigh
3. Epiphyseal
4. Epiphyseal (growth) plate

Fractures

1. A fracture in which skin, tissue, or muscle has been damaged
2. Compartment syndrome is a serious complication, occurring when swelling causes pressure to increase within the closed space of an extremity. The increased pressure compromises the circulation to the muscles and nerves, causing paralysis and necrosis.
3. Blood loss
4. Retention
5. Internal fixation

6. Nonaccidental
7. Ulna; clavicle; tibia; femur
8. Epiphyseal plate
9. Crush; long

Soft Tissue Injuries

1. d   2. c   3. b   4. a

Osgood–Schlatter Disease

1. Repetitive stress from sports, overuse of immature muscles and tendons, imbalance in strength of quadriceps muscle
2. a. Insidious onset of knee pain
   b. Swelling of the tibial tubercle
   c. Difficulty with weight bearing

Osteogenesis Imperfecta

1. An inherited disorder characterized by connective tissue and bone defects
2. Osteoporosis; bone fragility and fractures; blue sclerae; discolored teeth; deafness by 20 to 30 years of age; shorter-than-average adult height

Osteomyelitis

1. T   3. F   5. F
2. T   4. T

Juvenile Arthritis (JA)

1. An autoimmune inflammatory multisystem disease that affects the body's connective tissue
2. Inflammation of the eye structure in the uveal tract
3. When children with severe juvenile arthritis do not respond well to nonsteroidal anti-inflammatory drugs (NSAIDs)
4. Blindness and disability

Muscular Dystrophies

1. A group of degenerative, inherited disorders that affect the muscle cells of specific muscle groups, causing weakness and atrophy
2. Duchenne
3. Cardiopulmonary complications

Scoliosis, Kyphosis, and Lordosis

1. F   3. F   5. F   7. F
2. T   4. T   6. F   8. T

Review Questions

1. c   5. a   9. c   13. a
2. d   6. c   10. a   14. d
3. a   7. a   11. d
4. b   8. b   12. d

CHAPTER 51: THE CHILD WITH AN ENDOCRINE OR METABOLIC ALTERATION

Matching Key Terms

1. b   3. a   5. h   7. c
2. e   4. f   6. g   8. d

Review of the Endocrine System

1. b   3. a   5. b   7. a
2. a   4. a   6. a

Diagnostic Tests and Procedures

1. Laboratory testing
2. Height; weight

Neonatal Hypoglycemia

1. 40 mg/dL
2. Premature; small-for-gestational-age
3. Jitteriness; poor feeding; lethargy; seizures; hypotonia; high-pitched cry; bradycardia; cyanosis; temperature instability; respiratory alterations, including apnea
4. Feed the infant formula, breast milk, or D_5W. Monitor the response by performing glucose checks.
5. Gestational age assessment; infant's weight, length, and head circumference plotted on growth curve; blood glucose level by 2 hours of age
6. Infiltration of an intravenous site (IV) can cause severe extravasation.

Hypocalcemia

1. 7.0 mg/dL
2. Maternal diabetes causes immature parathyroid function in the neonate.
3. Oral supplements are administered with feedings because they can cause gastric irritation.

Phenylketonuria and Inborn Errors of Metabolism

1. Autosomal recessive
2. Central nervous system
3. Testing should be done after the infant is 48 hours old.
4. A special diet that restricts phenylalanine intake (low-phenylalanine diet)
5. F   6. T   7. F

Congenital Adrenal Hyperplasia

1. Glucocorticoid; androgens
2. Ambiguous genitalia
3. Glucocorticoid therapy

Congenital and Acquired Hypothyroidism

1. F   4. T   7. b   10. a
2. T   5. F   8. b   11. a
3. T   6. a   9. a
12. Administer one daily oral dose. Dissolve in a small amount of water and administer using a syringe or place into the nipple of a baby bottle with a small amount of formula. Do not put in a full bottle because the infant must drink all of the formula to receive a full dose. If the infant vomits within 1 hour, administer it again. Parents must observe the infant for both hypothyroidism and hyperthyroidism, so teach the parents about signs and symptoms.

Hyperthyroidism (Graves Disease)

1. Antithyroid therapy with propylthiouracil or methimazole

2. a. Neutropenia
   b. Hepatotoxicity
   c. Hypothyroidism
3. To determine whether the child has gone into remission

Diabetes Insipidus

1. Vasopressin or antidiuretic hormone (ADH)
2. a. Increased urination (polyuria)
   b. Excessive thirst (polydipsia)
3. The normal response to a water deprivation test is decreased urine output with high specific gravity and no change in serum sodium level. In diabetes insipidus, when fluid is restricted, the child continues to produce large amounts of dilute urine, and the serum sodium level may increase.
4. Synthetic vasopressin (DDAVP)
5. Intranasally or by subcutaneous injection

Syndrome of Inappropriate Antidiuretic Hormone (SIADH)

1. The kidneys reabsorb too much free water.
2. a. Decreased
   b. Increased
   c. Decreased
   d. Increased
3. Seizures

Precocious Puberty

1. A premature appearance of secondary sexual characteristics, accelerated growth rate, and advanced bone maturation
2. Rapid bone growth, which causes early fusion and ultimately results in short adult stature
3. Administration of a gonadotropin-releasing hormone (GnRH) agonist or blocker
4. It inhibits the binding of GnRH to the pituitary gland, causing a decrease in hormone production. This stops sexual development from progressing and slows down bone age advancement.

Growth Hormone (GH) Deficiency

1. F   2. T   3. T   4. T

Diabetes Mellitus

1. Glucose
2. Glycogen
3. To regulate blood glucose by controlling the rate of glucose uptake by cells
4. An autoimmune process that results in the destruction of the insulin-secreting cells of the pancreas
5. When glucose is unable to move into the intercellular space, hyperglycemia occurs.
6. Glucose spills into the urine via osmotic diuresis, causing increased urination.
7. Excess fluid is lost through polyuria, causing thirst.
8. Cellular starvation from the lack of glucose causes hunger.
9. Cellular starvation from the lack of glucose causes weight loss.
10. 126 mg/dl; 200 mg/dl
11. F   13. T   15. T   17. F
12. F   14. T   16. F   18. T
19. Four ounces of fruit juice; 6 oz of regular cola; 6 lifesavers; or a commercial glucose product
20. Hypoglycemia could result from a missed or delayed meal, too much insulin, or an unusual amount of exercise without increasing carbohydrate intake.
21. Place the unconscious child in a side-lying position. Rub a small amount of glucose gel on the child's inner cheek and gums, or subcutaneously or intramuscularly inject glucagon. If the child weighs more than 50 lb (22.75 kg), inject 1 mL. If the child weighs less than 50 lb (22.75 kg), inject 20 to 30 mcg/kg. The onset of action for glucagon is 10 to 15 minutes. When the child regains consciousness, replace the lost glycogen stores with a large snack.
22. It is necessary to replace fluids lost from diuresis, resulting from hyperglycemia. Fluids are essential for flushing ketones.
23. Regular insulin intravenously administered
24. Blood glucose is elevated; urinary ketones are present; arterial pH <7.25
25. Type 2 diabetes
26. The presence of diabetes, obesity, and a poor lipid profile
27. Acanthosis nigricans is a velvety darkening of the skin around the neck that may also be found on the inguinal folds, axillae, antecubital fossa, knees, or dorsum of the hand. It is a marker of hyperinsulinism.
28. At least 60 minutes a day

Review Questions

1. c   6. a   11. c
2. c   7. d   12. b
3. d   8. b   13. a
4. b   9. c   14. a
5. d   10. b   15. d

CHAPTER 52: THE CHILD WITH A NEUROLOGIC ALTERATION

Matching Key Terms

1. c   3. g   5. a   7. b
2. d   4. e   6. f

Review of the Central Nervous System

1. a. Fourth week
   b. 15 to 20 weeks
   c. 30 weeks
   d. 16 weeks
2. a. Cerebrum
   b. Cerebellum
   c. Brainstem

389

3. The cerebrospinal fluid (CSF) acts as a watery cushion surrounding and absorbing any shock to the brain, spinal cord, and meninges.

4. b	6. e	8. a
5. d	7. f	9. c

Increased Intracranial Pressure (ICP)

1. It compensates with decreased CSF production, increased CSF absorption, and reduced cerebral mass because of fluid displacement.
2. a. Bulging fontanel, high-pitched cry, poor feeding, vomiting, irritability, restlessness, distended scalp veins, eyes deviated downward, increased head circumference, separation of cranial sutures
   b. Headache, diplopia, mood swings, slurred speech, nausea and vomiting (especially in the morning), altered level of consciousness, papilledema (after 48 hours)
3. a. Eye opening
   b. Verbal response
   c. Motor response

4. b	7. f	10. T	13. F
5. d	8. a	11. F	
6. c	9. e	12. F	

Spina Bifida

1. Failure of the neural tube to close, resulting in incomplete closure of vertebrae
2. a. Sac-like protrusion filled with spinal fluid and meninges
   b. Sac filled with spinal fluid, meninges, nerve roots, and spinal cord
   c. Failure of the vertebrae to fuse

3. T	5. F	7. T
4. T	6. T	8. T

Hydrocephalus

1. Surgical placement of a ventriculoperitoneal shunt
2. Position the child off the shunt site so that no weight is on the valve for the first 2 days.
3. Poor feeding, nausea or vomiting, elevated temperature, redness or tenderness along the shunt tract

4. a	6. b	8. a	10. d
5. c	7. b	9. c	

Cerebral Palsy

1. F	2. T	3. T	4. T

5. Equipment includes suction, oxygen, bag-valve-mask device, and padding of side rails. Pillows should not be used to pad the side rails because they may cause suffocation.

Head Injury

1. Evaluation of the airway, breathing, and circulation (ABCs)
2. Notify the physician if bleeding does not stop after 10 minutes of holding pressure; if the wound requires sutures; if the child is younger than 1 year of age; if the child has a seizure after head injury; if the child is unconscious or confused; or if the child has any of the following: severe headache, vomiting, slurred speech, blurred vision, difficulty walking or crawling, blood or watery drainage from nose or ear, unequal pupils, or crossed eyes.

3. c	5. e	7. d
4. a	6. b	8. f

9. The child may become more easily upset and more irritable when tired or stressed as an aftereffect of a head injury.

Spinal Cord Injury

1. T	3. T	5. T
2. T	4. T	6. T

Seizure Disorders

1. a	2. d	3. b	4. c

5. A seizure occurs when there is an excessive disorderly discharge of neuronal activity in the brain. Epilepsy refers to recurrent seizure activity that does not occur in association with an acute illness.
6. Height; rapidity
7. Precipitating events, behavior before and immediately after the seizure, a detailed description of how the seizure progressed, and the duration of the seizure
8. Pad side rails; keep the bed in a low position; suction airway at the child's bedside; remove sharp objects or furniture from the area; do not put anything in the child's mouth; place child on his or her side; do not restrain the child; place on a soft surface if not in bed; and loosen clothing around the neck.
9. Gums may become swollen and tender; brush and floss teeth after every meal using a soft toothbrush, have a dental examination every 3 to 6 months, and have blood levels regularly monitored.
10. Prolonged seizure activity that may be a single seizure, lasting 10 minutes, or recurrent seizures, lasting more than 30 minutes, with no return to consciousness between seizures
11. Perinatal asphyxia

Meningitis

1. Lumbar puncture
2. Pain with an extension of the leg and knee
3. Flexion of head causes flexion of hips and knees.
4. Intravenous antibiotic therapy

5. T	6. F	7. T	8. F

Guillain–Barré Syndrome (GBS)

1. Inflammation is caused by the infiltration of lymphocytes into the peripheral nerves.
2. Bag-valve-mask device, oxygen, suction equipment, endotracheal tubes, laryngoscope
3. There is bilateral ascending muscle weakness or paralysis that progresses from the feet to the head, which reverses as healing occurs.

390

Headaches

1. Migraine headaches may be preceded by an aura. The most common symptoms include throbbing pain, often on both sides of the head; nausea and vomiting; irritability; abdominal pain; photophobia; and phonophobia. In tension-type headaches, the pain is more generalized than in migraines; pain is described as a band-like tightness or pressure. Other symptoms include tight neck muscles, soreness of the scalp, fatigue, and dizziness; nausea is rare.

Review Questions

1. b	6. c	11. b
2. d	7. a	12. c
3. a	8. a	13. d
4. c	9. d	14. c
5. d	10. a	15. c

CHAPTER 53: PSYCHOSOCIAL PROBLEMS IN CHILDREN AND FAMILIES

Overview of Childhood Psychopathology

1. F   2. T   3. T

Anxiety and Mood Disorders

1. b	5. e	9. j	13. T
2. f	6. a	10. g	14. F
3. c	7. i	11. F	
4. d	8. h	12. T	

15. Selective serotonin reuptake inhibitors (SSRIs)

Suicide

1. Using cryptic verbal messages; giving away personal items; changes in expected patterns of behavior; specific statements about suicide or self-harm; preoccupation with death; frequent risk-taking or self-abusive behaviors; use of drugs or alcohol to cope; overwhelming sense of guilt or shame; obsessional self-doubt; open signs of mental illness; history of physical or sexual abuse; homosexuality; significant change or life event that is internally disruptive
2. Have you ever thought of trying to hurt yourself? How might you do this? Have you ever thought of trying to kill yourself? How might you do this? Have you ever told anyone about wanting to kill yourself? How do you feel right now? Do you have access to firearms? Knives? (For more, see Box 53-1, "Questions to Assess Suicide Potential.")
3. Communicate with the adolescent in an empathetic and nonjudgmental way to decrease his or her sense of isolation and rejection. Use a clear, direct, and supportive tone of voice and demeanor. Be physically and emotionally present and offer opportunities for him or her to discuss feelings and thoughts. Remove any potentially harmful objects.
4. T   5. F   6. F   7. T

Eating Disorders: Anorexia Nervosa and Bulimia Nervosa

1. a. The deliberate refusal to maintain an adequate body weight
   b. Distorted body image
   c. Amenorrhea
2. Recurrent episodes of binge eating; a sense of lack of control over eating binges; self-induced vomiting or excessive use of laxatives, diuretics, and/or emetics to prevent weight gain; excessive exercise to prevent weight gain; a persistent overconcern with body image
3. T   4. T   5. F   6. F

Attention-Deficit/Hyperactivity Disorder (ADHD)

1. a. Attention and concentration
   b. Impulse control
   c. Overactivity
2. Based on reports by the child, parent(s), and teacher(s)
3. Teach the family about the disorder.
4. T   5. T   6. F

Substance Abuse

1. An increase in antisocial behavior; poor school performance; irregular school attendance; aggressive or rebellious behavior; excessive influence by peers; deterioration of relationships with family or former friends; history of a lack of parental support and supervision; rapid or extreme changes in mood; loss of interest in hobbies; changes in eating or sleeping patterns as manipulative behaviors increase
2. T   3. F   4. T

Childhood Physical and Emotional Abuse and Neglect

1. Isolation from community and social groups; intense competition for emotional resources within the family; low levels of differentiation among family members; distrust of outsiders and family members; unpredictable and unstable family environment (For more, see Box 53-3, "Characteristics of Abusive Family.")
2. Vigorous shaking while the infant is being held by the extremities or shoulders causes whiplash-induced intracranial or intraocular bleeding.
3. It is a form of physical abuse in which the caretaker (usually the mother) falsifies or produces an illness in the child and then takes the child in for medical care, claiming no knowledge of how the child became ill.
4. Have a nonjudgmental and supportive attitude, answer questions directly and specifically, and act as an advocate for the child and the family. Provide an accepting environment, use role modeling as a method of parent teaching, focus on the child's positive attributes, and encourage the parents to participate in the child's care and to reinforce positive behavior.
5. T   6. T   7. T   8. T

Review Questions

1. d	3. c	5. b	7. c
2. a	4. a	6. d	8. b

CHAPTER 54: THE CHILD WITH A DEVELOPMENTAL DISABILITY

Matching Key Terms

1. c   2. b   3. d   4. a

Intellectual and Developmental Disorders

1. Intellectual; adaptive
2. The term is limited to conditions that originate before 18 years of age, with significant evidence of intellectual functioning that is below average, as well as deficits in at least two areas, such as communication, home living, community use, health and safety, leisure, self-care, social skills, self-direction, functional academics, or work abilities.
3. Intellectual disability
4. A descriptive term that denotes a significant limitation in intellectual and functional capacity.
5. Severe and chronic disability that is attributable to mental or physical impairment or a combination of both that must be present before the individual turns 22 years old and is likely to continue. There must be substantial functional limitations in three or more areas, such as self-care, receptive and expressive language, learning, mobility, self-direction, capacity for independent living, or economic self-sufficiency.
6. Each child with a disability must have a written individualized education program (IEP) that outlines specialized instruction and services the school system must provide. It is designed by the child's parents and school personnel after an educational assessment.

Intellectual and Developmental Disorders

1. Intense stress experienced by families of disabled children, parental isolation, unrealistic expectations for the child's performance resulting from a lack of knowledge about normal growth and development
2. Delayed achievement of developmental milestones
3. a. Down syndrome
   b. Fragile X syndrome
4. T   5. T   6. F   7. T

Down Syndrome

1. Trisomy 21
2. Characteristic appearance
3. The child's typical coping patterns; daily routines; understanding of language; learning abilities; social and motor skills
4. T   5. F   6. F   7. T

Fragile X Syndrome

1. T   2. F   3. F

Fetal Alcohol Syndrome (FAS)

1. Persistent symmetric growth retardation, malformations of the face and skull, skeletal and cardiac malformations, central nervous system (CNS) deficits, intellectual and developmental disabilities
2. Maternal alcohol consumption during pregnancy

Autism Spectrum Disorders (ASDs)

1. The child has difficultly developing and maintaining social relationships; impaired communication ability; and the presence of stereotyped, repetitive, and fixated interests and behaviors.
2. Understand social cues; act according to social norms
3. F   4. F   5. F   6. F
7. A child with autism who has a highly developed intellectual skill in one particular area but otherwise has severe intellectual disabilities
8. In both instances, an initial period of normal development is followed by the emergence of autism symptoms, and development stops.

Failure to Thrive

1. An underlying physical condition
2. Poverty; maternal depression; poor social support systems; poor bonding or maladaptive interactions between the child and mother; an irritable, resistant-to-touch infant
3. Maladaptive parent–infant relationship

Review Questions

1. d   3. d   5. c   7. b
2. c   4. a   6. b   8. a

CHAPTER 55: THE CHILD WITH A SENSORY ALTERATION

Review of the Eye and the Ear

1. f   4. c   7. b
2. g   5. d   8. e
3. a   6. h   9. i
10. 22 to 50 days of gestation
11. 4 to 6 weeks of gestation
12. 6 months
13. 5 years

Disorders of the Eye

1. d   4. f   7. a
2. b   5. i   8. c
3. h   6. e   9. g
10. Squinting, head tilting, holding a book close to the eyes, decreased attention span, and poor school performance
11. Correction to 20/200 or less in the better eye or a visual field of 20 degrees or less
12. Amblyopia: decreased vision in the deviated eye
13. It strengthens the weak eye while the good eye is patched.
14. Excessive tearing, light sensitivity, muscle spasm causing involuntary closing of the eyelid, corneal enlargement, and haziness
15. Surgery
16. Pain, nausea and vomiting, and increased inflammation
17. Slightly elevate the head of the bed and avoid any position in which the affected eye is dependent because this would cause edema and pressure on the eye.

18. Itching; burning; light sensitivity; scratchy eyelids; redness; edema; discharge
19. Chemical irritation from eye prophylaxis
20. Practice good handwashing habits, do not share the child's linens or eye medication with other family members, and do not allow the child to return to school or daycare until he or she has received eyedrops for 24 hours.
21. Excessive tearing and crusting of eyelids on awakening; a small mass just below the inner aspect of the eye
22. It reduces the risk of rebleeding between 3 and 5 days following an injury.
23. Wearing protective eyewear, such as goggles and facemasks
24. Rebleeding, change in the size of the area, presence of bright red blood, signs of increased intraocular pressure (pain, nausea and vomiting, increased inflammation), and side effects from medication
25. Irrigate immediately with water or a saline solution. For a mild burn, use at least 2 L of fluid for 30 minutes; for a severe burn, use at least 10 L for 2 to 4 hours.

26. F	29. F	32. T
27. T	30. F	33. T
28. F	31. T	34. T

Hearing Loss in Children

1. b	2. d	3. a	4. c

5. Excessive cerumen; foreign bodies; perforated tympanic membrane; otitis media
6. Infection; heredity; exposure to loud noises; ototoxic medications; prematurity
7. Auditory brainstem response; evoked otoacoustic emissions test
8. Audiometry
9. Have the child use a hearing aid if he or she has one; look at the child when speaking; speak clearly and slightly slower; eliminate background noise; and use visual aids.

10. T	12. T	14. T
11. F	13. F	

Language Disorders

1. a	2. b	3. c

4. a. Pitch and intonation
   b. Articulation
   c. Fluency
5. Describe any activities to the child; expand on what the child says; add new information; build the child's vocabulary; and repeat the child's words using adult pronunciations.

6. T	7. F	8. T	9. T

Review Questions

1. b	4. b	7. b	10. d
2. a	5. c	8. c	11. d
3. c	6. a	9. d	

Answer Key